CT Angiography

Guest Editor

W. DENNIS FOLEY, MD

RADIOLOGIC CLINICS OF NORTH AMERICA

www.radiologic.theclinics.com

Consulting Editor
FRANK H. MILLER, MD

March 2010 • Volume 48 • Number 2

W.B. SAUNDERS COMPANY
A Division of Elsevier Inc.

1600 John F. Kennedy Boulevard • Suite 1800 • Philadelphia, Pennsylvania 19103-2899

http://www.theclinics.com

RADIOLOGIC CLINICS OF NORTH AMERICA Volume 48, Number 2
March 2010 ISSN 0033-8389, ISBN 13: 978-1-4377-1943-7

Editor: Barton Dudlick
Developmental Editor: Theresa Collier

Radiologic Clinics of North America (ISSN 0033-8389) is published bimonthly by Elsevier Inc., 360 Park Avenue South, New York, NY 10010-1710. Months of issue are January, March, May, July, September, and November. Periodicals postage paid at New York, NY and additional mailing offices. Subscription prices are USD 361 per year for US individuals, USD 545 per year for US institutions, USD 176 per year for US students and residents, USD 421 per year for Canadian individuals, USD 684 per year for Canadian institutions, USD 520 per year for international individuals, USD 684 per year for international institutions, and USD 253 per year for Canadian and foreign students/residents. To receive student and resident rate, orders must be accompanied by name of affiliated institution, date of term and the signature of program/residency coordinator on institution letterhead. Orders will be billed at individual rate until proof of status is received. Foreign air speed delivery is included in all Clinics subscription prices. All prices are subject to change without notice. **POSTMASTER:** Send address changes to Radiologic Clinics of North America, Elsevier Health Sciences Division, Subscription Customer Service, 3251 Riverport Lane, Maryland Heights, MO63043. **Customer Service: Telephone: 1-800-654-2452** (U.S. and Canada); **1-314-447-8871** (outside U.S. and Canada). **Fax: 1-314-447-8029. E-mail: journalscustomerservice-usa@ elsevier.com** (for print support); **journalsonlinesupport-usa@elsevier.com** (for online support).

Reprints. For copies of 100 or more of articles in this publication, please contact the Commercial Reprints Department, Elsevier Inc., 360 Park Avenue South, New York, New York 10010-1710. Tel.: (+1) 212-633-3812; Fax: (+1) 212-462-1935; E-mail: reprints@elsevier.com.

Radiologic Clinics of North America also published in Greek Paschalidis Medical Publications, Athens, Greece.

Radiologic Clinics of North America is covered in *MEDLINE/PubMed (Index Medicus), EMBASE/Excerpta Medica, Current Contents/Life Sciences, Current Contents/Clinical Medicine, RSNA Index to Imaging Literature, BIOSIS, Science Citation Index,* and *ISI/BIOMED.*

Contributors

CONSULTING EDITOR

FRANK H. MILLER, MD
Professor of Radiology; Chief, Body Imaging
Section and Fellowship Program and GI
Radiology; and Medical Director MRI,
Department of Radiology, Northwestern
University Feinberg School of Medicine,
Chicago, Illinois

GUEST EDITOR

W. DENNIS FOLEY, MD
Professor, Department of Radiology, Medical
College of Wisconsin, Milwaukee, Wisconsin

AUTHORS

SUHNY ABBARA, MD
Associate Professor, Harvard Medical
School; Director Cardiovascular Imaging,
Department of Radiology, Massachusetts
General Hospital, Harvard Medical School,
Boston, Massachusetts

JOSSER E. DELGADO ALMANDOZ, MD
Division of Neuroradiology, Massachusetts
General Hospital, Harvard Medical School,
Boston, Massachusetts;
Clinical Fellow in Diagnostic and
Endovascular Surgical Neuroradiology;
Division of Neuroradiology,
Mallinckrodt Institute of Radiology,
Washington University School of Medicine,
Saint Louis, Missouri

STEPHAN W. ANDERSON, MD
Assistant Professor of Radiology, Boston
Medical Center, Boston, Massachusetts

JOSEPH J. BUDOVEC, MD
Assistant Professor of Radiology, Body and Digital
Imaging Section, Department of Radiology,
Medical College of Wisconsin, Milwaukee,
Wisconsin

FRANDICS P. CHAN, MD, PhD
Associate Professor of Radiology; Director,
Cardiovascular Imaging, Department
of Radiology, Lucile Packard Children's
Hospital, Stanford University School
of Medicine, Palo Alto, California

JONATHAN H. CHUNG, MD
Cardiothoracic Imaging Fellow and Clinical
Assistant, Department of Radiology,
Massachusetts General Hospital, Boston,
Massachusetts

BHAVIKA R. DAVE, MD
Cardiovascular Imaging and Interventional Fellow,
Department of Radiology, Massachusetts General
Hospital, Boston, Massachusetts

MONICA EPELMAN, MD
Assistant Professor of Radiology;
Director, Neonatal Imaging,
Department of Radiology,
The Children's Hospital
of Philadelphia, University of
Pennsylvania School of Medicine,
Philadelphia, Pennsylvania

ELLIOT K. FISHMAN, MD
Professor, Department of Radiology, Johns
Hopkins Medical Institutions, Baltimore, Maryland

DOMINIK FLEISCHMANN, MD
Associate Professor of Radiology; Director,
Computed Tomography, Department of
Radiology, Stanford University Medical Center,
Stanford, California

W. DENNIS FOLEY, MD
Professor, Department of Radiology, Medical
College of Wisconsin, Milwaukee, Wisconsin

BRIAN B. GHOSHHAJRA, MD
Cardiac Imaging Fellow, Department of Radiology,
Massachusetts General Hospital, Boston,
Massachusetts

MICHAEL GROGAN, MD, JD
Resident, Department of Radiology, Medical
College of Wisconsin, Milwaukee, Wisconsin

JEFFREY C. HELLINGER, MD
Assistant Professor of Radiology and Cardiology;
Director, Cardiovascular Imaging and 3D Imaging
Laboratory, Department of Radiology, The
Children's Hospital of Philadelphia, University of
Pennsylvania School of Medicine, Philadelphia,
Pennsylvania

BERNICE E. HOPPEL, PhD
Toshiba Medical Research Institute, Vernon Hills,
Illinois

KAREN M. HORTON, MD
Professor, Department of Radiology, Johns
Hopkins Medical Institutions, Baltimore, Maryland

KANAKO K. KUMAMARU, MD
Department of Radiology, University of Tokyo
Hospital, Tokyo, Japan

DIPTI K. LENHART, MD
Division of Abdominal Imaging and Intervention,
Department of Imaging, Massachusetts General
Hospital, Harvard Medical School, Boston,
Massachusetts

MICHAEL H. LEV, MD
Associate Professor of Radiology; Director,
Emergency Neuroradiology and Neurovascular
Laboratory, Division of Neuroradiology,
Massachusetts General Hospital, Harvard Medical
School, Boston, Massachusetts

PETER S. LIU, MD
Clinical Lecturer, Department of Radiology,
University of Michigan Medical Center,
Ann Arbor, Michigan

RICHARD T. MATHER, PhD
Toshiba Medical Research Institute,
Vernon Hills, Illinois

ANDRES PENA, MD
Senior Research Fellow, Department
of Radiology, The Children's Hospital of
Philadelphia, University of Pennsylvania
School of Medicine, Philadelphia,
Pennsylvania

ROCIO PEREZ-JOHNSTON, MD
Division of Abdominal Imaging and Intervention,
Department of Imaging, Massachusetts General
Hospital, Harvard Medical School, Boston,
Massachusetts

JOEL F. PLATT, MD
Professor, Department of Radiology, University
of Michigan Medical Center, Ann Arbor,
Michigan

MATTHEW POLLEMA, MD
Instructor, Department of Radiology, Medical
College of Wisconsin, Milwaukee, Wisconsin

STUART R. POMERANTZ, MD
Instructor of Radiology; Associate Director,
Neuro-CT; Division of Neuroradiology,
Massachusetts General Hospital, Harvard
Medical School, Boston, Massachusetts

MICHAEL POON, MD
Professor of Radiology and Cardiology;
Director, Advanced Cardiovascular Imaging,
Department of Radiology, Stony Brook
University School of Medicine, Stony Brook,
New York

CARLOS A. ROJAS, MD
Cardiac Imaging Fellow, Department
of Radiology, Massachusetts General Hospital,
Boston, Massachusetts

JAVIER M. ROMERO, MD
Instructor of Radiology; Director, Ultrasound
Imaging Services; Associate Director,
Neurovascular Laboratory; Division of
Neuroradiology, Massachusetts General Hospital,
Harvard Medical School, Boston, Massachusetts

GEOFFREY D. RUBIN, MD
Professor of Radiology; Chief, Cardiovascular
Imaging, Department of Radiology, Stanford
University Medical Center, Stanford University
School of Medicine, Stanford, California

FRANK J. RYBICKI, MD, PhD
Applied Imaging Science Laboratory,
Department of Radiology, Brigham and
Women's Hospital, Harvard Medical School,
Boston, Massachusetts

DUSHYANT V. SAHANI, MD
Director of CT, Associate Professor of Radiology,
Division of Abdominal Imaging and Intervention,
Department of Imaging, Massachusetts General
Hospital, Harvard Medical School, Boston,
Massachusetts

OSAMU SAKAI, MD, PhD
Professor of Radiology, Boston Medical Center,
Boston, Massachusetts

JORGE A. SOTO, MD
Associate Professor of Radiology, Boston Medical
Center, Boston, Massachusetts

TROY STONELY, MD
Instructor, Department of Radiology, Medical
College of Wisconsin, Milwaukee, Wisconsin

JENNIFER W. UYEDA, MD
Radiology Resident, Boston Medical Center,
Boston, Massachusetts

Contents

Since 1958, catheter angiography has assumed the role of gold standard for vascular imaging, despite the invasive nature of the procedure. Less invasive techniques for vascular imaging, such as computed tomographic angiography (CTA), have been developed and have matured in conjunction with developments in catheter arteriography. In a few cases, such as imaging, the aorta and the pulmonary arteries, CTA has supplanted catheter angiography as the gold standard. The expanding role of CTA emphasizes the need for deep, broad-based understanding of physical principles. This review describes CT hardware and associated software for angiography. The fundamentals of CTA physics are complemented with several clinical examples.

CT scanner technology is continuously evolving, with scan times becoming shorter with each scanner generation. Achieving adequate arterial opacification synchronized with CT data acquisition is becoming increasingly difficult. A fundamental understanding of early arterial contrast medium dynamics is thus of utmost importance for the design of CT scanning and injection protocols for current and future cardiovascular CT applications. Arterial enhancement is primarily controlled by the iodine flux (injection flow rate) and the injection duration versus a patient's cardiac output and local downstream physiology. The technical capabilities of modern CT equipment require precise scan timing. Together with automated tube current modulation and weight-based injection protocols, both radiation exposure and contrast medium enhancement can be individualized.

Patients with thoracic aortic diseases may be completely asymptomatic (as in thoracic aortic aneurysms) or present acutely with severe chest pain (as in acute aortic dissections). Thoracic aortic disease is often occult until a life-threatening complication occurs or the disease is discovered incidentally on imaging. Multidetector-row computed tomography (MDCT) can be used to diagnose various acute and chronic abnormalities of the aorta, including aortic aneurysms, aortic dissection, intramural hematoma, penetrating atherosclerotic ulcer, traumatic aortic transection, and congenital malformations. This article reviews the MDCT appearance of various thoracic aortic diseases.

As a result of the development of multidetector row computed tomography (CT) technology, multidetector CT angiography is rapidly becoming the preferred examination for the initial evaluation of an increasing number of clinical neurovascular applications such as carotid artery steno-occlusive disease, acute ischemic and hemorrhagic stroke, subarachnoid hemorrhage, and cerebral vasospasm. This article reviews the most recent literature on these topics, provides the reader with useful clinical tips for performing and interpreting these increasingly complex diagnostic examinations, presents illustrative cases, and looks at future developments in this vibrant area of neuroradiology research.

Multidetector computed tomography angiography (MDCTA) allows high spatial resolution, including nearly isotropic submillimeter resolution in the X, Y, and Z planes, and rapid image acquisition in a single breath hold, with greatly enhanced diagnostic capabilities over conventional CT. MDCTA has largely replaced digital subtraction angiography because it is faster, less invasive, and provides more information. When technical parameters are optimized, it provides the radiologist with the information needed to diagnose life threatening diseases of the aortoiliac system, gives critical information for the vascular surgeon or interventional radiologist to treat that disease, and identifies subsequent complications related to therapy. This article briefly discusses the technical components and optimization of MDCTA of the abdominal aorta and iliac arteries (aortoiliac system) and examines the diseases of the aortoiliac system evaluated by MDCTA.

Multidetector computed tomography angiography (MDCTA) is an established, noninvasive, and effective imaging method to evaluate the liver and the pancreas primarily for neoplasm staging and presurgical planning. However, its role has also extended into a variety of other clinical indications. Technological advances in MDCT scanners and post processing now offer new opportunities with CTA, but the challenges of protocol optimization should be confronted appropriately to meet the new expectations. In this review, we focus on the technical details with MDCTA protocols for liver and pancreas and briefly discuss the common pathologic conditions where CTA is now considered integral to patient management.

Significant advancements in computed tomography (CT) scanner technology along with the development of powerful and affordable 3-dimensional (3D) software have resulted in new applications for CT imaging. The mesenteric vasculature was traditionally imaged with conventional angiography, but can now easily be imaged rapidly and safely using multidetector-row CT (MDCT) scanners and 3D imaging software. CT can now be used to visualize the normal mesenteric vasculature, both arteries and veins, identify important anatomic variants, and evaluate a wide range of pathology. This article examines the technique of MDCT and its role in imaging the mesenteric circulation.

Although catheter angiography remains the accepted gold standard for imaging of the renal vascular system, rapid progress in cross-sectional imaging techniques has caused a paradigm shift in many diagnostic algorithms toward noninvasive techniques such as computed tomographic angiography (CTA). CTA's cross-sectional imaging techniques provide an opportunity for comprehensive renal investigation that would be impossible with angiography alone. While other competing noninvasive technologies such as ultrasound and magnetic resonance angiography can be used successfully in renal imaging, the benefits of CTA are substantial, including high spatial and temporal resolution, widespread availability, implantable device compatibility, and easy technical reproducibility. This article describes the technical considerations relevant to CTA of the renal vascular system, postprocessing algorithms for volumetric data, and numerous specific applications.

CT Angiography of the Lower Extremities

W. Dennis Foley and Troy Stonely

CT angiography (CTA) of the lower extremities has evolved into a robust noninvasive angiographic technique with the advent of 16 and 64 multidetector computed tomographic systems and advances in system design. CTA has displaced conventional catheter arteriography in a large range of applications and is predominantly used in the evaluation of atherosclerotic peripheral arterial occlusive disease in symptomatic patients who are candidates for intervention. Other disease entities including atheroembolism andthromboembolism, aneurysmal disease, and arteritides including Buerger disease and Takayasu arteritis can be precisely evaluated by CTA. Particular applications include arterial vascular mapping for free flap transfers and fibular grafts and evaluation of trauma, before and following orthopedic and plastic surgery interventions. Patients with intravascular stents and arterial bypass grafts who usually undergo serial evaluation by noninvasive, nonangiographic testing are potential candidates for angiographic study when clinical findings of noninvasive tests are in disagreement. The key to a successful clinical application is in understanding how to acquire, display, and interpret high-quality CTA in diverse clinical circumstances.

Upper Extremity Computed Tomographic Angiography: State of the Art Technique and Applications in 2010

Jeffrey C. Hellinger, Monica Epelman, and Geoffrey D. Rubin

From technical and interpretative perspectives, upper extremity computed tomographic angiography (CTA) is one of the more challenging vascular CTA applications. Synchronizing the relatively large scan coverage with a single bolus of contrast medium requires precise selection of acquisition and contrast delivery parameters. To avoid multiple acquisitions and minimize radiation exposure and contrast medium volume, it is important to have fundamental knowledge on how to select these parameters. Equally important is knowing how to adeptly apply advanced workstation visualization techniques and tool functions for the upper extremity vascular tree. In this review, upper extremity arterial and venous anatomy is discussed, followed by a detailed overview on state-of-the-art upper extremity CTA technical considerations and strategies. The review concludes with discussion and illustration of upper extremity CTA clinical applications.

CT Angiography in Trauma

Jennifer W. Uyeda, Stephan W. Anderson, Osamu Sakai, and Jorge A. Soto

Rapid assessment and diagnosis of traumatic arterial injuries are critical in the evaluation of acutely injured patients. CT angiograms (CTAs) have become common imaging methods in busy trauma centers. CTA has largely replaced digital subtraction angiography because of its speed, noninvasive nature, accuracy, and widespread availability. This article reviews the current use of multidetector CTA in trauma with attention to technique and protocol considerations, illustrates findings of many commonly encountered injuries, and discusses the clinical implications of vascular trauma throughout the body.

Whether congenital or acquired, timely recognition and management of disease is imperative, as hemodynamic alterations in blood flow, tissue perfusion, and cellular oxygenation can have profound effects on organ function, growth and development, and quality of life for the pediatric patient. Ensuring safe computed tomographic angiography (CTA) practice and "gentle" pediatric imaging requires the cardiovascular imager to have sound understanding of CTA advantages, limitations, and appropriate indications as well as strong working knowledge of acquisition principles and image post processing. From this vantage point, CTA can be used as a useful adjunct along with the other modalities. This article presents a summary of dose reduction CTA methodologies along with techniques the authors have employed in clinical practice to achieve low-dose and ultralow-dose exposure in pediatric CTA. CTA technical principles are discussed with an emphasis on the low-dose methodologies and safe contrast medium delivery strategies. Recommended parameters for currently available multidetector-row computed tomography scanners are summarized alongside recommended radiation and contrast medium parameters. In the second part of the article an overview of pediatric CTA clinical applications is presented, illustrating low-dose and ultra-low dose techniques, with an emphasis on the specific protocols.

A revised version of this article can be found online at: www.radiologic.theclinics.com.

GOAL STATEMENT
The goal of the *Radiologic Clinics of North America* is to keep practicing radiologists and radiology residents up to date with current clinical practice in radiology by providing timely articles reviewing the state of the art in patient care.

ACCREDITATION
The *Radiologic Clinics of North America* is planned and implemented in accordance with the Essential Areas and Policies of the Accreditation Council for Continuing Medical Education (ACCME) through the joint sponsorship of the University of Virginia School of Medicine and Elsevier. The University of Virginia School of Medicine is accredited by the ACCME to provide continuing medical education for physicians.

The University of Virginia School of Medicine designates this educational activity for a maximum of 15 *AMA PRA Category 1 Credits*™ for each issue, 90 credits per year. Physicians should only claim credit commensurate with the extent of their participation in the activity.

The American Medical Association has determined that physicians not licensed in the US who participate in this CME activity are eligible for a maximum of *15 AMA PRA Category 1 Credits*™ for each issue, 90 credits per year.

Credit can be earned by reading the text material, taking the CME examination online at http://www.theclinics.com/home/cme, and completing the evaluation. After taking the test, you will be required to review any and all incorrect answers. Following completion of the test and evaluation, your credit will be awarded and you may print your certificate.

FACULTY DISCLOSURE/CONFLICT OF INTEREST
The University of Virginia School of Medicine, as an ACCME accredited provider, endorses and strives to comply with the Accreditation Council for Continuing Medical Education (ACCME) Standards of Commercial Support, Commonwealth of Virginia statutes, University of Virginia policies and procedures, and associated federal and private regulations and guidelines on the need for disclosure and monitoring of proprietary and financial interests that may affect the scientific integrity and balance of content delivered in continuing medical education activities under our auspices.

The University of Virginia School of Medicine requires that all CME activities accredited through this institution be developed independently and be scientifically rigorous, balanced and objective in the presentation/discussion of its content, theories and practices.

All authors/editors participating in an accredited CME activity are expected to disclose to the readers relevant financial relationships with commercial entities occurring within the past 12 months (such as grants or research support, employee, consultant, stock holder, member of speakers bureau, etc.). The University of Virginia School of Medicine will employ appropriate mechanisms to resolve potential conflicts of interest to maintain the standards of fair and balanced education to the reader. Questions about specific strategies can be directed to the Office of Continuing Medical Education, University of Virginia School of Medicine, Charlottesville, Virginia.

The faculty and staff of the University of Virginia Office of Continuing Medical Education have no financial affiliations to disclose.

The authors/editors listed below have identified no financial or professional relationships for themselves or their spouse/partner:
Stephan W. Anderson, MD; Joseph J. Budovec, MD; Jonathan H. Chung, MD; Bhavika R. Dave, MD; Josser E. Delgado Almandoz, MD; Barton Dudlick (Acquisitions Editor); Monica Epelman, MD; Brian B. Ghoshhajra, MD; Michael Grogan, MD, JD; Jeffrey C. Hellinger, MD; Theodore E. Keats, MD (Test Author); Kanako K. Kumamaru, MD; Dipti K. Lenhart, MD; Peter S. Liu, MD; Frank H. Miller, MD (Consulting Editor); Andres Peña, MD; Rocio Perez-Johnston, MD; Joel F. Platt, MD; Matthew Pollema, MD; Michael Poon, MD; Carlos A. Rojas, MD; Osamu Sakai, MD, PhD; Jorge A. Soto, MD; Troy Stonely, MD; and Jennifer W. Uyeda, MD.

The authors/editors listed below have identified the following financial or professional relationships for themselves or their spouse/partner:
Suhny Abbara, MD is an industry funded research/investigator for Bracco, is a consultant for Perceptive Informatics, Inc., is on the Speakers' Bureau for Siemens Medical, and is on the Advisory Committee/Board for Partners Imaging, Magellan Health.
Elliot K. Fishman, MD receives research support from and is on the Advisory Board of Siemens and GE.
Dominik Fleischmann, MD is an industry funded research/investigator for GE Health Care and Siemens Medical Solutions, and is on the Speakers' Bureau for Bracco Diagnostics.
W. Dennis Foley, MD (Guest Editor) is an industry funded research/investigator, is a consultant, and is a stockholder for GE Healthcare.
Bernice E. Hoppel, PhD is employed by Toshiba Medical Research Unit and GE Healthcare, and is a patent holder for GE Healthcare.
Karen M. Horton, MD is an industry funded research/investigator for Siemens.
Michael H. Lev, MD is an industry funded research/investigator for GE Healthcare and Vernalis, serves on the Advisory Committee for GE Healthcare and CoAxia and serves on the Speakers Bureau for GE Healthcare.
Richard T. Mather, PhD is employed by Toshiba Medical Systems Corporation.
Stuart R. Pomerantz, MD is an industry funded research/investigator, a consultant, and is on the Speakers' Bureau for GE Healthcare.
Javier M. Romero, MD is an industry funded research/investigator for General Electric.
Geoffrey D. Rubin, MD is on the Advisory Board for Fovia, and owns stock in Terarecon.
Frank J. Rybicki, MD, PhD serves on the Speakers Bureau for Toshiba Medical Systems, and is an industry funded research/investigator for Toshiba Medical Systems, Bracco Diagnostics, and Vital Images.
Dushyant V. Sahani, MD receives grant support from GE Healthcare.

Disclosure of Discussion of Non-FDA Approved Uses for Pharmaceutical Products and/or Medical Devices.
The University of Virginia School of Medicine, as an ACCME provider, requires that all faculty presenters identify and disclose any off-label uses for pharmaceutical and medical device products. The University of Virginia School of Medicine recommends that each physician fully review all the available data on new products or procedures prior to clinical use.

TO ENROLL
To enroll in the Radiologic Clinics of North America Continuing Medical Education program, call customer service at 1-800-654-2452 or sign up online at http://www.theclinics.com/home/cme. The CME program is available to subscribers for an additional annual fee USD 245.

Radiologic Clinics of North America

THE CLINICS ARE NOW AVAILABLE ONLINE!

Access your subscription at:
www.theclinics.com

Preface
CT Angiography

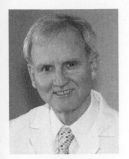

W. Dennis Foley, MD
Guest Editor

CT angiography has become a well-established method for noninvasive angiography and in conjunction with MR angiography has largely displaced catheter arteriography in the role of a preintervention angiographic technique. The clinical success of CT angiography is related to multidetector CT scanners, in particular scanners with 64-row or greater detectors, which have allowed wide area coverage in combination with submillimeter isotropic spatial resolution and rapid acquisition. In this issue of the *Radiologic Clinics of North America*, the technical basis of CT angiography, continued further improvements, and the appropriate integration of injection acquisition techniques to achieve good clinical results are detailed.

The article on imaging technology by Kanako Kumamaru and coauthors addresses the issue of spatial and temporal resolution and Z-axis coverage. Specialized acquisition modes, including gating and dual energy techniques, are explored. New developments in relation to wide area detector and dual-source acquisition are outlined with commentary on limitations related to x-ray scatter and cone-beam reconstruction. The discussion of EKG gating relates predominantly to cardiac imaging, although cardiac gating is increasingly used in CT angiography of the thoracic aorta.

The article on injection acquisition by Dominik Fleischmann outlines the physiologic and pharmacokinetic principles pertinent to arterial enhancement for imaging different anatomic regions. Successful implementation of CT angiography in clinical practice is ultimately dependent on adopting protocols that use the basic principles enumerated in this article.

The articles on clinical applications cover the full range of noncardiac CT angiography, illustrating the vascular and related organ system abnormalities that can be demonstrated by CT angiography. For each individual target area, the appropriate clinical indications and CT angiographic findings are described and discussed. Some new and evolving applications are explored. For all applications, emphasis is placed on the appropriate contrast material load and radiation dose, particularly in relation to pediatric applications of CT angiography.

In each application area, the authors provide their preferred method of injection/acquisition, information that should be of value for practicing radiologists. Variation in the approach to lower-extremity CT angiography between the fixed scan time strategy and a modification that may be considered velocity-compensated CT angiography illustrates some diversity in approach without losing sight of the basic goal of uniformly enhancing the vasculature throughout the display field of view.

A minor degree of overlap occurs in the articles on the abdominal aorta and lower extremities in relation to the pelvis. This is by intent to allow a comprehensive analysis in each article of the relevant findings for these 2 body areas.

This issue of *Radiologic Clinics of North America* should provide a useful basis for understanding the clinical applications of current state-of-the-art CT angiography and points the way to new developments, which will further enhance this clinically valuable technique.

W. Dennis Foley, MD
Department of Radiology
Medical College of Wisconsin
Froedtert Hospital East
9200 West Wisconsin Avenue, Milwaukee
WI 53226, USA

E-mail address:
dfoley@mcw.edu

Radiol Clin N Am 48 (2010) xiii
doi:10.1016/j.rcl.2010.04.001

CT Angiography: Current Technology and Clinical Use

Kanako K. Kumamaru, MD[a], Bernice E. Hoppel, PhD[b],
Richard T. Mather, PhD[b], Frank J. Rybicki, MD, PhD[c,*]

KEYWORDS

- Computed tomography • Angiography
- Vascular diseases • Coronary artery disease

Before Multidetector-row Computed Tomography (MDCT), the main barriers to the clinical implementation of Computed Tomographic Angiography (CTA) were acquisition speed and both spatial and temporal resolution. Imaging of any vascular bed requires rapid volume coverage coupled with the ability to resolve disease in small-diameter contrast-opacified vessels. One extreme for volume coverage is CTA for peripheral artery disease (PAD); imaging speed is mandated by blood velocity, on the order of 30 to 180 mm/s[1] from the abdominal aorta to the feet. The computed tomography (CT) acquisition must be synchronized with the contrast bolus throughout a large craniocaudal, or z-axis, field of view (FOV), which proves challenging in the presence of severe PAD; scans too fast will outrun the bolus. Scans too slow, that is, imaging after peak arterial enhancement, result in venous contamination. Another extreme in CTA is coronary angiography whereby superior temporal resolution is essential to decrease motion-related artifacts. As detailed later, faster gantry rotations, dual-source CT, and multisegment reconstruction have improved temporal resolution so that high-quality cardiac imaging is now routine.

Egas Moniz developed cerebral angiography in 1927, using x-rays and iodinated contrast material to allow him to diagnose brain disorders such as tumors, strokes, and injuries.[2] The first diagnostic coronary angiography was performed in 1958.[3]

Since then, catheter angiography has assumed the role of gold standard for vascular imaging, despite the invasive nature of the procedure, with 1.5% to 2% risk of significant morbidity and mortality, as well as high cost.[4] Less invasive techniques for vascular imaging have been developed, such as sonography with Doppler imaging,[5,6] magnetic resonance imaging (MRI),[7] and CTA,[8,9] and have matured in conjunction with developments in catheter arteriography. In many cases noninvasive imaging has become complementary to catheter angiography, such as Doppler imaging for the evaluation of patients with recurrent symptoms after angioplasty.[10] In many cases CT has been used in conjunction with catheter angiography, and in a few cases such as when imaging the aorta and the pulmonary arteries, CTA has supplanted catheter angiography as the gold standard. The expanding role of CTA emphasizes the need for deep, broad-based understanding of physical principles. The purpose of this review is to describe CT hardware and associated software for angiography. The fundamentals of CTA physics are complemented with several clinical examples.

METRICS FOR CT ANGIOGRAPHY

Three common, useful CT image quality metrics focus on the ability to resolve, or depict, differences between tissues, namely spatial resolution, temporal resolution, and volume coverage.

[a] Department of Radiology, University of Tokyo Hospital, 7-3-1 Hongo, Bunkyo-ku, Tokyo 113-8655, Japan
[b] Toshiba Medical Research Institute, 706 Deerpath Drive, Vernon Hills, IL 60061, USA
[c] Applied Imaging Science Laboratory, Department of Radiology, Brigham and Women's Hospital & Harvard Medical School, 75 Francis Street, Boston, MA 02115, USA
* Corresponding author.
E-mail address: frybicki@partners.org

Radiol Clin N Am 48 (2010) 213–235
doi:10.1016/j.rcl.2010.02.006
0033-8389/10/$ – see front matter © 2010 Elsevier Inc. All rights reserved.

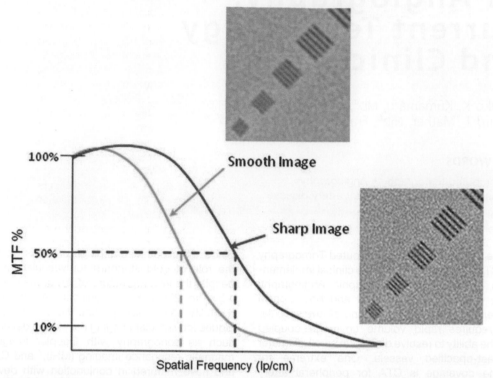

Fig. 1. Spatial resolution, described in units of line pairs per centimeter, determines the conspicuity of small objects. The ability to resolve the bar pattern gives an estimate of the spatial resolution of a system under prescribed conditions. Higher spatial frequencies allow smaller line pairs to be resolved and therefore will produce a sharper image.

Contrast media administration is also briefly reviewed because it is an essential part of the CTA acquisition.

Spatial resolution measures the smallest high-contrast object depicted by the CT system, and depends largely on the detector collimation and reconstruction kernel. Another key parameter is the size of the focal spot. Submillimeter slices generated from modern hardware has expanded the role of CTA from aortography to smaller vessels. Spatial resolution can be described in terms of the modulation transfer function (MTF)

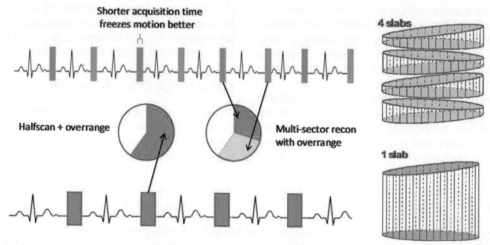

Fig. 2. Multisegment reconstruction. For a half-scan reconstruction and monosector reconstruction, data from a single heart beat are acquired over a longer temporal window and used to reconstruct the cardiac image at each z location. In multisegment reconstruction, data at each z-axis location are acquired from several heartbeats, each with a shorter temporal window, and then combined. (*Courtesy of* XiangYang Tang, Emory University.)

of the system (Fig. 1). Consider a set of equally spaced lines where the spaces have the same thickness as the lines. A "line pair" is defined as one line plus one space. The "spatial frequency" is measured in line pairs per centimeter. For example, 5 line pairs per centimeter would refer to lines and spaces each 1 mm thick, the total of the 5 line pairs and spaces would occupy exactly 1 centimeter. The MTF describes how well the CT scanner can separate objects with different spatial frequencies. Larger objects with poorly defined edges have predominantly low spatial frequencies; small objects with sharp edges have higher spatial frequencies. The CT scanner's spatial resolution is measured by the spatial frequency of the smallest, sharpest object it can see. CTA functions at roughly 8 to 15 line pairs per centimeter for a single focal spot, and higher with an in-plane dual focal spot. Although inferior to conventional catheter angiography, CTA can assess arteries as small as 1 mm in diameter. Because it is volumetric, CTA allows 3-dimensional visualization of the vasculature to separate superimposed structures. As illustrated in the applications described here, CT can image small, tortuous coronary arteries as well as the renal[11] and neurovascular circulation,[12,13] up to and including a comprehensive evaluation of the aorta.[14]

The second important metric for CTA, particularly for cardiac imaging, is temporal resolution. For cardiac imaging, superior temporal resolution is achieved from faster gantry rotation, dual-source CT, and multisegment reconstruction. Modern scanners have a gantry rotation time of 280 to 350 milliseconds. Therefore, a volume of data (3–4 cm on 64-detector row scanners) can be acquired with full scan mode in less than a half second. However, for cardiac imaging, faster imaging is needed to decrease motion artifacts associated with the beating heart. The half-scan technique[15] uses data from a little over 50% of a gantry rotation to improve temporal resolution to 175 milliseconds or less.

Dual-source CT provides the best temporal resolution available by using 2 radiation sources to simultaneously acquire different data projections.[16] This arrangement improves temporal resolution by a factor of 2[17]; in coronary imaging, image quality is improved with a temporal resolution of 82.5 milliseconds for higher heart rates.[18–20] Multisegment reconstruction[21] uses fewer data per cardiac cycle at each z-axis location, but acquires the additional projectional data at the same z-axis location for a full half-scan reconstruction from additional heartbeats. In essence, different sections of the image are obtained from different heartbeats (Fig. 2). Multisegment reconstruction increases patient radiation dose compared with single-segment reconstruction and is prone to artifacts from beat to beat variation.[22,23] Adaptive segmented reconstruction can compensate for some cardiac irregularity artifacts,[22,24,25] and improve sensitivity, specificity, and accuracy in the detection of

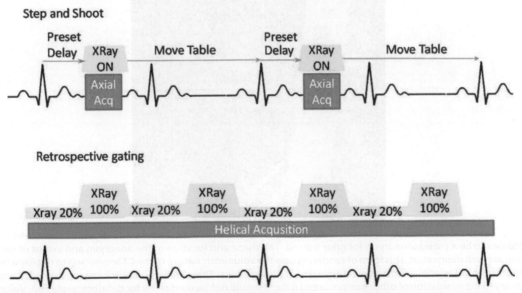

Fig. 3. Retrospective gating (*lower*) uses a helical acquisition with constant table motion throughout the cardiac cycle. The x-ray output is ramped up and down dependent on the phase of the cardiac cycle. Prospective gating, or the step and shoot method (*upper*), uses an axial acquisition at a predetermined delay time. During the following heart beat, the table is moved to the next location. Each data slab is acquired every other heart beat.

significant stenoses when compared with half-scan reconstructions of the same data.[26]

The z-axis coverage per gantry rotation plays a large role in the CTA acquisition. For example, 4 ×

1-mm detector-row CT requires the following trade-off between acquisition speed and slice thickness. With 0.5-second gantry rotation and a 1.25 pitch, a 30-cm cephalocaudad coverage typical of

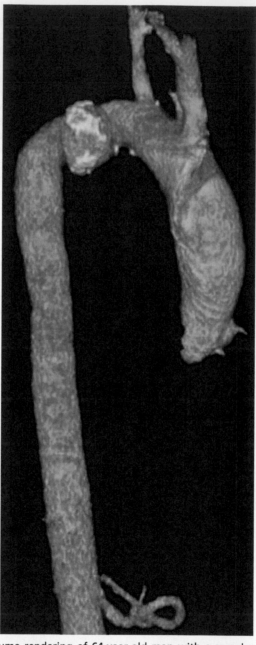

Fig. 4. Three-dimensional volume rendering of 64-year-old man with a saccular aneurysm of the aortic arch, presumed to be a pseudoaneurysm for prior trauma. The shape and location of the aneurysm and extent of calcification are well delineated. This form of rendering uses the volumetric nature of the CT acquisition to display a large data set from any spatial orientation. A single view is shown above. Three-dimensional volume rendering is complementary to the evaluation of other postprocessed data; it should not be used alone for data interpretation. Volumes are highly desirable to illustrate findings for referring clinicians and can be particularly important for surgical planning. (*From* Gasparovic H, Rybicki FJ, Millstine J, et al. Three dimensional computed tomographic imaging in planning the surgical approach for redo cardiac surgery after coronary revascularization. Eur J Cardiothorac Surg 2005;28(2):244–9; with permission.)

aortoiliac or mesenteric CTA requires a 30-second acquisition. Using a 4 × 3-mm detector row configuration, scan time is reduced to 10 seconds. Such trade-offs are not necessary with 16- or greater detector row systems because of larger volume coverage. In fact, 4 cm or greater coverage per gantry rotation from larger detectors introduces the problem of imaging too quickly and thus outrunning the iodinated contrast bolus. Wide-area detector systems (8–16 cm per rotation) can image axially, that is, without table motion, and may have advantages for dynamic perfusion imaging.[27]

The injection of contrast medium is essential to delineate the vascular lumen and, when possible, to discriminate the lumen from the vessel wall. Because high patient tolerance and lumen opacification are paramount, the ideal agent for CTA is nonionic, iso- or low osmolar, and has high iodine concentration. In the United States, the maximum concentration is 370 mg of iodine per mL; in Europe 400 mg of iodine per mL is available. Viscosity can impede high injection rates but is decreased by injection of contrast media warmed close to physiologic temperatures. Streak artifact

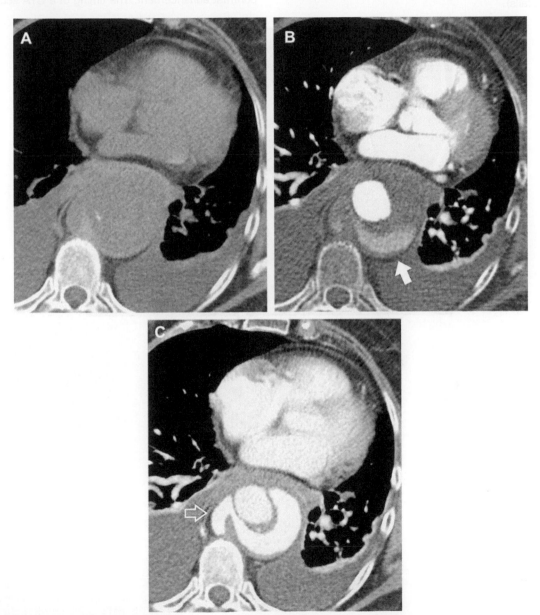

Fig. 5. Axial images from a 79-year-old woman with type B aortic dissection and rupture. (A) Noncontrast; (B) 30 seconds after intravenous injection; (C) 60 seconds after intravenous injection. The false lumen partially enhances after 30 seconds (*solid arrow*) with extravasation (*open arrow*) at the later point of enhancement.

emanating from the superior vena cava and right atrium, as seen with high iodine concentrations and large volumes, reflect suboptimized imaging protocols; saline flush injection following contrast should avoid this problem. Protocols must be tailored to the vascular bed and typically require rapid contrast administration (3–6 mL/s). Biphasic injection can provide a more homogeneous enhancement profile over time.[28,29] Faster acquisitions enable smaller contrast volumes because peak enhancement is required for shorter acquisition times (Appendix 1 gives imaging parameter details).

IMAGE ACQUISITION

The large majority of CTA uses helical CT[30] with continuous gantry rotation and table motion. Along with the rotation time, the helical pitch determines the table speed, and therefore the speed at which the volume is scanned. Care must be taken to match the helical pitch and table speed with the first circulation of contrast material through the anatomic region of interest. Acquisitions with too high a helical pitch and table speed outrun the iodine bolus and do not acquire data during peak contrast enhancement. The timing of a CTA scan

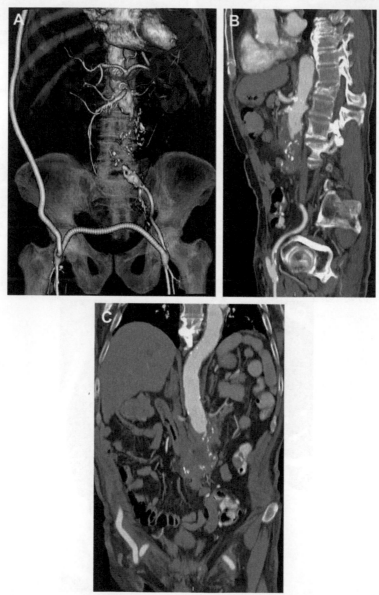

Fig. 6. A 73-year-old man status post axillobifemoral bypass graft for an occluded distal aorta. (A) Patency of the entire graft is illustrated on a single 3-dimensional volume-rendered image. (B) Sagittal and (C) coronal maximum-intensity projections demonstrate the occluded distal aorta and mesenteric vessels.

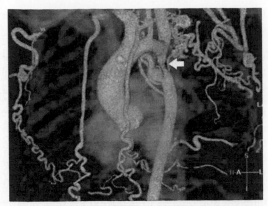

Fig. 7. Three-dimensional volume-rendered image of 54-year-old man with severe coarctation (*arrow*). In this patient, the single image provides a good overview of extensive collaterals through intercostal, internal thoracic, and axillary arteries.

is of critical importance so that the data are acquired during peak enhancement and not before or after the contrast has arrived. To ensure proper circulation timing, scanners use either a mini test bolus or automatic bolus-tracking software. With the test bolus approach, a small amount of contrast is injected and low radiation dose scans are acquired as a separate series to time the contrast arrival. Subsequently, a CTA scan is acquired with the full dose of contrast material, with a scan delay as determined by the test bolus. The second, more common approach is automatic tracking of the main bolus arrival with subsequent automatic initiation of the acquisition. This "bolus tracking" is accomplished by starting the main injection of contrast with the scanner taking intermittent low radiation dose scans. When contrast opacification reaches a preset threshold, the scanner automatically moves to the start position and begins the CTA helical acquisition.

Retrospective electrocardiograph (ECG) gating with helical CT can be used to freeze motion, either from the aortic root in CT aortography or for coronary CTA. Retrospective gating is not required for evaluation of the descending aorta, and should not be used because retrospective gating inherently has a higher radiation dose than helical imaging without gating. When retrospective gating is used, image reconstruction uses only the data acquired during a short segment of the cardiac cycle (Fig. 3). The data are then postprocessed to correlate with the ECG and assign cardiac phase to each segment of the reconstructed data. For coronary imaging, the entire circulation can be imaged in 4 to 8 seconds using 64-detector row scanners. Image quality is degraded by blurring secondary to rapid heart rates and misregistration artifacts secondary to heart rate variability and arrythmia.[19–21,23,31] For single-source x-ray systems, β-blockers should be used to decrease the heart rate, dependent on patient tolerance. Motion compensation algorithms allow for more consistent image quality.[32]

Prospective helical ECG-gated CT has been implemented primarily for coronary CTA to lower dose when compared with retrospective

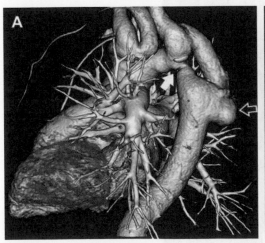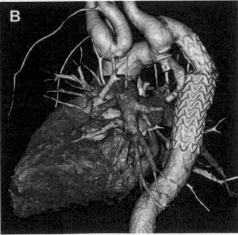

Fig. 8. A 60-year-old woman with right aortic arch, coarctation (*solid arrow*), and saccular pseudoaneurysm (*open arrow*) before (*A*) and after (*B*) endovascular stent graft placement. Three-dimensional volume rendering provides anatomic mapping for surgical planning as well as posttreatment follow-up. Images of this patient demonstrate how CT has assumed the role of gold standard in aortography. Conventional angiography cannot delineate 3-dimensional relationships between structures preoperatively. It is also invasive and impractical for follow-up. MR aortography typically provides relatively comparable image quality but is limited by susceptibility artifact in many stent graft patients.

gating.[33–35] Both helical and axial prospective acquisitions reduce the patient radiation dose dramatically.[36–38] Prospective gating uses information from prior heartbeats to estimate the correct time to turn the x-rays on and off during the acquisition R-R intervals (see Fig. 3). Helical acquisitions are similar to the retrospective approach, except that the x-rays are turned completely off except during the acquisition phases in diastole. For an axial acquisition, the scanner acquires an axial slab during one heartbeat, repositions the patient during the next heartbeat, and acquires another axial slab in the next heartbeat. This acquisition spans several heartbeats with 64-detector rows[39] or can be achieved in a single heartbeat with wide-area detector CT.[40,41]

Multiple-energy CTA with bone subtraction software is a potentially important tool that is either under investigation or just entering the clinical arena. The long-term goal of multienergy imaging is additional anatomic and physiologic information based on the energy dependence of tissue attenuation differences.[42,43] Tissue components can be determined via postprocessing of images collected at 2 energies,[44,45] or via direct analysis within the raw CT projection data simultaneously acquired at separate energies.[46] There are several different approaches to acquiring the dual-energy data. Slow kV switching uses 2 rotations at

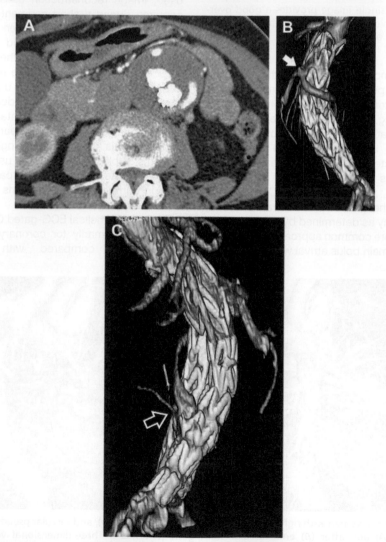

Fig. 9. An 85-year-old woman, status post endovascular stent repair for an abdominal aortic aneurysm. (A) Contrast-enhanced axial image shows enhancement outside of the round stent limbs but within the aneurysm; this is the criterion for an endoleak. (B, C) Three-dimensional volume-rendered images illustrate the source of the abnormal contrast enhancement; the type II endoleak is shown with flow from the enhanced inferior mesenteric artery (*solid arrow*) and fifth lumbar arteries (*open arrow*).

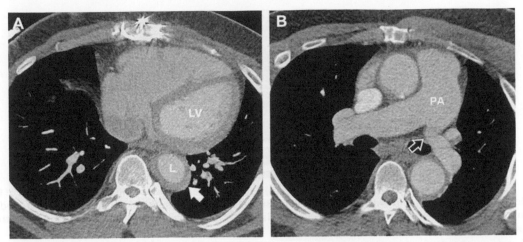

Fig. 10. A 41-year-old man with known Takayasu arteritis. (*A*) Axial image at the level of the left ventricle (LV) shows a thickened aortic wall (*solid arrow*) identified between the iodinated contrast filled lumen (L) and the surrounding lung parenchyma. (*B*) Axial image at the level of the main pulmonary artery (PA) show less prominent thickening of aortic wall plus stenosis of the left pulmonary artery (*open arrow*).

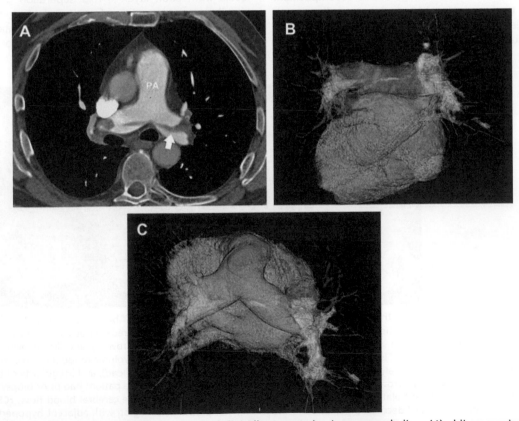

Fig. 11. An 80-year-old man with dyspnea and clinically suspected pulmonary embolism. (*A*) oblique maximum-intensity projection oriented to optimally demonstrate the bifurcation of the main pulmonary artery (PA) shows a saddle-type pulmonary embolism, characterized by filling defects (*arrow*). (*B, C*) Three-dimensional volume-rendered images use segmentation to illustrate the extent of the thrombus in yellow.

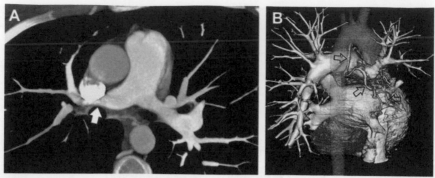

Fig. 12. A 24-year-old woman with known vasculitis. (*A*) Contrast-enhanced axial image shows the stenosis of the right pulmonary artery (*solid arrow*). (*B*) Three-dimensional volume-rendered image (aorta is demonstrated as translucent) enables the visualization of many small collaterals (*open arrow*) from the bronchial arteries and their relationship to surrounding tissues.

different kV settings, but cannot be used for CTA. Dual-source CT has been clinically realized, with each tube operating at a different kV and acquiring data 90° apart. Each tube can operate different currents to equalize the noise between the different energies.[47–49] Both slow kV switching and dual source use image-based decomposition. To use raw data based decomposition, each projection must be acquired at both energies simultaneously. Fast kV switching allows the energy to be changed for each adjacent projection, which approximates simultaneous acquisition and has the potential for plaque characterization.[50] A spectrally sensitive detector, such as a sandwich detector, uses distinct detector materials[51] to separate different energy levels from each layer.[52] This separation gives simultaneous acquisition of each projection, but is challenged by poor energy discrimination. Energy-sensitive, photon-counting detectors[53]

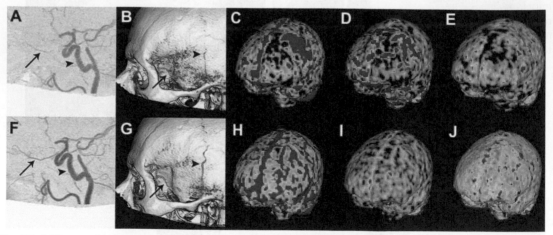

Fig. 13. A 39-year-old man with giant cell arteritis imaged with 320-detector row CT before (*top row*) and after (*bottom row*) corticosteroid therapy. (*A*) CTA shows beading and stenosis of the precavernous, cavernous, and supraclinoid portions of the internal carotid artery (*arrowhead*). There is narrowing and irregularity of ophthalmic artery (*arrow*) that is resolved after treatment (*F*). (*B*) Three-dimensional volume rendering shows narrowing and beading of parietal branch of the left superficial temporal artery (*arrowhead*), and irregularity of the remaining frontal branch (*arrow*) that are improved after therapy (*G*). Note that the patient had prior biopsy of the frontal branch. (*C, H*) (relative cerebral blood volume: rCBV) and (*D, I*) (relative cerebral blood flow: rCBF) maps illustrate a region of decreased perfusion in the left frontal parasagittal region with adjacent hypoperfusion that returned to normal symmetric perfusion after therapy. (*E*) Mean transit time (MTT) map shows left frontal decreased transit time that resolved following treatment (*J*). (*From* Yahyavi-Firouz-Abadi N, Wynn BL, Rybicki FJ, et al. Steroid-responsive large vessel vasculitis: application of whole-brain 320-detector row dynamic volume CT angiography and perfusion. AJNR Am J Neuroradiol 2009;30(7):1409–11; with permission.)

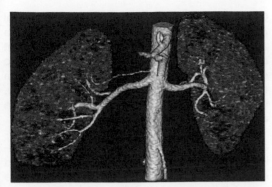

Fig. 14. Three-dimensional volume-rendered image for the planning of kidney transplant, showing normal renal arteries. Note the clearly visualized right accessory renal artery.

are fast enough to determine the energy of every photon absorbed, allowing true simultaneous multienergy imaging, but these are not yet fast enough to read data at clinical CT acquisition speeds.

Bone subtraction software[54] is particularly important for neurovascular imaging at the skull base or discrimination between the anterior tibia and the anterior tibial artery. In the skull, this can be accomplished via image subtraction using 2 helical or wide-volume scans.[22,55] Dual-energy CT may enhance current bone removal algorithms.[56] Complete bone removal in the transcranial region and in the limbs is expected to improve vascular interpretation.[48,57,58] At present, residual fragments from incomplete separation must be manually sculpted using postprocessing tools, which is tedious and prone to human error.

Dual-energy CT has additional potential benefits of removing blooming and beam hardening effects that may overlap and conceal stenoses.[51,59]

NEW DEVELOPMENTS IN CT ANGIOGRAPHY

Until recently, state of the art CT was defined by "64-generation" scanners that produced 64-slices, either 64-detector rows or 32-detector rows, and a strategy to double the slice number by alternate deflection of the focal spot of the x-ray source. More modern CT scanners make up the "post-64 era"[60] and improve on the fundamental CT parameters.

Wide-area detector CT extends craniocaudal coverage to 16 cm and enables simultaneous large-volume craniocaudal imaging either with no table motion (axial imaging) or via helical acquisition. For smaller volumes such as the heart and kidneys, imaging can be shortened to 1 second or less. As noted earlier, with very rapid imaging, careful timing of the contrast media is needed to optimize image quality.

The main advantage of wide-area detector scanning is temporal uniformity. With helical or "step-and-shoot" axial scanning, the total z-axis volume is the combination of subvolumes, each acquired at a different time point. For imaging with no anatomic motion and no temporal variation, for example, noncontrast thoracic CT with a perfect breath hold, there is no benefit of temporal uniformity because the combination of slabs is identical to imaging with the larger z-axis coverage. However, CTA

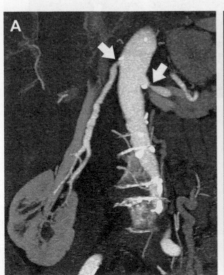
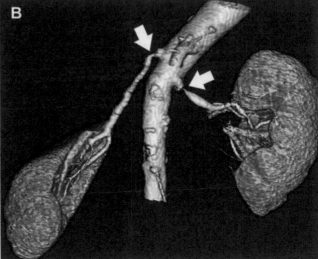

Fig. 15. An 85-year-old woman with bilateral renal artery stenosis (arrows). (A) Coronal maximum-intensity projection focused on the right renal artery. (B) Three-dimensional volume rendering also demonstrates the relationship of the renal arteries and the kidneys.

introduces flowing contrast media that always varies during subvolume acquisition. Wide-area detector CT decreases the variation in contrast enhancement to the limit of scanning the entire z-axis FOV axially so that the volume has temporal uniformity, without step or misregistration artifacts. Furthermore, simultaneous axial acquisition of the entire volume eliminates overscan, reducing dose when compared with a comparable helical acquisition.[61–63] The future applications of stationary table CTA include the evaluation of contrast flow dynamics.[64–67]

One advantage of dual-source CT is high temporal resolution achieved from 2 coplanar x-ray tubes and detector arrays.[16] The temporal resolution can be reduced to one-quarter of a gantry rotation, with the greatest advantage being coronary imaging with reduced motion artifact. The second advantage is that the system can operate at two energies, one at a low kVp and the other at a high kVp, to achieve a dual-energy acquisition.[42] The ability to provide material decomposition imaging can be applied to CTA with removal of vessel wall calcium and decrease of blooming artifact. However, regarding removal of coronary calcifications, it is important to note that a dual-source CT system cannot provide simultaneous dual-energy capability with quarter rotation temporal resolution. Another new application of 64-detector row (128-slice) vascular

CT is dual-source imaging with a very high helical pitch. This technique provides rapid large-area z-axis volume acquisition, and single heartbeat coronary imaging has been shown under specific conditions of very low heart rate.[68] The application for vascular imaging will likely be aortography, whereby very fast acquisitions can cover the entire aorta.

There are several technical challenges associated with CT technology. One of the primary challenges is x-ray scatter. Ideally, an x-ray should either pass completely through the subject or be completely absorbed. When incompletely absorbed, the x-ray loses energy and changes direction.[69,70] This phenomenon is known as scatter. If the scattered x-ray is not detected, the effect is the same as if it were completely absorbed. However, if the scatter angle is small or if the detector is wide, there is an increased chance that the x-ray will be detected. For dual-source CT, cross-scatter occurs when x-rays from one source are scattered and detected by the other detector. When any of these happen, the x-ray is misregistered with the photons that reached the same point by passing entirely though the subject. Misregistered x-rays introduce image noise and decrease image quality. To minimize scatter, CT scanners typically have small metal septa between detector elements. Because scattered photons approach the detector from directions other than

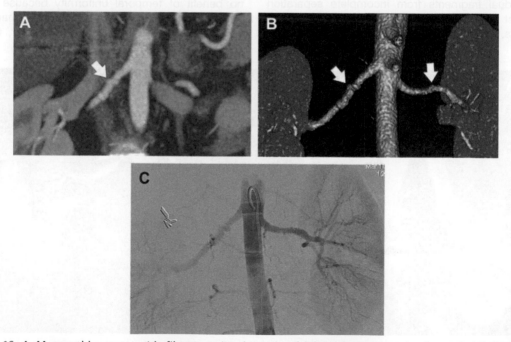

Fig. 16. A 44-year-old woman with fibromuscular dysplasia of bilateral renal arteries (*arrows*). (*A*) Coronal maximum-intensity projection and (*B*) 3-dimensional volume-rendered image have sufficient spatial resolution, showing beaded appearance of proximal renal arteries consistent with the finding on (*C*) catheter angiogram.

the focal spot, these septa are aligned with a line between the detector element and the x-ray focal spot, thus eliminating nearly all x-rays that approach the detector from an incorrect angle.[71] These septa typically are only along the x-y plane, but some wide-area detector scanners have septa along the z-direction.

The cone angle issue is inherent to MDCT. Conventional reconstruction algorithms assume that the x-ray source, the detector, and the slice of interest all lie within the same plane. Furthermore, these algorithms assume that all projections for a slice fall on the same detector row.[72,73] These assumptions are only valid for single-slice, axial CT. Interpolation between projections is designed to approximate detector row geometries, but larger interpolations introduce cone beam artifacts requiring sophisticated algorithms to minimize artifacts.

For helical scanning, as detectors increase in size there is an additional challenge. To reconstruct images at either end of the helical volume, the algorithm requires additional raw data before and after the volume, leading to a longer beam-on time and additional patient radiation. The extra rotations are called "over-ranging" or helical overscan. The relative contribution of the overscan region to the total patient radiation dose is a function of the length of the acquired volume, the helical pitch, and the detector configuration.[74,75] The percentage contribution of the overscan region increases with shorter volumes. Because the required extra data are based on angular projections and not distance, the detector configuration is significant; wider configurations have a larger overscan area. This circumstance is partially mitigated by dynamic collimators to

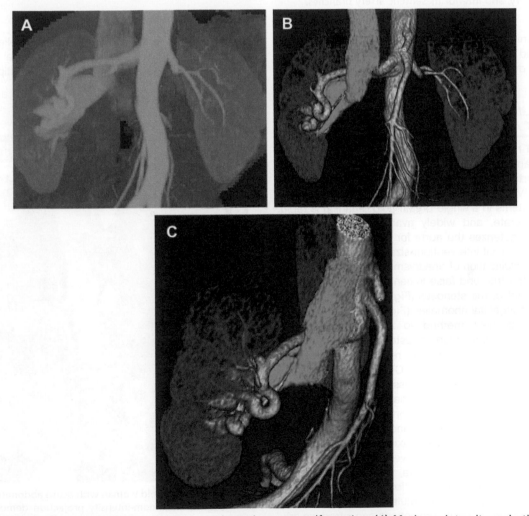

Fig. 17. A 39-year-old woman with right renal arteriovenous malformation. (A) Maximum-intensity projection shows early venous filling, an important finding in this diagnosis. (B, C) Three-dimensional volume-rendered images (venous system is segmented in blue) illustrate the shape and position of tortuous arteries or veins.

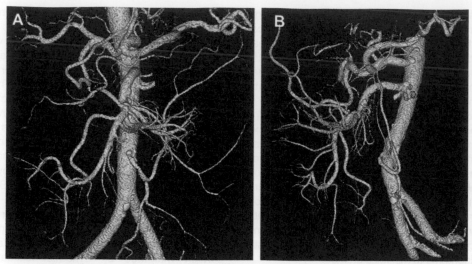

Fig. 18. (*A, B*) Three-dimensional volume-rendered images in a patient with normal celiac, superior mesenteric artery, and inferior mesenteric artery branches.

minimize the effect[76]; however, high helical pitch and fast rotation times can limit the effectiveness of dynamic collimation.

CLINICAL CT ANGIOGRAPHY
CT Aortography

CT has replaced catheter angiography as the gold standard for imaging the aorta.[77,78] The entire aorta can be imaged in seconds, and the z-axis FOV can be extended to the carotid and/or iliac systems in a single breath hold. Imaging is rapid, accurate, and widely available. CT completely characterizes the aorta for either catheter-based or surgical intervention: size, shape, and severity of calcification of aneurysms (**Fig. 4**), morphology of the true and false lumen in dissection (**Fig. 5**), extent of the stenoses (**Fig. 6**), and the anatomy of congenital anomalies (**Figs. 7** and **8**). CT is the overall best method to detect posttreatment complications such as restenosis, thrombosis, or endoleak after aneurysm repair (**Fig. 9**). In addition, contrast-enhanced CT can provide useful insights into the thickness and composition of the vessel wall by differentiating lumen and arterial wall, allowing the evaluation of vasculitis (**Fig. 10**). Image postprocessing includes 3-dimensional volume rendering and maximum-intensity projections. The latter can be very accurate for larger vessels such as the aorta, with adequate intraluminal contrast concentration. Smaller vessels are best analyzed with multiplanar reformations; maximum-intensity projections can introduce artifact in smaller vessels once the image thickness approaches or exceeds the diameter of the

vessel. Volume rendering provides an excellent overview of large vessels such as the aorta as well as the spatial orientation of multiple structures.

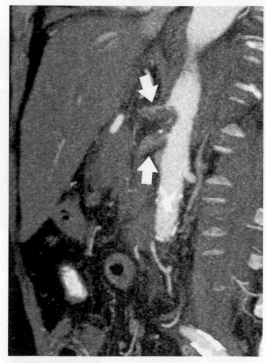

Fig. 19. An 84-year-old woman with acute abdominal pain. Sagittal maximum-intensity projection demonstrates thrombosis with occlusion of the celiac artery with near occlusion of the superior mesenteric artery (*arrows*).

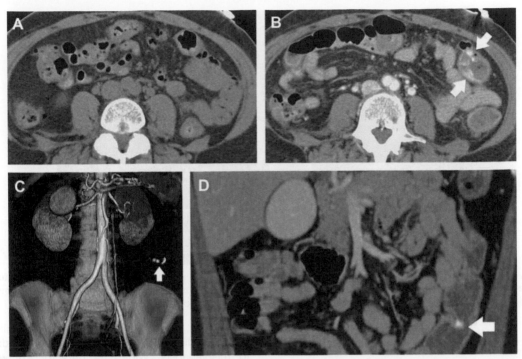

Fig. 20. A 54-year-old woman with abdominal pain and rectal bleeding. Comparison between (*A*) noncontrast and (*B*) contrast-enhanced image shows extravasation of contrast media (*arrows*) into the lumen of the distal transverse colon, indicating active bleeding. Reformation of the CT data as (*C*) a 3-dimensional volume rendering or (*D*) coronal maximum-intensity projection shows the high attenuation of the contrast indicating hemorrhage (*arrows*).

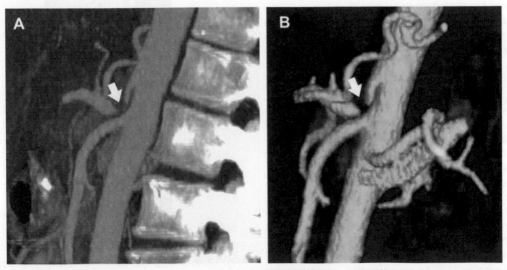

Fig. 21. A 50-year-old man with abdominal pain and high clinical suspicion for median arcuate ligament compression (*arrow*). (*A*) Sagittal maximum-intensity projection and (*B*) 3-dimensional volume rendering are essential to detail the relationship between the compressed celiac axis and the aorta. Note the normal superior mesenteric artery, a characteristic finding in these patients.

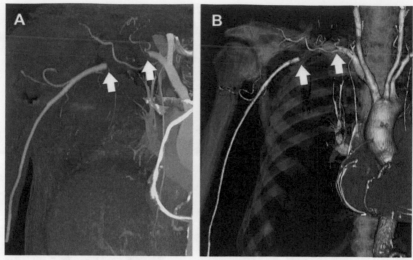

Fig. 22. A 91-year-old man with right shoulder and arm pain. Upper extremity CTA displayed as (A) maximum-intensity projection and (B) 3-dimensional volume rendering shows acute subclavian artery thrombosis (arrows). Patients with more long-standing obstruction are expected to have more collateral flow.

CT Pulmonary Angiography

CT pulmonary angiography (CTPA) has replaced catheter angiography as the gold standard for imaging the pulmonary arteries. The only role for other modalities is patients with a contraindication to CT. Breath-hold imaging of the entire thorax is routine because multidetector rows dramatically increase the z-axis coverage per gantry rotation, and because gantry rotation speeds are less than 0.5 second. CTPA has high sensitivity and specificity in detecting pulmonary embolism (Fig. 11).[79,80] Long-term changes in patients with pulmonary embolism or pulmonary artery stenosis include the development of small collateral arteries that can be characterized with volume rendering to show the relationship with surrounding structures (Fig. 12).

Neurovascular CT Angiography

CTA of the head and neck provides high-quality, 3 dimensional image data sets to study cerebrovascular anatomy in any arbitrary plane. CT enjoys increasing use with respect to MR and catheter angiography [81–83]; the noninvasive nature saves both procedure time and patient discomfort. Furthermore, in complicated patients CTA can often be performed using less iodinated contrast media than catheter angiography, an advantage for patients at high risk for contrast-induced nephropathy.[84,85] As noted earlier, neurovascular CTA has challenges near the skull base, such as in the petrous carotid region. These vessels travel very close to the surrounding bone and can be easily obscured or distorted, potentially leading to misdiagnosis. Wide-area detector CT with 16-cm z-axis coverage can image the whole brain axially, enabling angiography images to be obtained in conjunction with whole-brain perfusion

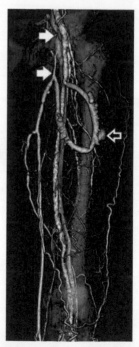

Fig. 23. A 38-year-old man with left thigh arteriovenous hemodialysis graft. Three-dimensional volume rendering shows stenosis (solid arrows) in the left saphenous and femoral veins cranial to the anastomosis. There is a small graft aneurysm (open arrow).

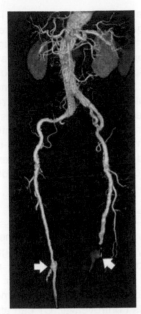

Fig. 24. An 82-year-old man status post endovascular stent graft placement. Note that the tortured bilateral iliac and femoral arteries with distal aneurysms (*arrows*) are well visualized on 3-dimensional volume-rendered image.

images obtained with no table motion and no artifact from the postacquisition combination of sub-volumes (Fig. 13).

Coronary CT Angiography

Calcium scoring images are acquired without intravenous contrast to optimally visualize and quantify calcified plaque, a strong indicator of coronary artery disease.[86] However, this is not considered angiography because the lumen is not evaluated for stenosis. For CTA, artifacts such as calcium blooming[87,88] and beam hardening[89,90] can be problematic in the interpretation of stenosis, particularly when there are metal stents[91,92] and heavily calcified coronary arteries. Coronary imaging differs from CTA of other body parts because ECG gating is needed to freeze cardiac motion. When retrospective ECG gating is used, ejection fraction and wall motion evaluation can be added to the interpretation. However, the trend in current cardiac CT is to perform prospective ECG gating to lower radiation dose.

New data are beginning to support the use of CT data beyond the interpretation of coronary stenosis. For example, plaque characterization in its early stages (fatty and fibrous) may be possible.[93,94] Coronary events may be predicted from the type and distribution of plaque or estimation of the endothelial shear stress along the coronary tree.[95,96] At present, such assessment relies on intravascular ultrasound (IVUS), which has the disadvantages that only a single-vessel study can be performed at a time and that there is a known albeit relatively small rate of complications.[97–99]

Renal and Mesenteric CT Angiography

Renal arteries are common sites of atherosclerosis with associated stenosis, aneurysms, or occlusion. Because the average renal artery diameter is approximately 4 to 5 mm and accessory arteries are considerably smaller, up to 15% of vessels can be missed by 1- to 4-detector row CTA.[100]

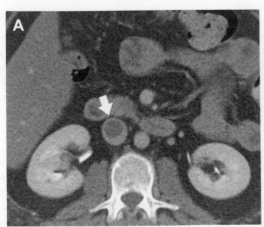
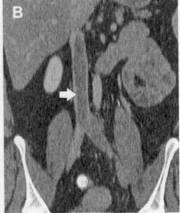

Fig. 25. A 39-year-old woman with extensive thrombus in inferior vena cava. (*A*) Contrast-enhanced axial image shows the filling defect in inferior vena cava (*arrow*). (*B*) Coronal maximum-intensity projection can depict long segments of thrombus (*arrow*).

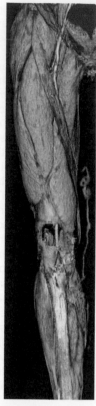

Fig. 26. Three-dimensional volume rendering of a 58-year-old man with varicose veins. CT venography provides the interventionist with a comprehensive view of the varicose veins (segmented in blue) with clear anatomic landmarks such as muscle and bone.

Submillimeter isotropic resolution from more modern hardware improves spatial resolution; these scanners also have shorter acquisition times to better visualize normal (Fig. 14) and atherosclerotic (Fig. 15) renal arteries. CT can also be used for other diagnoses such as fibromuscular dysplasia (Fig. 16). Three-dimensional volume rendering and maximum-intensity projections are important in the planning of therapy (Fig. 17).

Mesenteric arteries are very small, with distal branches measuring 1 mm or less in diameter (Fig. 18). CT for mesenteric ischemia (Fig. 19) can be acquired at multiple phases of contrast enhancement to evaluate arteries, veins, and the bowel wall. A dynamic protocol can also be used to pinpoint the location of a gastrointestinal bleed (Fig. 20). CT can also be used as an imaging modality of choice for clinically suspected median arcuate ligament syndrome (Fig. 21).

Peripheral CT Angiography

Patients with PAD (Fig. 22), acute embolic events, trauma, and complications after procedures

(Fig. 23) can be evaluated with CT. As noted earlier, adequate enhancement requires an understanding of the scanner speed and kinetics of the iodinated contrast medium. In patients with severe PAD, the speed of the contrast bolus can be 30 mm per second.[1] While outrunning the bolus is highly unlikely with a 4-detector row CT, the risk increases with faster table speeds associated with 64 (or more) slices per gantry rotation. Maximum-intensity projections and 3-dimensional volume rendering provide a good overview of the vessel anatomy, patency, and the development of collateral vessels (Fig. 24).

CT Venography

Imaging during venous enhancement, or CT venography, can be used to diagnose deep venous thrombosis (Fig. 25). The role of CT venography in the pelvis and lower extremities acquired in combination with CT pulmonary angiography[101] is controversial. CT can also be used to evaluate varicose veins, although it is not a first-line imaging modality for this condition (Fig. 26). Lower extremity CT venography is usually acquired roughly 180 to 240 seconds after antecubital vein contrast injection. Although there is no standard protocol to visualize inferior vena cava, the portal phase (60–70 seconds after contrast injection) or equilibrium phase (90–120 seconds) can be used.

SUMMARY

Recent advances in technology have moved CT to the front line for many vascular diseases, dramatically changing clinical evaluation pathways. Understanding CT technology is critical for optimizing protocols.

APPENDIX 1: CT IMAGING PARAMETERS

Scan parameters influence image quality and patient dose in CTA.[102–105] Factors such as kV, mAs, pitch, detector configuration, and rotation time are interrelated. Understanding these relationships enables design of optimal protocols for a particular CT system and a given application.

kV (Kilovolts)

Tube potential, or kV, represents the voltage between the anode and cathode of the x-ray CT tube and thus determines the energy of the emitted x-rays. When compared with lower energies, higher energy x-rays have a greater probability of passing through the body to reach a detector and creating a signal. All else being equal, higher kVp means less noise but also less contrast between materials because contrast is generated by x-rays absorbed by the body.[106] However, higher energy x-rays absorbed by the body deposit more energy than those with lower energy and thus gives greater dose. Furthermore, the higher tube potential causes more x-rays to be generated for the same tube current. For the same scan parameters, changing the kVp from 120 to 135 increases the dose by about 33%.[107] Because of the higher dose and poorer contrast,[88] 135 to 140 kVp is clinically used for better penetration of obese patients or dense anatomy, for example, bone or metal.[108]

mAs (Milliampere Seconds)

The tube current, or mA, determines the number of x-rays the tube produces. Combined with the gantry rotation time, this represents the total x-ray output of the tube per rotation, or mAs. Changing the mAs is the most common method of adjusting dose and noise level. Halving the mAs will reduce patient dose twofold but will also halve the number of x-rays reaching the detector. Image noise increases and low contrast detectability will be diminished.[109]

Helical Pitch

Helical pitch is the distance the CT table travels in a rotation divided by the total active detector width in the z-direction. Higher pitch lowers dose because of faster table movement and subsequent lower beam-on time at each z-axis location. Because of redundant data with 64-detector row CT, good reconstruction algorithms prevent the slice sensitivity profile (a curve showing the relationship between the CT number and slice position along the patient's z-axis in helical CT) from broadening with pitches between 1 and 2. However, as the pitch increases, there are fewer projection data for a given slice and thus noise increases. To compensate, the mA is typically increased. Higher pitch value may also introduce more helical artifact. Thus, increased pitch values are clinically relevant for studies requiring fast acquisition with decreased scan time.

mAs_eff (Effective mAs)

The mAs_eff is the mAs divided by the pitch, and has been used as a dose surrogate that is appropriate for comparing dose between protocols on a single-scanner model.[110] However, mAs_eff is not an appropriate value for comparing dose between scanners because of differences in geometry and filtration.

Collimation

Many combinations of slice width and number can be acquired. The actual x-ray beam is slightly wider than the nominal beam width, defined as the number of detector rows multiplied by detector element width. This situation ensures that detectors on the edge of the array receive uniform x-ray coverage, resulting in a small amount of unused radiation called penumbra.[22] The total amount of penumbra typically is the same regardless of the nominal beam width. Therefore, with larger beams, the extra radiation from the penumbra is a smaller percentage of the overall useful beam width. The combination of a wide beam and thinner slices optimizes image quality and dose efficiency.

Acquired and Reconstructed Slice Width

The acquired slice width depends on the detector configuration and thus determines the minimum reconstructed image width. For example, images from a 16×1-mm detector configuration can be reconstructed at 1 mm or greater; a 16×0.5-mm configuration enables 0.5-mm slice reconstruction. At equal radiation dose, thicker slices have less noise because proportionately more photons are used. However, the trade-off is poorer z-axis resolution and subsequent partial volume artifacts[111] that comprise vascular imaging and image reformation.[112] Thus, to resolve small image detail in routine CTA, optimum image quality and dose efficiency use the thinnest slices available.[113]

Reconstruction Kernel

The acquired data are filtered by the reconstruction kernel, which largely influences the perceived spatial resolution, image noise, and dose needed for clinically useful images. Sharper kernels improve in-plane spatial resolution with the trade-off of greater noise; smoother kernels reduce noise at the expense of in-plane resolution. Kernels for most CT examinations are relatively sharp, reflecting the need for spatial detail in small vessels. The sharpest kernels used in clinical practice are for evaluation of in-stent luminal diameter and detection of in-stent stenoses.[22,114]

REFERENCES

1. Fleischmann D, Rubin GD. Quantification of intravenously administered contrast medium transit through the peripheral arteries: implications for CT angiography. Radiology 2005;236(3):1076–82.
2. Ligon BL. Biography: history of developments in imaging techniques: Egas Moniz and angiography. Semin Pediatr Infect Dis 2003;14(2):173–81.

3. Mueller RL, Sanborn TA. The history of interventional cardiology: cardiac catheterization, angioplasty, and related interventions. Am Heart J 1995; 129(1):146–72.

4. Waugh JR, Sacharias N. Arteriographic complications in the DSA era. Radiology 1992;182(1):243–6.

5. Scoutt LM, Zawin ML, Taylor KJ. Doppler US. Part II. Clinical applications. Radiology 1990;174(2): 309–19.

6. Krnic A, Vucic N, Sucic Z. Duplex scanning compared with intra-arterial angiography in diagnosing peripheral arterial disease: three analytical approaches. Vasa 2006;35(2):86–91.

7. Wardlaw JM, Chappell FM, Best JJ, et al. Non-invasive imaging compared with intra-arterial angiography in the diagnosis of symptomatic carotid stenosis: a meta-analysis. Lancet 2006;367(9521): 1503–12.

8. Heijenbrok-Kal MH, Kock MC, Hunink MG. Lower extremity arterial disease: multidetector CT angiography meta-analysis. Radiology 2007;245(2):433–9.

9. Schoenhagen P, Halliburton SS, Stillman AE, et al. Noninvasive imaging of coronary arteries: current and future role of multi-detector row CT. Radiology 2004;232(1):7–17.

10. Rybicki FJ, Nallamshetty L, Yucel EK, et al. ACR appropriateness criteria on recurrent symptoms following lower-extremity angioplasty. J Am Coll Radiol 2008;5(12):1176–80.

11. Leiner T, de Haan MW, Nelemans PJ, et al. Contemporary imaging techniques for the diagnosis of renal artery stenosis. Eur Radiol 2005; 15(11):2219–29.

12. Arora S, Chien JD, Cheng SC, et al. Optimal carotid artery coverage for carotid plaque CT-imaging in predicting ischemic stroke. J Neuroradiol 2010;37(2):98–103.

13. Rozie S, de Weert TT, de Monye C, et al. Atherosclerotic plaque volume and composition in symptomatic carotid arteries assessed with multidetector CT angiography; relationship with severity of stenosis and cardiovascular risk factors. Eur Radiol 2009;19(9):2294–301.

14. Buckley O, Rybicki FJ, Gerson DS, et al. Imaging features of intramural hematoma of the aorta. Int J Cardiovasc Imaging 2010;26(1):65–76.

15. Hsieh J. Computed tomography: principles, design, artifacts, and recent advances. Bellingham (WA): SPIE Optical Engineering Press; 2003.

16. Flohr TG, McCollough CH, Bruder H, et al. First performance evaluation of a dual-source CT (DSCT) system. Eur Radiol 2006;16(2):256–68.

17. McCollough CH, Schmidt B, Yu L, et al. Measurement of temporal resolution in dual source CT. Med Phys 2008;35(2):764–8.

18. Araoz PA, Kirsch J, Primak AN, et al. Optimal image reconstruction phase at low and high heart rates in dual-source CT coronary angiography. Int J Cardiovasc Imaging 2009;25(8):837–45.

19. Xu L, Yang L, Zhang Z, et al. Low-dose adaptive sequential scan for dual-source CT coronary angiography in patients with high heart rate: comparison with retrospective ECG gating. Eur J Radiol 2009. [Epub ahead of print].

20. Blankstein R, Shah A, Pale R, et al. Radiation dose and image quality of prospective triggering with dual-source cardiac computed tomography. Am J Cardiol 2009;103(8):1168–73.

21. Blobel J, Baartman H, Rogalla P, et al. [Spatial and temporal resolution with 16-slice computed tomography for cardiac imaging]. Rofo 2003;175(9): 1264–71 [in German].

22. Herzog C, Arning-Erb M, Zangos S, et al. Multidetector row CT coronary angiography: influence of reconstruction technique and heart rate on image quality. Radiology 2006;238(1):75–86.

23. Leschka S, Wildermuth S, Boehm T, et al. Noninvasive coronary angiography with 64-section CT: effect of average heart rate and heart rate variability on image quality. Radiology 2006;241(2):378–85.

24. Wintersperger BJ, Nikolaou K, von Ziegler F, et al. Image quality, motion artifacts, and reconstruction timing of 64-slice coronary computed tomography angiography with 0.33-second rotation speed. Invest Radiol 2006;41(5):436–42.

25. Hein I, Taguchi K, Silver MD, et al. Feldkamp-based cone-beam reconstruction for gantry-tilted helical multislice CT. Med Phys 2003;30(12):3233–42.

26. Dewey M, Laule M, Krug L, et al. Multisegment and halfscan reconstruction of 16-slice computed tomography for detection of coronary artery stenoses. Invest Radiol 2004;39(4):223–9.

27. Klingebiel R, Siebert E, Diekmann S, et al. 4-D Imaging in cerebrovascular disorders by using 320-slice CT: feasibility and preliminary clinical experience. Acad Radiol 2009;16(2):123–9.

28. Fleischmann D, Rubin GD, Bankier AA, et al. Improved uniformity of aortic enhancement with customized contrast medium injection protocols at CT angiography. Radiology 2000; 214(2):363–71.

29. Halpern EJ. Triple-rule-out CT angiography for evaluation of acute chest pain and possible acute coronary syndrome. Radiology 2009;252(2):332–45.

30. Kalender WA, Seissler W, Klotz E, et al. Spiral volumetric CT with single-breath-hold technique, continuous transport, and continuous scanner rotation. Radiology 1990;176(1):181–3.

31. Nieman K, Rensing BJ, van Geuns RJ, et al. Noninvasive coronary angiography with multislice spiral computed tomography: impact of heart rate. Heart 2002;88(5):470–4.

32. Mather R, Boedeker K, Nicholson T. Automatic cardiac phase selection for motion-free coronary

imaging. Second Annual Meeting of the SCCT [abstract 65]. Washington, DC, July 5–8, 2007.

33. Budoff MJ, Achenbach S, Blumenthal RS, et al. Assessment of coronary artery disease by cardiac computed tomography: a scientific statement from the American Heart Association Committee on Cardiovascular Imaging and Intervention, Council on Cardiovascular Radiology and Intervention, and Committee on Cardiac Imaging, Council on Clinical Cardiology. Circulation 2006;114(16):1761–91.

34. Fazel R, Krumholz HM, Wang Y, et al. Exposure to low-dose ionizing radiation from medical imaging procedures. N Engl J Med 2009;361(9):849–57.

35. Arnoldi E, Johnson TR, Rist C, et al. Adequate image quality with reduced radiation dose in prospectively triggered coronary CTA compared with retrospective techniques. Eur Radiol 2009;19(9):2147–55.

36. Shuman WP, Branch KR, May JM, et al. Prospective versus retrospective ECG gating for 64-detector CT of the coronary arteries: comparison of image quality and patient radiation dose. Radiology 2008;248(2):431–7.

37. Martini C, Palumbo A, Maffei E, et al. Dose reduction in spiral CT coronary angiography with dual-source equipment. Part I. A phantom study applying different prospective tube current modulation algorithms. Radiol Med 2009;114(7):1037–52.

38. Hirai N, Horiguchi J, Fujioka C, et al. Prospective versus retrospective ECG-gated 64-detector coronary CT angiography: assessment of image quality, stenosis, and radiation dose. Radiology 2008; 248(2):424–30.

39. Earls JP, Berman EL, Urban BA, et al. Prospectively gated transverse coronary CT angiography versus retrospectively gated helical technique: improved image quality and reduced radiation dose. Radiology 2008;246(3):742–53.

40. Steigner ML, Otero HJ, Cai T, et al. Narrowing the phase window width in prospectively ECG-gated single heart beat 320-detector row coronary CT angiography. Int J Cardiovasc Imaging 2009;25(1):85–90.

41. Dewey M, Zimmermann E, Laule M, et al. Three-vessel coronary artery disease examined with 320-slice computed tomography coronary angiography. Eur Heart J 2008;29(13):1669.

42. Alvarez RE, Macovski A. Energy-selective reconstructions in X-ray computerized tomography. Phys Med Biol 1976;21(5):733–44.

43. Avrin DE, Macovski A, Zatz LE. Clinical application of Compton and photo-electric reconstruction in computed tomography: preliminary results. Invest Radiol 1978;13(3):217–22.

44. Maass C, Baer M, Kachelriess M. Image-based dual energy CT using optimized precorrection functions: a practical new approach of material decomposition in image domain. Med Phys 2009; 36(8):3818–29.

45. Schmidt TG. Optimal "image-based" weighting for energy-resolved CT. Med Phys 2009;36(7):3018–27.

46. Zou Y, Silver M. Analysis of Fast kV-switching in dual energy CT using a pre-reconstruction decomposition technique. SPIE Medical Imaging 2008: Physics of Medical Imaging session, vol 6931, 691313. San Diego (CA), February 17–21, 2008.

47. Johnson TR, Krauss B, Sedlmair M, et al. Material differentiation by dual energy CT: initial experience. Eur Radiol 2007;17(6):1510–7.

48. Uotani K, Watanabe Y, Higashi M, et al. Dual-energy CT head bone and hard plaque removal for quantification of calcified carotid stenosis: utility and comparison with digital subtraction angiography. Eur Radiol 2009;19(8):2060–5.

49. Barreto M, Schoenhagen P, Nair A, et al. Potential of dual-energy computed tomography to characterize atherosclerotic plaque: ex vivo assessment of human coronary arteries in comparison to histology. J Cardiovasc Comput Tomogr 2008; 2(4):234–42.

50. Mendonca P, Bhotika R, Thomsen B, et al. Multi-material decomposition of dual-energy CT. SPIE Medical Imaging 2009: Physics of Medical Imaging session, 7622–67. Vista (FL), February 7–12, 2009.

51. Roessl E, Ziegler A, Proksa R. On the influence of noise correlations in measurement data on basis image noise in dual-energylike x-ray imaging. Med Phys 2007;34(3):959–66.

52. Heismann B, Wirth S. SNR performance comparison of dual-layer detector and dual-kVp spectral CT. Nuclear Science Symposium Conference Record, 2007. NSS '07. IEEE 2007;5:3820–2.

53. Schlomka JP, Roessl E, Dorscheid R, et al. Experimental feasibility of multi-energy photon-counting K-edge imaging in pre-clinical computed tomography. Phys Med Biol 2008;53(15):4031–47.

54. Henrich G, Mai N, Backmund H. Preprocessing in computed tomography picture analysis: a "bone-deleting" algorithm. J Comput Assist Tomogr 1979;3(3):379–84.

55. Li Q, Lv F, Li Y, et al. Subtraction CT angiography for evaluation of intracranial aneurysms: comparison with conventional CT angiography. Eur Radiol 2009;19(9):2261–7.

56. Morhard D, Fink C, Graser A, et al. Cervical and cranial computed tomographic angiography with automated bone removal: dual energy computed tomography versus standard computed tomography. Invest Radiol 2009;44(5):293–7.

57. Deng K, Liu C, Ma R, et al. Clinical evaluation of dual-energy bone removal in CT angiography of the head and neck: comparison with conventional bone-subtraction CT angiography. Clin Radiol 2009;64(5):534–41.

58. Meyer BC, Werncke T, Hopfenmuller W, et al. Dual energy CT of peripheral arteries: effect of automatic

bone and plaque removal on image quality and grading of stenoses. Eur J Radiol 2008;68(3):414–22.

59. Boll DT, Merkle EM, Paulson EK, et al. Calcified vascular plaque specimens: assessment with cardiac dual-energy multidetector CT in anthropomorphically moving heart phantom. Radiology 2008;249(1):119–26.

60. Otero HJ, Steigner ML, Rybicki FJ. The "post-64" era of coronary CT angiography: understanding new technology from physical principles. Radiol Clin North Am 2009;47(1):79–90.

61. Dewey M, Zimmermann E, Deissenrieder F, et al. Noninvasive coronary angiography by 320-row computed tomography with lower radiation exposure and maintained diagnostic accuracy: comparison of results with cardiac catheterization in a head-to-head pilot investigation. Circulation 2009;120(10):867–75.

62. Hoe J, Toh KH. First experience with 320-row multidetector CT coronary angiography scanning with prospective electrocardiogram gating to reduce radiation dose. J Cardiovasc Comput Tomogr 2009;3(4):257–61.

63. Geleijns J, Salvado Artells M, de Bruin PW, et al. Computed tomography dose assessment for a 160 mm wide, 320 detector row, cone beam CT scanner. Phys Med Biol 2009;54(10):3141–59.

64. Rybicki FJ, Otero HJ, Steigner ML, et al. Initial evaluation of coronary images from 320-detector row computed tomography. Int J Cardiovasc Imaging 2008;24(5):535–46.

65. Siebert E, Bohner G, Dewey M, et al. 320-slice CT neuroimaging: initial clinical experience and image quality evaluation. Br J Radiol 2009;82(979):561–70.

66. Kandel S, Kloeters C, Meyer H, et al. Whole-organ perfusion of the pancreas using dynamic volume CT in patients with primary pancreas carcinoma: acquisition technique, post-processing and initial results. Eur Radiol 2009;19(11):2641–6.

67. Steigner ML, Mitsouras D, Whitmore AG, et al. Iodinated contrast opacification gradients in normal coronary arteries imaged with prospectively ECG-gated single heart beat 320-detector row computed tomography. Circ Cardiovasc Imaging 2010;3(2):179–86.

68. Achenbach S, Marwan M, Schepis T, et al. High-pitch spiral acquisition: a new scan mode for coronary CT angiography. J Cardiovasc Comput Tomogr 2009;3(2):117–21.

69. Joseph PM, Spital RD. The effects of scatter in x-ray computed tomography. Med Phys 1982;9(4):464–72.

70. Haykin SS, Justice JH. Array signal processing. Englewood Cliffs (NJ): Prentice-Hall; 1985.

71. Endo M, Mori S, Tsunoo T, et al. Magnitude and effects of x-ray scatter in a 256-slice CT scanner. Med Phys 2006;33(9):3359–68.

72. Feldkamp L, Davis L, Kress J. Practical cone-beam algorithm. J Opt Soc Am A 1984;1(6):612–9.

73. Wang G, Lin TH, Cheng P, et al. A general cone-beam reconstruction algorithm. IEEE Trans Med Imaging 1993;12(3):486–96.

74. Tzedakis A, Damilakis J, Perisinakis K, et al. The effect of z overscanning on patient effective dose from multidetector helical computed tomography examinations. Med Phys 2005;32(6):1621–9.

75. van der Molen AJ, Geleijns J. Overranging in multisection CT: quantification and relative contribution to dose—comparison of four 16-section CT scanners. Radiology 2007;242(1):208–16.

76. Deak PD, Langner O, Lell M, et al. Effects of adaptive section collimation on patient radiation dose in multisection spiral CT. Radiology 2009;252(1):140–7.

77. Yoshida S, Akiba H, Tamakawa M, et al. Thoracic involvement of type A aortic dissection and intramural hematoma: diagnostic accuracy—comparison of emergency helical CT and surgical findings. Radiology 2003;228(2):430–5.

78. Hayter RG, Rhea JT, Small A, et al. Suspected aortic dissection and other aortic disorders: multidetector row CT in 373 cases in the emergency setting. Radiology 2006;238(3):841–52.

79. Winer-Muram HT, Rydberg J, Johnson MS, et al. Suspected acute pulmonary embolism: evaluation with multi-detector row CT versus digital subtraction pulmonary arteriography. Radiology 2004;233(3):806–15.

80. Stein PD, Fowler SE, Goodman LR, et al. Multidetector computed tomography for acute pulmonary embolism. N Engl J Med 2006;354(22):2317–27.

81. Kershenovich A, Rappaport ZH, Maimon S. Brain computed tomography angiographic scans as the sole diagnostic examination for excluding aneurysms in patients with perimesencephalic subarachnoid hemorrhage. Neurosurgery 2006;59(4):798–801 [discussion: 801–2].

82. Silvennoinen HM, Ikonen S, Soinne L, et al. CT angiographic analysis of carotid artery stenosis: comparison of manual assessment, semiautomatic vessel analysis, and digital subtraction angiography. AJNR Am J Neuroradiol 2007;28(1):97–103.

83. Sakamoto S, Kiura Y, Shibukawa M, et al. Subtracted 3D CT angiography for evaluation of internal carotid artery aneurysms: comparison with conventional digital subtraction angiography. AJNR Am J Neuroradiol 2006;27(6):1332–7.

84. Katzberg RW, Haller C. Contrast-induced nephrotoxicity: clinical landscape. Kidney Int 2006;69(Suppl 100):S3–7.

85. Solomon R, Dumouchel W. Contrast media and nephropathy: findings from systematic analysis

and Food and Drug Administration reports of adverse effects. Invest Radiol 2006;41(8):651–60.

86. Agatston AS, Janowitz WR, Hildner FJ, et al. Quantification of coronary artery calcium using ultrafast computed tomography. J Am Coll Cardiol 1990; 15(4):827–32.

87. Liang Z, Karl W, Do S, et al. Calcium de-blooming in coronary CT image. BIBE 2007. Proceedings of the 7th IEEE International Conference on Bioinformatics and Bioengineering. Boston (MA), October 14–17, 2007. p. 257–62.

88. Prat-Gonzalez S, Sanz J, Garcia MJ. Cardiac CT: indications and limitations. J Nucl Med Technol 2008;36(1):18–24.

89. Dey D, Lee CJ, Ohba M, et al. Image quality and artifacts in coronary CT angiography with dual-source CT: initial clinical experience. J Cardiovasc Comput Tomogr 2008;2(2):105–14.

90. Zhang S, Levin DC, Halpern EJ, et al. Accuracy of MDCT in assessing the degree of stenosis caused by calcified coronary artery plaques. AJR Am J Roentgenol 2008;191(6):1676–83.

91. Kong LY, Jin ZY, Zhang SY, et al. Assessment of coronary stents by 64-slice computed tomography: in-stent lumen visibility and patency. Chin Med Sci J 2009;24(3):156–60.

92. Lettau M, Sauer A, Heiland S, et al. Carotid artery stents: in vitro comparison of different stent designs and sizes using CT angiography and contrast-enhanced MR angiography at 1.5T and 3T. AJNR Am J Neuroradiol 2009; 30(10):1993–7.

93. Motoyama S, Sarai M, Harigaya H, et al. Computed tomographic angiography characteristics of atherosclerotic plaques subsequently resulting in acute coronary syndrome. J Am Coll Cardiol 2009;54(1):49–57.

94. Cyrus T, Gropler RJ, Woodard PK. Coronary CT angiography (CCTA) and advances in CT plaque imaging. J Nucl Cardiol 2009;16(3):466–73.

95. Rybicki F, Melchionna S, Mitsouras D, et al. Prediction of coronary artery plaque progression and potential rupture from 320-detector row prospectively ECG-gated single heart beat CT angiography: Lattice Boltzmann evaluation of endothelial shear stress. Int J Cardiovasc Imaging 2009; 25(Suppl 2):289–99.

96. Ramkumar PG, Mitsouras D, Feldman CL, et al. New advances in cardiac computed tomography. Curr Opin Cardiol 2009;24(6):596–603.

97. Kordish I, Philipp S, Boese D, et al. [Dissection of the right coronary artery as a complication after the IVUS procedure]. Herz 2007;32(7):573–7 [in German].

98. Valgimigli M, Agostoni P, Serruys PW. Acute coronary syndromes: an emphasis shift from treatment to prevention; and the enduring challenge of

vulnerable plaque detection in the cardiac catheterization laboratory. J Cardiovasc Med (Hagerstown) 2007;8(4):221–9.

99. Tobis J, Azarbal B, Slavin L. Assessment of intermediate severity coronary lesions in the catheterization laboratory. J Am Coll Cardiol 2007;49(8): 839–48.

100. Patil UD, Ragavan A, Nadaraj, et al. Helical CT angiography in evaluation of live kidney donors. Nephrol Dial Transplant 2001;16(9):1900–4.

101. Saad WE, Saad N. Computer tomography for venous thromboembolic disease. Radiol Clin North Am 2007;45(3):423–45, vii.

102. Johns HE, Cunningham JR. The physics of radiology. 4th edition. Springfield (IL): Charles C. Thomas; 1983.

103. Bushberg JT. The essential physics of medical imaging. 2nd edition. Philadelphia: Lippincott Williams & Wilkins; 2002.

104. Seeram E. Computed tomography: physical principles, clinical applications & quality control. Philadelphia: Saunders; 1994.

105. McNitt-Gray MF. AAPM/RSNA physics tutorial for residents: topics in CT. Radiation dose in CT. Radiographics 2002;22(6):1541–53.

106. Kalender WA, Deak P, Kellermeier M, et al. Application- and patient size-dependent optimization of x-ray spectra for CT. Med Phys 2009;36(3):993–1007.

107. Downes P, Jarvis R, Radu E, et al. Monte Carlo simulation and patient dosimetry for a kilovoltage cone-beam CT unit. Med Phys 2009;36(9):4156–67.

108. Horiguchi J, Fujioka C, Kiguchi M, et al. Prospective ECG-triggered axial CT at 140-kV tube voltage improves coronary in-stent restenosis visibility at a lower radiation dose compared with conventional retrospective ECG-gated helical CT. Eur Radiol 2009;19(10):2363–72.

109. Huda W. Dose and image quality in CT. Pediatr Radiol 2002;32(10):709–13 [discussion: 751–4].

110. Mahesh M. MDCT physics: the basics-technology, image quality and radiation dose. 1st edition. Philadelphia (PA): Lippincott Williams & Wilkins; 2009.

111. Shiraishi J, Tsuda K, Inoue Y, et al. Measurement of CT section thickness by using the partial volume effect. Radiology 1992;184(3):870–2.

112. Lu MT, Ersoy H, Whitmore AG, et al. Reformatted four-chamber and short-axis views of the heart using thin section (</=2 mm) MDCT images. Acad Radiol 2007;14(9):1108–12.

113. McCollough CH, Zink FE. Performance evaluation of a multi-slice CT system. Med Phys 1999;26(11): 2223–30.

114. Sirineni GK, Kalra MK, Pottala K, et al. Effect of contrast concentration, tube potential and reconstruction kernels on MDCT evaluation of coronary stents: an in vitro study. Int J Cardiovasc Imaging 2007;23(2):253–63.

CT Angiography: Injection and Acquisition Technique

- Computed tomography • CT angiography
- Contrast medium enhancement

The era of CT angiography (CTA) was initiated by the introduction of spiral or helical CT, which allowed the acquisition of volumetric CT datasets within a single breath-hold in the early 1990s.[1] These unprecedented short scan times also allowed intravenous contrast medium (CM) to be injected in less time and thus at higher injection flow rates, which, if timed correctly, resulted in strong arterial opacification. The acquired datasets could then be displayed as CT angiograms using two- and three-dimensional postprocessing techniques.[2]

The evolution of CT technology over the past 15 years could not have been more dramatic. More powerful and sophisticated x-ray tubes and advances in detector design with increasing numbers of detector rows mounted on ever-faster rotating gantry systems have led to substantial gains in spatial and temporal resolution, volume coverage, and acquisition speed. These technical advancements together with improved image postprocessing have expanded the applicability of modern-day CTA to virtually all vascular territories.

Although some of the fundamental limitations of early CTA, notably the trade-offs between spatial resolution, volume coverage, and scan speed, were gradually eliminated by new technology, CM delivery became seemingly more difficult and less forgiving from one scanner generation to the next. Injection protocol design often limped behind faster scanning capabilities, and was typically based on empiric trial and error adaptations of existing injection protocols rather than on a firm understanding of enhancement dynamics. Synchronizing the CT data acquisition with adequate arterial enhancement, and designing

integrated scanning and injection protocols for CTA requires integration of several technical factors—most importantly scan time—with patient physiology. Additionally, recognizing how a patient's time-attenuation response to intravenous contrast administration can be altered by changing injection parameters is essential.

This article provides a durable conceptual framework for CM injection technique and CTA protocol design, based on a few fundamental principles of early CM dynamics. CT technology continues to evolve with new scanner capabilities, including dual-energy data acquisition, scanning at lower kVp (for stronger x-ray attenuation of iodine), and new implementations of iterative reconstruction (which lowers background noise). The nuances of CM injection will be affected with these developments.

The underlying physiology governing contrast dynamics, however, is unlikely to change in the foreseeable future. A solid understanding of the basic concepts of early CM dynamics is a prerequisite for being able to construct effective injection strategies, which can then be implemented broadly across various scanners and adapted accordingly to upcoming scanner or technological advancement.

CONTRAST MEDIUM FOR VASCULAR OPACIFICATION IN COMPUTED TOMOGRAPHY ANGIOGRAPHY

All x-ray–based angiographic imaging methods require use of intravascular CM to overcome the lack of inherent attenuation differences between

Department of Radiology, Stanford University Medical Center, 300 Pasteur Drive, S-072, Stanford, CA 94305-5105, USA
E-mail address: d.fleischmann@stanford.edu

Radiol Clin N Am 48 (2010) 237–247
doi:10.1016/j.rcl.2010.02.002
0033-8389/10/$ – see front matter © 2010 Published by Elsevier Inc.

radiologic.theclinics.com

blood and surrounding soft tissue. Angiographic x-ray contrast media are water-soluble derivates of iodinated benzene (triiodobenzene), and their diagnostic use is based exclusively on the physical ability of iodine to absorb x-rays. For a given x-ray energy, the increase in CT numbers observed in a given vessel or tissue after CM administration is directly proportional to the local iodine concentration.[3]

All CM injection strategies for CTA have the ultimate goal of achieving an adequate iodine concentration within the vasculature of interest. Although the relationship between CT attenuation and intravascular iodine concentration is well defined, no quantitative definition of "adequate enhancement" exists. The optimal intensity of arterial opacification depends on many interrelated factors, such as the technical quality of the dataset, specifically spatial resolution and noise, but also on the diameter of the arteries of interest, and thus ultimately on the clinical context. The actual standard of reference for adequate arterial opacification therefore remains human perception: the viewer's ability to visually extract the diagnostically relevant information from the CT datasets.

Arterial opacification in CTA is not a static but rather a dynamic process achieved through intravenous CM injection into the flowing blood stream. Arterial opacification is therefore a time-dependent phenomenon: the time-attenuation response, which is described later.

PHARMACOKINETICS AND PHYSIOLOGY OF ARTERIAL ENHANCEMENT

Pharmacokinetically, all angiographic x-ray contrast media are extracellular fluid markers, which are rapidly distributed between the intravascular and extravascular interstitial spaces after intravenous injection.[4] Traditional pharmacokinetic studies on CM have concentrated on the phase of elimination (ie, after complete distribution within the extracellular space) rather than on early kinetics. For the timeframe relevant to CTA, however, this particularly complex early phase of rapid CM distribution and redistribution determines vascular enhancement.

Vascular enhancement differs significantly from parenchymal (organ or soft tissue) enhancement. In nonvascular CT, the degree of organ opacification correlates closely with the total volume of CM (iodine) administered, and is inversely related to a patient's body weight (a surrogate parameter for extracellular space). Arterial enhancement, however, does not specifically rely on total CM volume, but rather on two particular key components: (1) the amount of iodinated CM delivered

per unit of time, which for a given iodine concentration is the *injection flow rate* (mL/s); and (2) the *injection duration*, measured in seconds. The resulting product of injection flow rate and injection duration is, of course, CM volume, and most power injectors require that a CM injection protocol is keyed into the interface as CM volume and flow rate. Practically, however, it is more useful in CTA injection protocols to consider CM injection as *injection flow rate × injection duration*. For example, an intravenous CM injection described as "100 mL @ 5 mL/s" should be understood as "5 mL/s for 20 s." Decomposing injection protocols into *injection flow rate × injection duration* is the most important step to an intuitive understanding of cardiovascular CT injection protocols. This point cannot be overemphasized and is reflected in the first two key rules of early arterial CM dynamics (**Box 1**).

Early Arterial Contrast Medium Dynamics

The time-attenuation response to intravenously injected CM varies among individuals, between vascular beds, and often even within the same vascular territory. In a given individual, the time-attenuation response varies in the thoracoabdominal aorta compared with the lower extremity arteries. Even for the relatively small coronary arterial tree, this response may differ in the proximal coronary segments versus the distal segments, with the smaller peripheral segments requiring up to several additional heartbeats for adequate filling.

All arterial enhancement responses, however, share the same basic principles.[5] **Fig. 1** schematically illustrates the early arterial CM dynamics observed in the abdominal aorta after intravenous injection of a 16-mL test bolus. The interval needed for the CM to arrive in the arterial territory of interest is referred to as the CM transit time (t_{CMT}), which is an important landmark for scan timing.

The arterial time attenuation response itself consists of two phases. The first peak of the time attenuation response is referred to as the *first pass* effect, followed by the recirculation phase, characterized by the observation that the tail of the time-attenuation curve does not return to zero after the first pass, but undulates or rebounds above the baseline. This tail is only partly caused by true recirculation of opacified blood from highly perfused organs such as the brain and the kidney, but is mostly a consequence of bolus broadening. Although the recirculation phase is deliberately ignored in indicator-dilution–based methods to calculate cardiac output (eg, using gamma variate

Key rules controlled by the user

1. Arterial enhancement is proportional to the iodine administration rate

Arterial opacification can be increased by

- Increasing the injection flow rate
- Increasing the iodine concentration of the contrast medium

2. Arterial enhancement increases cumulatively with the injection duration

- Longer contrast medium injections increase arterial enhancement
- A minimum injection duration of approximately 10 seconds is usually needed to achieve adequate arterial enhancement

Key rules controlled by patient physiology or pathology

3. Individual enhancement is controlled by cardiac output

- Cardiac output is inversely proportional to arterial opacification
- Increasing or decreasing both the injection rate and the injection volumes to body weight reduces the interindividual variability of arterial enhancement

4. Arterial filling times may be delayed physiologically or pathologically

- Even normal coronary arteries need several heartbeats to fully opacify
- Mixing of opacified and nonopacified blood in aneurysms delays enhancement
- Bolus propagation in diseased lower-extremity arteries tree may be substantially delayed

fitting[6]), it cannot be ignored here because it explains the somewhat unintuitive effect of the injection duration on vascular enhancement.

Early arterial CM dynamics can be broken down into four basic key rules. The first two key rules describe the effect of user-selectable parameters on arterial enhancement (rules 1 and 2), and the following two summarize the physiologic observations that are beyond the control of the user (rules 3 and 4).

Effect of injection flow rate on arterial enhancement: rule 1

For a given patient and vascular territory, the degree of arterial enhancement is directly proportional to the rate of iodine administration. **Fig. 1** shows that when the injection rate is doubled from 4 to 8 mL/s, or more precisely, if the rate of iodine administration is increased from 1.2 to 2.4 g of iodine per second (if a 300 mg I/mL CM is used), the corresponding enhancement response is twice as strong. Changing the iodine concentration of the contrast agent has the same proportional effect on arterial enhancement as changing the injection flow rate.

Increasing the injection flow rates has physiologic and practical limitations, however. Injection flow rates of 8 mL/s or greater have been shown to no longer directly translate into stronger enhancement,[7] possibly because of pooling in the central venous system with reflux into the inferior vena cava. This phenomenon can be observed with even moderate or low flow rates in patients with significantly decreased right ventricular function or reduced cardiac output. High injection flow rates are also limited by the size of the intravenous cannula, most of which preclude injection rates of greater than 5 and 6 mL/s for 20- and 18-gauge cannula, respectively. This limitation exists even if CM is warmed and therefore less viscous (upper limit of 10 mL/s for a 17-gauge cannula).

Effect of injection duration on arterial enhancement: rule 2

The effect of increasing (or shortening) the injection duration is more difficult to understand than the direct relationship of the iodine administration rate, but it is equally important. One intuitive way to think about the effect of the injection duration is shown in **Fig. 1**. A longer injection duration of 32 seconds (128 mL total volume), for example, can be considered as the sum of eight subsequent injections of small "test boluses" of 4 seconds (16 mL each). Each of these eight test boluses has its own effect (first pass and recirculation) on arterial enhancement. Under the assumption of a time-invariant linear system,[8] the cumulative enhancement response to the entire 128-mL injection is equal to the sum (time integral) of each enhancement response to its respective test bolus (total of eight).[5] The recirculation effects of the prior test boluses overlap (and thus sum up) with the first pass effects of following test boluses. The result is an invariable continuous increase in arterial enhancement over the duration of the injection, rather than a constant plateau of enhancement.

These first two key rules sufficiently describe how user-selectable parameters can alter arterial opacification, and underscore the importance of decomposing injection protocols into the injection flow rate and the injection duration, rather than

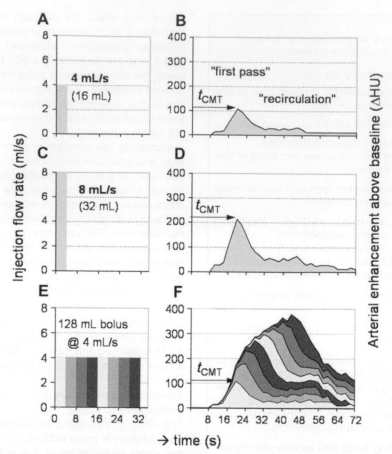

Fig. 1. Simple "additive model" illustrating the effects of injection flow rate and injection duration on arterial enhancement. Intravenous contrast medium (CM) injection (A) causes an arterial enhancement response (B), which consists of an early "first pass" peak and a lower "recirculation" effect. Doubling the injection flow rate (doubling the iodine administration rate) (C) results in approximately twice the arterial enhancement (D). The effect of the injection duration (E) can be regarded as the sum (time integral) of several enhancement responses (F). Note that because of the asymmetric shape of the test-enhancement curve and caused by recirculation effects, arterial enhancement after an injection of 128 mL (the "time integral of 8 consecutive injections of 16 mL") increases continuously over time. (Adapted from Fleischmann D. Present and future trends in multiple detector-row CT applications: CT angiography. Eur Radiol 2002;12:S11; with kind permission from Springer Science+Business Media.)

thinking in terms of injection volume and flow rate, which obscures the underlying physiology.

Effect of cardiac output on vascular enhancement: rule 3

The degree of arterial enhancement after the same intravenous CM injection is highly variable between individuals. Even in patients with normal cardiac output, mid-aortic enhancement may range from 140 to 440 HU (a factor of three).[9] If body weight is taken into account, the average aortic enhancement ranges from 92 to 196 HU/mL/kg (a factor of two).[10] Adjusting the CM injection rates (and volumes) to body weight will therefore reduce interindividual differences of arterial enhancement, but will not completely eliminate

them. Nevertheless, this adjustment is recommended and should at least be applied to patients with small (<60 kg) and large (>90 kg) body size. The authors' CT protocols account for variability in body size by grouping individuals into five categories (Tables 1 and 2). This practical approach allows for individualization of CM delivery while avoiding the need of a calculator.

The fundamental physiologic parameter affecting arterial enhancement is cardiac output and, to a lesser extent, central blood volume. Cardiac output is inversely related to the degree of arterial enhancement, particularly in first pass dynamics.[11] This relationship can be understood intuitively when thinking about a CM injection as flow of iodine (iodine molecules per second)

Table 1
Integrated 64-channel computed tomography acquisition and injection protocol for abdominal computed tomography angiography

Acquisition	64 × 0.6 mm (number of channels × channel width); automated tube current modulation (250 quality reference mAs)		
Pitch	Variable (depends on volume coverage, usually <1.0)		
Scan time	Fixed to 10 s (in all patients)		
Injection duration	Fixed to 18 s (in all patients)		
Scanning delay	t_{CMT} + 8 s (scan starts 8 s after CM arrives in the aorta, as established with automated bolus triggering)		
Contrast medium	High concentration (350–370 mg I/mL)		
Injection flow rates and volumes	Individualized to body weight		
	Body Weight	**CM Flow Rate**	**CM Volume**
	<55 kg	4.0 mL/s	72 mL
	56–65 kg	4.5 mL/s	81 mL
	66–85 kg	5.0 mL/s	90 mL
	86–95 kg	5.5 mL/s	99 mL
	>95 kg	6.0 mL/s	108 mL

Abbreviations: CM, contrast medium; t_{CMT}, contrast medium transit time.

injected into a larger flow of blood (milliliters of blood per second). The relative amount of flow of iodine into the flow of blood will determine the iodine concentration in the blood, and thus its CT attenuation. Arterial enhancement is therefore lower in patients with high cardiac output but is stronger in patients with low cardiac output (despite the delayed t_{CMT} in the latter).

Effect of local flow kinetics on vascular enhancement: rule 4

The first three key rules provide a basic framework for understanding early CM dynamics. Rules 1 and 2 explain the two user-selectable parameters (injection flow rate and injection duration) that dictate arterial opacification. Rule 3 explains the global effect of a patient's cardiac output. For specific CT angiographic applications, however,

Table 2
Integrated 64-channel CT acquisition and injection protocol for lower-extremity computed tomography angiography

Acquisition	64 × 0.6 mm (number of channels × channel width); automated tube current modulation (250 quality reference mAs)	
Pitch	Variable (depends on volume coverage, usually <1.0)	
Scan time	Fixed to 40 s (in all patients)	
Injection duration	Fixed to 35 s (in all patients)	
Scanning delay	t_{CMT} + 3 s (minimum delay)	
Contrast medium	High concentration (350–370 mg I/mL)	
Injection flow rates and volumes (biphasic)	Maximum flow rate for first 5 s of injection, continued with 80% of this flow rate for 30 s, followed by 30 mL saline flush	
	Body Weight	**CM Volumes and Biphasic Flow Rates**
	<55 kg	20 mL (4.0 mL/s) + 96 mL (3.2 mL/s)
	56–65 kg	23 mL (4.5 mL/s) + 108 mL (3.6 mL/s)
	66–85 kg	25 mL (5.0 mL/s) + 120 mL (4.0 mL/s)
	86–95 kg	28 mL (5.5 mL/s) + 132 mL (4.4 mL/s)
	>95 kg	30 mL (6.0 mL/s) + 144 mL (4.8 mL/s)

Abbreviations: CM, contrast medium; t_{CMT}, contrast medium transit time.

additional local physiologic and pathologic factors must be accounted for when designing injection strategies, and even more so when scan times become short relative to the time it takes to fill a given vascular territory of interest. For current state-of-the art scanners, this consideration is important if (1) a vascular territory is anatomically large or diseased (such as in peripheral arterial occlusive disease), and (2) when subsecond acquisitions are applied (particularly for coronary CTA). In both instances, the time required to fill the vascular territory cannot be ignored. The implication of this consideration is that even with subsecond scan times, an injection protocol must aim for an opacification that is long enough to allow filling of the entire arterial territory of interest.

Contrast Medium Transit Time and Scan Timing

The t_{CMT} varies among patients, ranging from as short as 8 to as long as 40 seconds in patients with cardiovascular diseases. Cardiovascular CT data acquisition therefore must be timed relative to the t_{CMT} of the vascular territory of interest. Transit times can be easily determined using either a test-bolus injection or automatic bolus triggering. In the era of single-slice CTA, the t_{CMT} was often used directly as the scanning delay, which is defined as the interval between the beginning of CM injection and the initiation of CT data acquisition. With faster scanners and shorter scan times, however, the t_{CMT} is instead a landmark relative to which the scanning delay can be individualized.

Depending on the vessels of interest, an additional delay relative to the t_{CMT} can be chosen. In CTA, this additional delay may be as short as 2 seconds ("t_{CMT} + 2s"), but often slightly longer delays of 5 or 8 seconds are used ("t_{CMT} + 8 s"). The notation "t_{CMT} + 8 s" means that the scan is initiated 8 seconds after the CM has arrived in the target vasculature.

Test Bolus

The injection of a small test-bolus (15–20 mL) while acquiring a low-dose dynamic (nonincremental) CT acquisition is a reliable means to determine the t_{CMT} from the intravenous injection site to the arterial territory of interest.[12] The t_{CMT} equals the time-to-peak enhancement interval measured in a region-of-interest (ROI) placed within a reference vessel (see Fig. 1). The advantage of using a test bolus is its reliability and accuracy in predicting the t_{CMT}, notably for cardiac and coronary CTA even in patients with substantially altered hemodynamics. If preprogrammed into the scanner, the workflow is not noticeably slower than automated bolus triggering. The main disadvantage of using a test-bolus for scan timing is the need for an additional amount of CM.

Automated Bolus Triggering

For automated bolus triggering, a circular ROI is placed into the target vessel on a nonenhanced image.[13] While CM is injected, a series of low-dose nonincremental scans are obtained and the attenuation within the ROI is monitored. The t_{CMT} equals the time when a predefined enhancement threshold ("trigger level") is reached (eg, 100 ΔHU). Automated bolus triggering causes a slight delay relative to the true t_{CMT}, which depends on the scanner model and other factors, such as the longitudinal distance between the monitoring-series and the starting position of the scan. Also, when a prerecorded breath-holding command is programmed into the CT acquisition, this increases the minimal delay before a scan can be initiated.

When using automated bolus triggering, the minimal trigger delay after CM arrival is usually 2 seconds, which can be ignored when designing an injection protocol for a 10-second or longer acquisition. If a longer trigger delay is necessary or intentionally chosen, such as 8 seconds ("t_{CMT} + 8 s"), the injection duration must be increased accordingly to guarantee a long enough enhancement phase within the vascular territory of interest. Bolus triggering is a very robust and practical technique for routine use and has the advantage of not requiring an additional test-bolus injection, thus decreasing the total amount of contrast used. It also eliminates unwanted organ enhancement (eg, renal collecting system) in the subsequent full-bolus study.

Mathematical Modeling

Accurate individual prediction and controlling of time-dependent arterial enhancement is highly desirable for CTA, especially for fast scanners. One attempt to individualize contrast delivery based on patient physiology is the black-box model approach by Hittmair,[8] which is based on a linear system theory and mathematical analysis of a patient's characteristic time–attenuation response to a small test-bolus injection.[14,15] Each individual's extracted response function ("patient factor") is used to individually tailor biphasic injection protocols to achieve uniform, prolonged arterial enhancement at a predefined level.[15] The model has been successfully used for individualizing injections for relatively long scan times (30 seconds)[10,15] but cannot be directly used for today's short and very short scan times without major modification.[16] The greatest practical value of mathematical modeling lies in its ability to explain the complex early CM dynamics, as illustrated throughout this article.

SCANNING AND INJECTION PROTOCOL DESIGN

CT protocols have the goal of standardizing the sequence of events for repeatedly acquired CT studies on a daily basis. Protocols are tailored to the organ of interest and optimized for a given scanner. The sequence of acquisitions (eg, digital radiograph for selecting the scanning range; pre-contrast-, angiographic-, and delayed acquisitions) with their respective technical acquisition and reconstruction parameters (eg, kVp, mAs, detector configuration, pitch, rotation time, slice thickness/interval, reconstruction kernel) are pre-programmed into the scanner menu. Injection parameters are either kept as a separate protocol book or electronic file. In the future, injection protocols may be stored in the memory of power injectors or on the scanner console.

The most important technical CTA parameter to be considered when developing a scanning and injection protocol is the scan time. The dramatic increase in scan speed is nicely illustrated when comparing acquisition times for abdominal CTA, which was between 30 and 40 seconds in the single-slice era. The same anatomic territory can now be scanned in only 3 to 4 seconds, and the latest scanners allow cardiac and thoracic CTA acquisitions in a fraction of a second.

Advantages and Disadvantages of Fast Computed Tomography Acquisitions

All modern CT scanners (64-channel systems and beyond) allow very fast data acquisitions with very short scan times, which has several obvious advantages. Shorter scan times allow for easier breath-holding and are the prerequisite for imaging during phases of maximum enhancement. Fast gantry rotations are also fundamental for cardiac imaging because the gantry rotation time directly translates into temporal resolution. In the setting of cardiovascular CT, shorter scan times also allow for the use of less total CM volumes and larger anatomic coverage.

However, fast scan times also come with potential disadvantages. First, short scan times usually need faster CM injections, and the traditional strategy of selecting the injection duration equal to the scan time is no longer appropriate. Second, fast data acquisitions may in fact be too fast when vascular opacification is delayed because of

pathologic conditions (rule 4). For example, opacification of large aneurysms may take several seconds because of slow mixing of opacified blood with nonopacified blood (Fig. 2), and filling of arteries distal to significantly diseased vessels may also substantially delay the propagation of an intravenously injected bolus downstream. This condition is most commonly encountered in lower-extremity CTA for peripheral arterial disease (Fig. 3).[17] Even normal vessel trees require a few seconds to fill completely, implying that to achieve the desired enhancement in the territory of interest, the target enhancement must be maintained for several seconds even if the scan time could be infinitely short. Very short injection protocols result in extremely short peak enhancement, which does not allow for desired enhancement of the distal tree.

In contrast with the single-detector CT era, when the goal was always to select the fastest possible acquisition speed, this is not necessarily the best choice with modern CT equipment. Deliberately scanning at a moderate table speed or allowing the bolus a head start is a more reliable strategy. Another benefit of not using the fastest possible acquisition speed is that slower scans

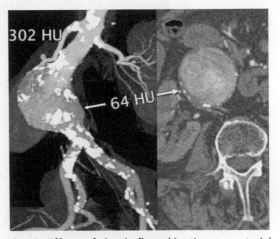

Fig. 2. Effect of local flow kinetics on arterial enhancement. Abdominal CT angiogram in a patient with an abdominal aortic aneurysm. Scan time was 6 seconds, and scan was initiated immediately after bolus arrival in the suprarenal aorta using automated bolus triggering (not shown). Note that adequate enhancement is achieved in the nondiseased segment of the abdominal aorta (302 HU). Just 2 seconds into the scan, however, the contrast medium has not mixed adequately with the blood pool contained within the aneurysms, resulting in poor opacification (64 HU) in the distal portion of the aneurysm and in the iliac arteries. This issue can be avoided through increasing the scanning delay relative to bolus arrival or deliberately scanning slower.

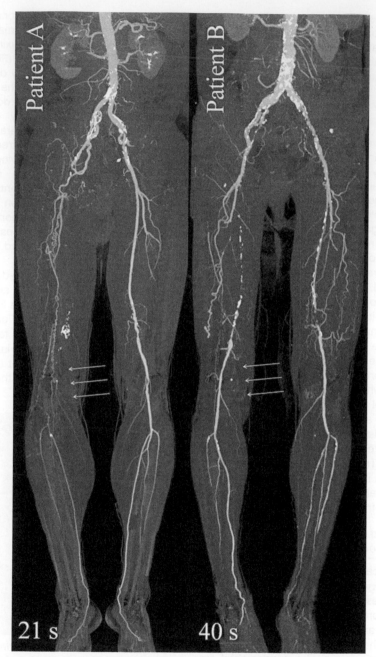

Fig. 3. Delayed opacification in peripheral arterial disease. Maximum-intensity projection (MIP) lower-extremity CT angiograms in two patients with long femoral arterial occlusions. In patient A (*left panel*), scan time was too fast (21 seconds) to allow adequate filling of reconstituted vessels (*arrows*). In patient B (*right panel*), scan time was deliberately slow (40 seconds) and injection duration was 35 seconds, allowing for adequate filling of reconstituted arteries (*arrows*) distal to the occluded segment.

(with submaximal gantry rotation speed and submaximal pitch) provide a considerable tube power reserve, which may be needed in large and obese patients to maintain acceptable image noise.

Contrast Medium Injection Strategies for Cardiovascular Computed Tomography

Given the wide variety of CT scanners currently available and the broad range of scan times for different vascular territories, it is not surprising that no universal strategy of CM injection exists for cardiovascular CT. The following strategies reflect the historic evolution of CTA as much as the increase in scan speed with the necessary adaptations.

Basic Computed Tomography Angiography Injection Strategy: Injection Time Equals Scan Time

The traditional injection strategy for CTA, derived in the era of single-slice CT, was to inject CM for a duration equal to the scan time. For a 40-second abdominal CTA acquisition, the injection duration would also be 40 seconds, resulting in a fairly large CM dose of 160 mL if a typical injection flow rate of 4 mL/s was used. Scan timing was determined either by using a test-bolus or with bolus tracking.

This basic strategy is still useful for many relatively slow CTA applications and for cardiac or gated thoracic CT, whenever scan times range

from 10 to 20 seconds. Over the years of CT evolution with increasingly shorter scan times, the injection flow rates have increased from 4 to 5 and even 6 mL/s. At the same time, the iodine concentration of the CM used has also increased from the traditional 300 mg I/mL to 350, 370, or 400 mg I/mL at most institutions. This evolution is not surprising, because the lower opacification from shorter injections (a consequence of rule 2) must be compensated for through increasing the iodine flux (rule 1) (**Fig. 4**). Through increasing the injection flow rate from 4 to 5 mL/s and using a contrast agent of 350 rather than 300 mg I/mL concentration, the iodine flux, and thus arterial enhancement, increases by 45%.

Basic strategy with additionally increased scanning delay

Use of even faster scanners showed that the basic strategy (injection duration equals scan time) alone is not applicable for scan times well below 10

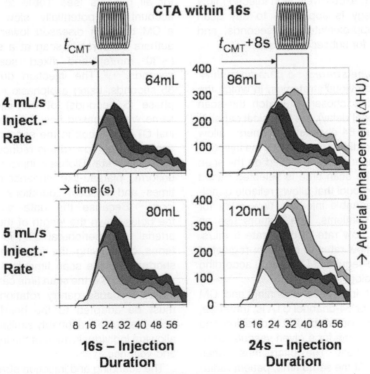

Fig. 4. Strategies to improve arterial enhancement with fast CT acquisitions. Two strategies to increase arterial enhancement compared with what can be achieved from a 16-second injection at 4 mL/s (*upper left panel*) can be used either alone or in combination. Increasing the injection rate from 4 to 5 mL/s increases the enhancement approximately 20% (*lower left panel*). Alternatively, the injection duration and scanning delay can also be increased, taking advantage of the fact that enhancement increases with longer injection durations (*right upper panel*). Maximum enhancement can be achieved when the injection rate (and or the iodine concentration) and injection duration are increased (*right lower panel*) simultaneously. (*From* Fleischmann D. Contrast-medium administration. In: Catalano C, Passariello R, editors. Multidetector-row CT angiography. Berlin, Heidelberg, New York: Springer 2005. p. 41–54; with kind permission from Springer Science+Business Media.)

seconds. A 4-second injection for a 4-second scan would not result in reliable enhancement in most patients. The obvious solution is simply to increase the injection duration and scanning delay accordingly; in other words, use rule 2. With this approach, the injection duration is no longer equal to but longer than the scan time, and the scanning delay is not equal to but longer than the t_{CMT} (see Fig. 4). The goal of this strategy is to build up arterial enhancement and not scan at contrast arrival but at the peak of arterial enhancement, which occurs later than the arrival time.

In addition to achieving stronger enhancement, the increased scanning delay strategy has another advantage. A longer scanning delay with an adequately prolonged injection duration will also allow a more reliable filling of the vasculature distal to the site of scan initiation (rule 4), such as downstream of an aneurysmal thoracic or abdominal aorta.

The tradeoff of this strategy is to use slightly more CM than in an injection-time-equals-scan time strategy, but with more reliable enhancement and while avoiding excessively high injection flow rates. This strategy is applicable to any scan time less than approximately 10 seconds, and can also be used for subsecond scans.

The fixed scan time strategy: a paradigm shift

Opposed to the previous strategies, in which the injection duration is chosen to match the scan time (± an additional delay), the technical capabilities of modern 64-channel scanners allow a reversal of the traditional paradigm; the injection duration is no longer selected based on the scan time, but rather the scan time is selected based on an injection protocol that allows reliable opacification with reasonable injection flow rates for a wide range of patients. The authors use an average injection flow rate of moderate 5 mL/s, which allows the flow rates to be down-regulated (≤4 mL/s) and up-regulated (≥6 mL/s) according to patients' physiology.

Authors current integrated scanning and CM injection strategy for 64-channel CTA is, therefore, to deliberately slow down the CT acquisition and use the same scan time for a given vascular territory for every patient. The pitch thus varies between patients. At the same time, patient radiation exposure is controlled by automated tube current modulation.

When the same scan time is used for all patients, the same injection duration can also be used, which simplifies individualizing the flow rates (and volumes) for different patient sizes. For example, the authors use a fixed scan time of 10 seconds for abdominal CTA, with an injection duration of 18 seconds and a scanning delay of t_{CMT} + 8 seconds, as determined by bolus triggering (see Table 1). This strategy allows breath-holding for virtually all patients, and results in reliably strong arterial enhancement because of high iodine flux and increased scanning delay relative to the t_{CMT}, while avoiding excessive injection flow rates. The relatively long scanning delay may avoid inadequate downstream opacification in the presence on aneurysms or flow obstructions (see Fig. 2).

Image noise is controlled within and across individuals using automated tube current modulation. A similar approach can be used for other vascular territories, including CTA of the chest or, with a fast enough scanner, even the chest, abdomen, and pelvis. This approach allows for the same weight-based injection protocol for many common CTA applications.

Only slight modifications are needed for lower-extremity CTA and cardiac CT. The authors' lower-extremity CTA protocol also uses a constant scan time and injection duration for all patients (see Table 2; see Fig. 3). To account for potentially slow propagation of a CM bolus in diseased lower extremities, the authors deliberately scan at a slow table speed (~30 mm/s) and fixed scan time of 40 seconds.[17,18] The injection duration is always 35 seconds, using a biphasic injection. The first phase (5 seconds) of the injection uses the same weight-based flow rates as in the abdominal CTA protocol; in the second phase (next 30 seconds), the flow rate is reduced to 80% of the initial flow rate. Biphasic injections lead to more uniform, plateau-like enhancement when scan times and injection durations are comparably long.[12] Because the data acquisition follows the bolus down the length of the lower extremity arterial tree, peripheral CTA is an exception in terms of allowing the injection duration to be shorter than the scan time (see Table 2).

In cardiac CT, the scan time cannot be predetermined, because gantry rotation time and pitch must be adapted to the heart rate. However, scan times are reasonably similar across patients, allowing individualization of the injection flow rates and volumes.

The scanning and injection strategies described earlier are not meant as rigid templates for CTA protocols, but as examples of how evolving technical scanner capabilities may be integrated with known physiologic constraints of arterial enhancement to effectively design practical injection protocols for cardiovascular CT. Alternative scanning and injection protocols may be equally effective, recognizing that the underlying physiology and key rules of enhancement dynamics remain constant.

SUMMARY

CM delivery remains an integral part of state-of-the art cardiovascular CT. Although CT technology continues to evolve, the physiologic and pharmacokinetic principles of arterial enhancement will remain unchanged in the foreseeable future. A basic understanding of early CM dynamics thus provides the foundation for designing current and future CT scanning and injection protocols, independent of the rapid evolution of CT technology. These tools allow CM use to be optimized for a wide variety of clinical CT applications, and for each patient while exploiting the full capabilities of this powerful imaging technology.

REFERENCES

1. Kalender WA, Seissler W, Klotz E, et al. Spiral volumetric CT with single-breath-hold technique, continuous transport, and continuous scanner rotation. Radiology 1990;176:181.
2. Rubin GD, Dake MD, Napel SA, et al. Three-dimensional spiral CT angiography of the abdomen: initial clinical experience. Radiology 1993;186:147.
3. Dawson P, Blomley MJ. Contrast media as extracellular fluid space markers: adaptation of the central volume theorem. Br J Radiol 1996;69:717.
4. Dawson P, Blomley MJ. Contrast agent pharmacokinetics revisited: I. Reformulation. Acad Radiol 1996; 3(Suppl 2):S261.
5. Fleischmann D. Present and future trends in multiple detector-row CT applications: CT angiography. Eur Radiol 2002;12:S11.
6. Thomson HK, Starmer F, Whalen RE, et al. Indicator transit time considered as a gamma variate. Circ Res 1964;14:502.
7. Claussen CD, Banzer D, Pfretzschner C, et al. Bolus geometry and dynamics after intravenous contrast-medium injection. Radiology 1984;153:365.
8. Fleischmann D, Hittmair K. Mathematical analysis of arterial enhancement and optimization of bolus geometry for CT angiography using the discrete fourier transform. J Comput Assist Tomogr 1999; 23:474.
9. Sheiman RG, Raptopoulos V, Caruso P, et al. Comparison of tailored and empiric scan delays for CT angiography of the abdomen. AJR Am J Roentgenol 1996;167:725.
10. Hittmair K, Fleischmann D. Accuracy of predicting and controlling time-dependent aortic enhancement from a test bolus injection. J Comput Assist Tomogr 2001;25:287.
11. Bae KT, Heiken JP, Brink JA. Aortic and hepatic contrast medium enhancement at CT. Part II. Effect of reduced cardiac output in a porcine model. Radiology 1998;207:657.
12. Van Hoe L, Marchal G, Baert AL, et al. Determination of scan delay-time in spiral CT-angiography: utility of a test bolus injection. J Comput Assist Tomogr 1995; 19:216.
13. Birnbaum BA, Jacobs JE, Langlotz CP, et al. Assessment of a bolus-tracking technique in helical renal CT to optimize nephrographic phase imaging. Radiology 1999;211:87.
14. Fleischmann D, Paik D, Napel S, et al. Quantitative CT angiography of the abdominal aorta in healthy adults. Eur Radiol 1999;9:S548.
15. Fleischmann D, Rubin GD, Bankier AA, et al. Improved uniformity of aortic enhancement with customized contrast medium injection protocols at CT angiography. Radiology 2000;214:363.
16. Kopeinigg D, Fleischman D, Stollberger R, et al. LST-based optimization of contrast enhancement profiles for CR-MRA: validation studies in phantoms and volunteers. Presented at the 20th Annual International Conference on Magnetic Resonance Angiography (MRA-Club'08). Graz, Austria, October 15–17, 2008.
17. Fleischmann D, Koechl A, Lomoschitz E, et al. Aorto-popliteal bolus transit times in peripheral CTA: can fast acquisitions outrun the bolus. Eur Radiol 2003; 13S:268.
18. Fleischmann D, Hallett RL, Rubin GD. CT Angiography of peripheral arterial disease. J Vasc Interv Radiol 2006;17:3.

CT Angiography of the Thoracic Aorta

Jonathan H. Chung, MD[a], Brian B. Ghoshhajra, MD[b],
Carlos A. Rojas, MD[b], Bhavika R. Dave, MD[c],
Suhny Abbara, MD[d],*

KEYWORDS

- Thoracic aortic aneurysm • Aortic dissection
- Aortic transection • Intramural hematoma
- Aortic coarctation • CT angiography • MDCT

The aorta is the largest artery in the human body, pumping up to 200 million liters of blood through the body in an average lifetime. Thoracic aortic disease presentation ranges from asymptomatic (as in an aneurysm incidentally detected on imaging) to severe acute chest pain (as in acute aortic dissection). The recent increased prevalence of aortic disease in western countries is a result of increased clinical awareness and longer life spans. Multidetector-row computed tomography (MDCT) of the aorta can be used to diagnose various acute and chronic conditions of the aorta, including aortic aneurysms, aortic dissections, intramural hematomas, penetrating atherosclerotic ulcers, traumatic injuries, inflammatory disorders, and congenital abnormalities.

In the early 1990s, single-detector spiral computed tomography (CT) was introduced into routine clinical imaging, allowing excellent visual assessment of vessels from any angle as opposed to catheter-based projectional angiography.[1–3] However, single-detector spiral CT had limitations, such as long breath holds, motion artifacts from slow gantry rotation time, and limited coverage in z-dimension.[1–3] In the late 1990s, MDCT was introduced. MDCT significantly improved image quality with improved resolution in the z-dimension, faster gantry rotation, increased coverage in the z-dimension, and increased table speed.[4]

Modern 64 detector-row and newer-generation CT scanners can evaluate the entire aorta, including its smaller branches, with one short breath hold. Compared with angiography, extravascular structures are also well assessed with MDCT.[4] MDCT provides superior image quality by acquiring isovolumetric subcentimeter voxels, which allow two-dimensional and three-dimensional reconstructions in any orientation.[5]

This article reviews the spectrum of MDCT imaging findings in thoracic aortic diseases. Although discussion focuses on the thoracic aorta, initial examination of the aorta should include the entire aorta and iliac arteries; aortic diseases such as aneurysm or dissection frequently affect the whole aorta or may affect multiple regions of the aorta.

CT IMAGING PROTOCOL
Noncontrast CT

Inclusion of a noncontrast CT scan is imperative in aortic imaging for suspected acute aortic syndrome, because aortic intramural hematomas are more evident without intra-arterial contrast. Radiation dose is often reduced during this phase by increasing collimation, decreasing kVp, or increasing the noise index with concomitant reduction in effective mAs.

[a] Department of Radiology, Massachusetts General Hospital, 55 Fruit Street, FND-202, Boston, MA 02114, USA
[b] Department of Radiology, Massachusetts General Hospital, 165 Cambridge Street, CPZ-4-400, Boston, MA 02114, USA
[c] Department of Radiology, Massachusetts General Hospital, 55 Fruit Street, GRB 290A, Boston, MA 02114, USA
[d] Department of Radiology, Massachusetts General Hospital, Harvard Medical School, 55 Fruit Street, GRB-290, Boston, MA 02114, USA
* Corresponding author.
E-mail address: sabbara@partners.org

Radiol Clin N Am 48 (2010) 249–264
doi:10.1016/j.rcl.2010.02.001
0033-8389/10/$ – see front matter © 2010 Elsevier Inc. All rights reserved.

CT Angiography

Nongated thoracic aortic CT angiography is usually performed with a pitch of 1 to 1.5, a collimation of 0.5 to 1.0 mm, and reconstruction of 1.0- to 1.5-mm slices with spacing of 0.75 to 1 mm. The kVp is usually set at 120 to 140. Lower kVp (80–100) may be used in thin patients. Automated tube current modulation should be used when available.

With this method of scanning, tube current is automatically reduced when scanning regions of lower attenuation, and increased for areas of higher attenuation.[6] A desired noise index is entered, defined as the standard deviation of Hounsfield units in the center of an image using soft tissue kernel reconstruction. A threshold-based bolus tracking algorithm with a region of interest in the ascending aorta is typically used.

The contrast is injected at rates of 3 to 5 mL/s and the overall contrast volume should be approximately the injection rate (in mL/s) multiplied by the scan duration in seconds plus 5 to 10 seconds. Adding 5 to 10 seconds to the contrast injection duration is necessary to compensate for the difference in position between the tracking position in the ascending aorta and the top of the chest. A small field of view can be selected to optimize spatial resolution. However, a full field of view must be reconstructed to detect incidental findings. Initial examination of the thoracic aorta should include the abdominal aorta and iliac arteries, because thoracic aortic pathology commonly involves these vessels.

Delayed Scan

Delayed scans 1 to 2 minutes after injection are obtained to assess for late filling of a false lumen in dissections, slow endoleaks in endovascular stent repair (more often used in the abdominal aorta), or contrast extravasation from aortic rupture.

Postprocessing

Multiplanar maximum intensity projections in the sagittal, sagittal–oblique (ie, candy cane view), coronal planes, aortic short axis, and aortic root long axis are routinely acquired. Three-dimensional volume–rendered images at multiple viewing angles may also be created. However, the source data (axial images) and interactive multiplanar reformations are clinically more useful than are static postprocessed images.

Normal Anatomy and Normal Variants

The thoracic aorta extends proximally from the aortic annulus to the diaphragmatic crura distally.[7] The thoracic aorta is subdivided into three parts: the ascending aorta, the arch, and the descending aorta. The ascending thoracic aorta comprises the aortic root and the tubular ascending aorta. The aortic root lies between the aortic annulus and the sinotubular junction (Fig. 1). The sinuses of Valsalva arise from the aortic root. The tubular ascending aorta extends from the sinotubular junction to the brachiocephalic trunk. Approximately 3 cm of the proximal ascending aorta is within the pericardium. The coronary arteries are the only branches of the ascending aorta.

The aortic arch extends from the brachiocephalic trunk to the origin of the left subclavian artery. The isthmus extends from the left subclavian artery to the ligamentum arteriosum. Three branches usually arise from the aortic arch: the brachiocephalic trunk (occasionally referred to as the *brachiocephalic artery* or *innominate artery*), the left common carotid artery, and the left subclavian artery. The brachiocephalic trunk divides into the right subclavian artery and the right common carotid artery.

Currently published normal measurements of the thoracic aorta are listed in Table 1. Most of currently accepted aortic dimensions are either

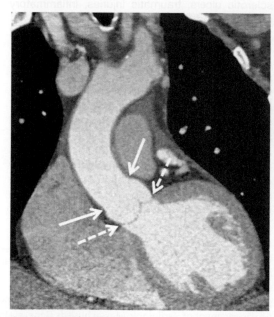

Fig. 1. Normal aorta on coronal contrast-enhanced CT. The aortic root extends from the aortic annulus (*dashed arrows*) to the sinotubular junction (*solid arrows*). The coronary arteries—the only branches of the ascending aorta—arise from the aortic root.

Table 1
Normal values for the thoracic aorta

Aorta	Normal Values	References
LVOT	20.3 ± 3.4 mm (2 SD)	Lu et al[79]
Aortic annulus	25–37 mm (95% CI) (end-diastolic) 26.3 ± 2.8 mm (coronal) 23.5 ± 2.7 mm (sagittal)	Lin et al[80] Tops et al[81]
Sinus of Valsalva	34.2 ± 4.1 mm (2 SD) 36.9 ± 3.8 mm (2 SD) (end-diastolic, gated)	Lu et al[79] Ocak et al[82]
Sinotubular junction	29.7 ± 3.4 mm (2 SD)	Lu et al[79]
Ascending aorta	32.7 ± 3.8 mm (2 SD) 33.6 ± 4.1 mm (2 SD) (male/intraluminal/end-systolic) 31.1 ± 3.9 mm (2 SD) (female/intraluminal/end-systolic) 21–35 mm (95% CI) (end-diastolic)	Lu et al[79] Mao et al[8] Mao et al[8] Lin et al[80]
Descending thoracic aorta	17–26 mm (95% CI) (end-diastolic)	Lin et al[80]

Abbreviations: CI, confidence interval; LVOT, left ventricular outflow tract; SD, standard deviation.

based on other imaging modalities (which may measure the aorta differently) or on nongated MDCT (often derived from body axial [x–y plane] rather than from true aortic short axis images). Therefore, some uncertainty exists as to the true normal size of the thoracic aorta. Electrocardiogram (ECG)-gated MDCT is poised to become the reference standard method for assessing the thoracic aorta, allowing for reproducible measurements not reliant on operator skill. Furthermore, variations in the size of the aorta during different portions of the cardiac cycle could also be documented.[8]

In 6.6% of people, the left vertebral artery arises directly from the arch (Fig. 2).[9] The bovine arch is another normal variant in which the left common carotid artery arises from the brachiocephalic trunk (Fig. 3) rather than the aorta, occurring in up to one fourth of the population.[9] Although ingrained in the medical literature, the bovine arch is a misnomer for this aortic variant; cows actually have a single brachiocephalic trunk that splits into the bilateral subclavian arteries and a bicarotid trunk.[10] Another arch variant is the ductus diverticulum—a focal bulge along the inner aspect of the isthmus representing a remnant of the ductus arteriosus (Fig. 4). Traumatic aortic transection also occurs in this location and can occasionally be difficult to differentiate from a ductus diverticulum. However, the ductus diverticulum has smooth margins with obtuse angles relative to the adjacent aorta. Aortic transection has irregular margins with acute angles relative to the adjacent aorta.

The descending thoracic aorta extends from the isthmus to the diaphragmatic crura. In contrast to the ascending aorta, the descending thoracic aorta has multiple branches, including the bronchial, intercostal, spinal, superior phrenic arteries, and various small mediastinal branches. Pseudocoarctation is a normal variant of the aortic arch

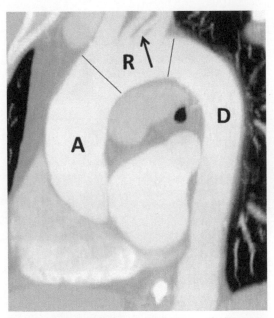

Fig. 2. Normal oblique sagittal view of the aorta (candy cane view) on contrast-enhanced CT. The thoracic aorta has three main subdivisions: the ascending aorta (A), the aortic arch (R), and the descending thoracic aorta (D). Incidental note is made of a four-vessel aortic arch in which the left vertebral artery arises directly from the aortic arch rather than from the proximal left subclavian artery (*arrow*).

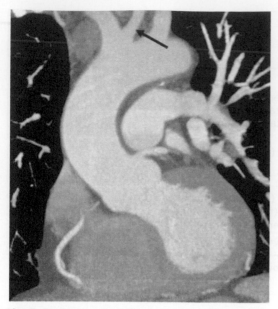

Fig. 3. Bovine aortic arch on contrast-enhanced CT. Coronal view of the aorta from CT angiography shows common origin of the brachiocephalic and left common carotid arteries (*arrow*) consistent with a bovine arch. Although believed to mirror normal cow anatomy, bovine arch is a misnomer.

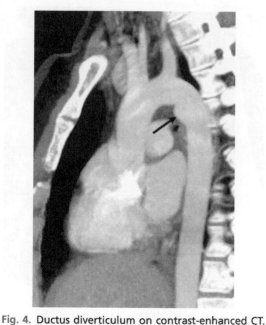

Fig. 4. Ductus diverticulum on contrast-enhanced CT. Oblique sagittal image of the aorta on contrast-enhanced CT shows a smooth protrusion along the inferior inner aspect of the isthmus of the aorta with obtuse margins with the adjacent aorta. This is in contradistinction to traumatic transections of the aorta, which has abrupt acute transitions and irregular margins with the adjacent aorta.

and proximal descending artery that occurs when the third to seventh embryonic dorsal segments fail to fuse appropriately; the resultant high proximal arch leads to pseudokinking of the redundant aorta where it is tethered to the pulmonary artery by the ligamentum arteriosum (**Fig. 5**). No hemodynamically significant luminal aortic narrowing exists in pseudocoarctation.

Acute Aortic Syndrome

Acute aortic syndrome is a group of aortic pathologies that are acute emergencies. Underlying aortic diseases include penetrating atherosclerotic ulcer, intramural hematoma, aortic dissection, rupturing aneurysms, and traumatic aortic injury. MDCT is the preferred examination because of its rapid acquisition and high definition of the aorta, its wall, and the end organs. ECG-gated CT is preferred, if readily available, especially if ascending aortic involvement is suspected. Nongated MDCT of the ascending aorta is limited by motion artifact, which can be misinterpreted as a dissection.[11] Motion artifact can be entirely eliminated by ECG gating.

AORTIC DISSECTION

Aortic dissection results from an intimal tear extending into the inner layer of the aortic media; the false and true lumens are separated by an intimal flap. The blood within the false lumen may be free-flowing or thrombosed. Acute aortic dissection is potentially life-threatening, with a reported incidence of 2.9 per 100,000 persons per year.[12] Risk factors for aortic dissection include preexisting thoracic aortic aneurysm, chronic hypertension, Marfan syndrome, bicuspid aortic valve, and prior cardiovascular surgery. Dissections most commonly originate in the ascending aorta (approximately 65% of cases); 20% occur in the descending thoracic aorta, 10% in the aortic arch, and 5% in the abdominal aorta.[13] The dissected aorta can be dilated or normal in caliber.

Aortic dissections can be classified according to involvement of the ascending aorta or arch. This involvement implies a worse prognosis and usually requires surgical management.[14] The DeBakey and Stanford classification systems are the most commonly used systems to categorize aortic dissections and are based on location. In type I DeBakey dissections, the intimal flap involves both the ascending and descending thoracic aorta; in type II, the intimal flap involves the ascending aorta only; and in type III the intimal flap is isolated to the descending thoracic aorta. In Stanford type A dissections, the intimal flap involves the ascending thoracic aorta (with

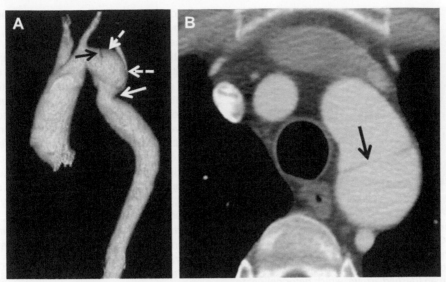

Fig. 5. Pseudocoarctation of the aorta on contrast-enhanced CT. (*A*) Three-dimensional volume-rendered image of contrast-enhanced CT shows redundancy of the aortic arch resulting in a kinked appearance at the level of the ligamentum arteriosum (*solid white arrow*). Longstanding aberrant flow dynamics through the redundant aorta and resultant axial stress has resulted in a focal aneurysm along the distal aortic arch (*dashed arrows*) and a localized dissection (*black arrow*). More commonly, aneurysms related to pseudocoarctations develop beyond the area of aortic pseudokinking. (*B*) Axial image from the same study redemonstrates the dissection flap (*arrow*). No significant collateral arteries are present, implying that no hemodynamically significant stenosis is present at the level of the pseudocoarctation.

or without extension into the descending aorta) (Fig. 6), whereas in type B, the flap does not involve the ascending thoracic aorta or arch (Fig. 7).

Dissections involving the ascending aorta (Stanford A; DeBakey I and II) are surgical emergencies, because dissections in this area are prone to rupture or other critical complications, including

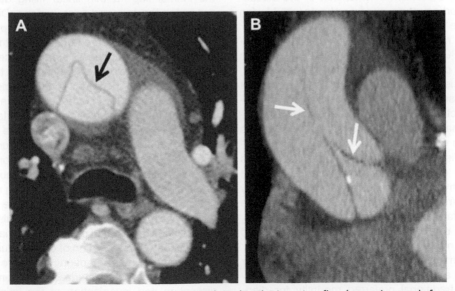

Fig. 6. Type A aortic dissection on contrast enhanced CT. (*A, B*) Dissection flap (*arrows*) extends from the aortic root to the proximal ascending aorta. Involvement of the aortic root puts this patient at risk for rupture into the pericardial sac and resultant cardiac tamponade, or aortic insufficiency as well as extension of the dissection flap into the coronary arteries.

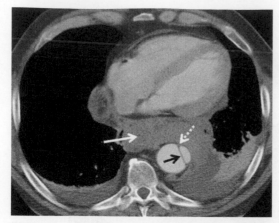

Fig. 7. Type B aortic dissection on axial contrast-enhanced CT. A dissection flap (*black arrow*) is isolated to the descending thoracic aorta. Focal low-density thrombus is present in the beaked margin of the false lumen (*dashed arrow*), which helps delineate the false from the true lumen. As in most cases, the false lumen is larger than the true lumen. A large high-density mediastinal hematoma is also noted; incidental note is made of lower attenuation pleural effusions with associated relaxation atelectasis.

development of hemopericardium, pericardial tamponade, and death. Other potential complications of ascending aortic dissections include aortic valve rupture, aortic insufficiency, coronary artery dissection, stroke, and myocardial infarction. Surgery in type B dissection is reserved for patients who have occlusion of major aortic branches, expansion or extension of the dissection, or aortic rupture, and for patients with Marfan syndrome who have an acute distal dissection.[15] Mortality rates for untreated Stanford A dissections is 1% to 2% per hour during the first 24 hours and 80% during the first 2 weeks.[16]

MDCT is the most common modality to detect aortic dissections.[17] Its high sensitivity for detecting dissection, wide availability, and ability to identify alternative diagnoses for chest pain makes MDCT an excellent first choice in evaluating suspected dissection.[18–20] MDCT rapidly delineates extension of the intimal flap, allowing for efficient preoperative planning. It can also help identify the entry/reentry sites, relationships between the true and false lumens, flow in the aortic branches, perfusion of end organs, aortic insufficiency, and coronary artery involvement.

Other imaging modalities may also be used for analyzing aortic dissection. Catheter aortography was the traditional preferred modality for diagnosing aortic dissection (sensitivity, 77%–90%; specificity, 90%–100%).[21] However, the risks associated with catheter manipulation and high-flow contrast injection makes this modality less attractive.

Transesophageal echocardiogram (TEE) is currently the second most frequently used modality, and can be considered an alternative that is especially useful in unstable patients. This modality has good accuracy, with a sensitivity of 90% to 100% and specificity of 77% to 100%.[22] However, TEE is limited by reliance on operator skill, ultrasound artifacts, and inconsistent visualization of the distal ascending aorta and proximal arch. Similarly, although MRI is highly accurate in detecting aortic dissections (sensitivity as high as 100%), widespread use of this modality has been hampered by long acquisition times, which is undesirable in the emergent setting. Furthermore, many medical devices are ferromagnetic, which are contraindications to MRI.

Currently, no available data compare the utility of modern MDCT and MRI/TEE. Modern MDCT can image the entire aorta from supra-aortic branches to femoral arteries within a few seconds, can eliminate pulsation artifact with gating (which otherwise could mimic type A dissections), and provides isovolumetric imaging, allowing reconstruction of images in any plane.[23] Furthermore, CT offers high-resolution images of the aortic wall.[24] However, MDCT should be used prudently, given its use of ionizing radiation. In addition, aortic evaluation on MDCT may suffer from streak artifacts, volume averaging with periaortic structures, and patient motion artifacts.[25]

The main MDCT finding in aortic dissection is the intimal flap—a thin linear filling defect that separates the true and false lumens. Differentiation of the false and true lumens is imperative in surgical repair and percutaneous treatment with endografts. In most cases, the true lumen can be identified by determining continuity with the undissected portion of the aorta. The true lumen spirals through the aortic arch (anterior in the ascending aorta and medial in the descending aorta).

The cross-sectional area of the false lumen is also often larger than that of the true lumen. The cobweb sign is insensitive but specific for the false lumen.[26] Thin linear areas of low attenuation are present in the false lumen, representing remnants of the media. Finally, the beak sign (see **Fig. 7**) is another helpful diagnostic sign of the false lumen. It represents the section of hematoma that cleaves a space for the propagation of the false lumen.[26,27] Intimo-intimal intussusception is a rare type of aortic dissection characterized by circumferential dissection and invagination of the intimal layer, likened to a windsock.[28] Neurologic impairment from occlusion of the aorta or arch branches may be more common in this entity.[29]

Presence of identifiable flow in the false lumen and patency have prognostic implications and can be evaluated on MDCT. Slow flow in the false lumen eventually leads to thrombus formation.[27] A patent false lumen has a higher 3-year mortality rate (32%) compared with a partially thrombosed lumen (14%) among the survivors of type B dissection.[18]

Evaluation of Aortic Dissection After Surgical Repair

After aortic dissection repair, patients require regular screening to exclude signs of impending aortic rupture. Aortic rupture is usually preceded by rapid expansion. Therefore, early detection of aortic enlargement is imperative. Other findings to exclude include prosthetic graft degeneration, infection, malfunction of aortic valve prosthesis, and aneurysm formation in other portions of the aorta. Each institution should have a postoperative CT follow-up schedule after dissection repair to detect early aortic growth. For example, initial postprocedural CT could be obtained at discharge. Subsequently, patients with an absolute aortic diameter less than 5 cm would undergo CT once a year; those with an absolute diameter greater than 5 cm would undergo CT every 6 months.[30]

Intramural Hematoma

Intramural hematoma (IMH) is hemorrhage localized to the aortic media in the absence of a visible intimal tear. IMH is considered equivalent to aortic dissection regarding prognostic and therapeutic implications because an intramural hematoma may progress to aortic dissection and rupture. IMH may develop secondary to spontaneous rupture of vasa vasorum of the medial aortic layer, penetrating aortic ulceration, or blunt trauma.[31] Hypertension is the most common predisposing risk factor.

Unenhanced CT is extremely valuable in identifying intramural hematomas. Typically, circumferential or crescent-shaped high attenuation thickening of the aortic wall is present, representing hematoma within the medial wall of the aorta (Fig. 8), which sometimes narrows the aortic lumen.[32]

Several findings help differentiate IMH from a thrombosed false lumen of an aortic dissection: IMHs do not enhance, no intimal tear is seen, and IMHs maintain a constant circumferential relationship with the aortic wall; the false lumen of a dissection has a longitudinal spiral geometry.[33] Involvement of the ascending aorta, pericardial or pleural effusion, and an aortic diameter of

greater than 5 cm may predict progression of an IMH to a true dissection.[34,35]

PENETRATING AORTIC ULCER

Penetrating aortic ulcer (PAU) represents an ulcerated atheroma disrupting the aortic intima.[36] PAU occurs when an atheromatous plaque ruptures, disrupting the elastic lamina, with variable extension into the media. Hypertension and advanced age are the most common risk factors. The descending aorta is most often affected.[37] CT commonly shows extensive aortic atherosclerosis. On CT, a discrete contrast-filled "collar button" is often seen outpouching beyond the expected confines of the aorta[36] (see Fig. 8; Fig. 9). PAUs are often multifocal, which is not surprising considering the diffuse nature of atherosclerosis.

PAU can be difficult to differentiate from ulcerated atherosclerotic plaque. The presence of contour deformity of the vessel is highly suggestive of PAU. Extension of the aortic ulcer into the medial layer can result in an IMH, localized aortic dissection, saccular pseudoaneurysm, or mediastinal hematoma.[38] Invasive intervention (surgery or endovascular repair) should be considered in patients with pain, hemodynamic instability, or signs of aortic expansion.[39] Asymptomatic patients can be followed closely with optimization of medical management.

Traumatic Aortic Transection

Traumatic aortic transection is a tear involving all layers of the aortic wall, usually caused by rapid deceleration (high-speed motor vehicle accident or fall from significant height). The mortality rate is high, with most patients dying on the field.[40,41] Survival is highest for tears at the aortic isthmus. Aortic injury also occurs at the aortic root and at the diaphragmatic hiatus. Proposed mechanisms for aortic injury include shearing and hydrostatic forces secondary to rapid deceleration, and osseous pinching. Given its accuracy, rapid acquisition, and wide availability, CT is usually the preferred imaging modality for suspected aortic transection.

MDCT imaging findings include small contained periaortic hematomas, traumatic pseudoaneurysm (Fig. 10), mediastinal hematoma, focal contour abnormality, abrupt change in aortic caliber, or an intraluminal ridge, flap, or thrombus.[42] A residual ductus diverticulum can mimic traumatic pseudoaneurysm. Absence of mediastinal hemorrhage, smooth contours, and obtuse margins with the adjacent aorta are more suggestive of a ductus diverticulum (see Fig. 4) than an acute injury.

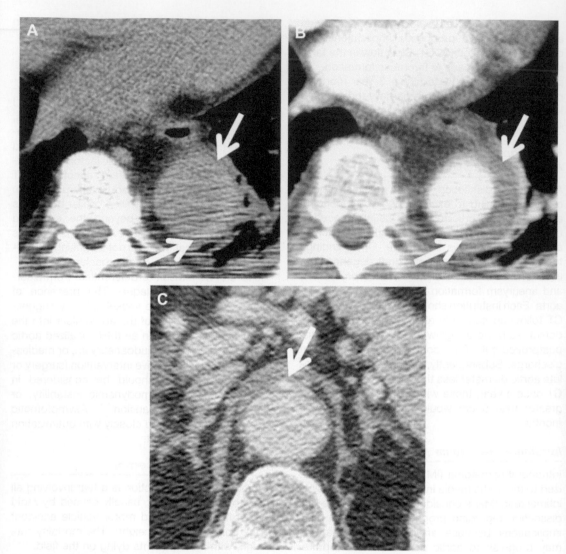

Fig. 8. Type B intramural hematoma from a penetrating aortic ulcer on axial noncontrast and contrast-enhanced CT. (*A*, *B*) Axial image from noncontrast CT shows a rind of hyperdense attenuation (*arrows in A*) around the descending thoracic aorta, which does not enhance after the administration of contrast (*arrows in B*). (*C*) In the upper abdominal aorta, focal outpouching is seen along the anterior aorta, beyond the expected confines of the lumen, consistent with a penetrating aortic ulceration (*arrow*).

THORACIC AORTIC ANEURYSM

A true aortic aneurysm represents greater than 50% dilation of the aorta; the wall of a true aneurysm comprises the intima, media, and adventitia.[43] Aortic aneurysms are the 13th most common cause of death in the United States. The incidence and prevalence of aortic aneurysms have increased concomitantly with life expectancy. The incidence of thoracic aortic aneurysms is currently 10.4 cases per 100,000 persons per year.[44] Affected individuals are most often in their 60s, and men are affected 2 to 4 times more often than women. Hypertension is present in 60% of cases. Thoracic aortic aneurysms are less common than abdominal aortic aneurysms. Up to 25% of patients with thoracic aneurysm will also have an abdominal aortic aneurysm.[45]

The aortic root and ascending aorta (aortic valve to innominate artery) are affected in 60% of patients with thoracic aneurysm (see **Fig. 11**), the arch in 10%, the descending thoracic aorta (distal to left subclavian artery) in 40%, and the thoracoabdominal aorta in 10%.[46] The extent, location, and size of the aneurysm should be documented on MDCT. Size should be obtained in aortic short

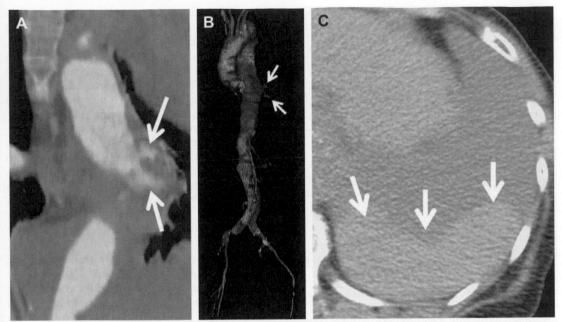

Fig. 9. Ruptured penetrating aortic ulceration on contrast-enhanced and noncontrast CT. (*A*) Coronal reformation from contrast-enhanced CT shows two focal irregular outpouchings (*arrows*) along the left lateral aspect of the aorta, consistent with penetrating aortic ulcerations. (*B*) Three-dimensional reformat from the same study demonstrates the irregularity of the ruptured aortic ulcerations (*arrows*). Aortoiliac stent graft is also present from previous abdominal aortic aneurysm repair. (*C*) Axial image from noncontrast CT shows a large left pleural effusion with increased density in the dependent aspect of the collection (hematocrit sign), highly suggestive of hemothorax from rupture of the penetrating aortic ulceration.

axis (orthogonal to the aortic segment long axis). In addition to evaluating aortic aneurysm morphology, MDCT can accurately detect the presence of complications such as rupture, infection, and fistulas. MDCT is ideal for postsurgical surveillance and surveillance in patients being treated medically. Furthermore, CT can detect involvement of aortic branches, which is essential for preoperative surgical evaluation.[47]

Thoracic aortic aneurysms can be classified based on extent or morphology. The Crawford classification includes four types of thoracoabdominal aneurysms.[48] Type I aneurysms extend from the left subclavian artery to the renal artery. Type II extend from the left subclavian artery to the aortic bifurcation; these have the worst postsurgical outcome. Type III aneurysms extend from the mid-thorax to the aortic bifurcation, and type IV extend from the diaphragm to the aortic bifurcation. Morphologically, thoracic aneurysms are divided into fusiform (uniform, symmetric dilation of the entire circumference of the aorta), saccular (localized outpouching of the aorta), and pseudoaneurysm (contained rupture of the aortic wall with disruption of the intima and media, with usually a narrow mouth).

Size is the only established risk factor predicting aortic rupture. No significant risk for aortic rupture is associated with aneurysms smaller than 4.0 cm. Risk for aortic rupture increases incrementally with aneurysm size; aneurysms 4.0 to 5.9 cm have a 16% risk for rupture and those greater than 6.0 cm have a 31% risk for rupture.[44] Thoracic aneurysms grow 1.0 to 10 mm per year.[49]

Descending midaortic aneurysms have the fastest growth rate, and ascending aneurysms have the slowest despite larger initial diameter.[49] In general, larger aneurysms grow faster. Aneurysms larger than 5.0 cm in diameter grow on average 7.9 mm per year versus 1.7 mm per year for smaller aneurysms.[50]

Risk for dissection is also related to the size of the aneurysm. The dissection risk per year is 2% for aneurysms smaller than 5.0 cm and 3% for aneurysms 5.0 to 5.9 cm. Aneurysms larger than 6.0 cm in diameter have a dissection risk per year of more than 7%, and these patients have a 5-year survival rate of only 54% without surgery.[51]

In patients with Marfan syndrome and Ehlers-Danlos syndrome, aortic root aneurysms may efface the sinotubular junction (annuloaortic ectasia), resulting in a classic tulip bulb configuration[52]

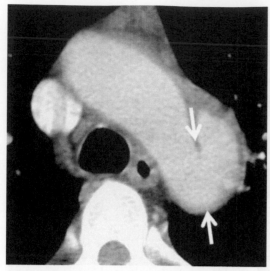

Fig. 10. Traumatic aortic pseudoaneurysm on contrast-enhanced CT. Axial image from contrast-enhanced CT shows irregular focal outpouching of the isthmic aorta with a narrow neck (*arrows*), consistent with partial aortic transection and pseudoaneurysm formation in this patient who has a history of a high-speed motor vehicle collision. No mediastinal hematoma is present. This site is the most common location of traumatic aortic injury identified by imaging; individuals with injuries in other regions of the thoracic aorta, such as the aortic root, seldom survive to receive medical attention.

(Fig. 12). Aortic root aneurysms may also occur in the setting of bicuspid aortic valves and familial thoracic aortic aneurysm syndrome (FTAAS). Most aneurysms of the tubular ascending aorta are idiopathic but may also occur with bicuspid aortic valve, FTAAS, giant cell arteriitis, and Syphilis.[53–56] Bicuspid aortic valve is known to be an independent predictor of ascending aortic aneurysm formation after surgical correction of coarctation.[54] Furthermore, normally functioning bicuspid aortic valves have been associated with enlargement of the aortic root or ascending aorta in 52% of patients.[53] Thoracic aortic aneurysms have a hereditary component—19% of patients with thoracic aneurysms have a family history independent of Marfan or Ehlers-Danlos syndromes.[55]

Aneurysms of the ascending aorta or the aortic arch may cause hoarseness from left vagus or left recurrent laryngeal nerve compression, hemidiaphragmatic paralysis from phrenic nerve compression, asthma-like symptoms from tracheobronchial compression, dysphasia from esophageal compression, and facial swelling from superior vena cava compression. Thoracic aortic aneurysms also predispose patients to thromboembolism, aortoesophageal fistula, and aortic dissection.

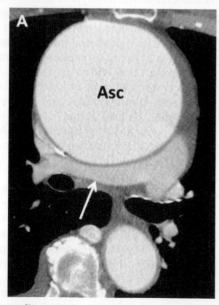

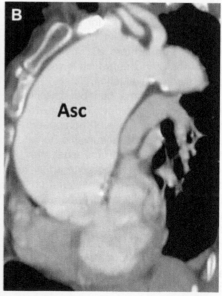

Fig. 11. Ascending aortic aneurysm on contrast-enhanced CT. Axial (*A*) and coronal (*B*) images from contrast-enhanced CT show a massive ascending aortic aneurysm (Asc). The right pulmonary artery is extrinsically narrowed by the aneurysm (*arrow*).

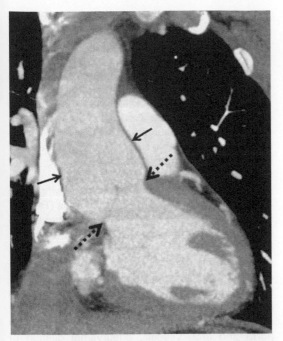

Fig. 12. Annuloaortic ectasia on contrast-enhanced CT. Multiplanar reformation in the aortic root long axis shows aortic root aneurysm with effacement and dilatation of the sinotubular junction (*solid arrows*), and widening of the aortic annulus (*dashed arrows*), indicating annuloaortic ectasia in this patient with Marfan syndrome.

Surgery is usually recommended for ascending aneurysm greater than 5 to 6 cm and descending aneurysm greater than 6 to 7 cm.[57] Aortic size index (ratio of aortic diameter over body surface area in m^2) greater than 2.75 cm/m^2 is an indication for surgery,[58] as is accelerated growth (>10 mm/y growth in aneurysms <5 cm).[59] Aortic regurgitation, in conjunction with an aortic root or ascending aortic aneurysm, requires aortic valve replacement plus aortic root repair if the aneurysm is 5 cm or greater.[60,61] Furthermore, in functional bicuspid aortic valves, aortic root repair or replacement of the ascending aorta is indicated if the root or ascending aorta is greater than 5.0 cm in diameter or is growing faster than 0.5 cm/y.[60]

SINUS OF VALSALVA ANEURYSM

Sinuses of Valsalva aneurysms are rare congenital anomalies resulting from failure of proper development of elastic components in the aortic media. The right coronary sinus of Valsalva is most commonly affected, followed by the noncoronary sinus.[62] These aneurysms usually rupture into right heart (right atrium or ventricle), causing left to right shunting. Rupture into the pericardial sac can lead to cardiac tamponade.

Sinus of Valsalva aneurysms may protrude into or obstruct the right ventricular outflow tract. Ventricular septal defect, aortic insufficiency, aortic coarctation, and bicuspid aortic valve are all associated with sinus of Valsalva aneurysms.[63] CT will show asymmetric dilatation of one or more of the sinuses of Valsalva (Fig. 13). Progressive increases in size rather than absolute size is more frequently used when determining proper surgical timing in asymptomatic patients.[64]

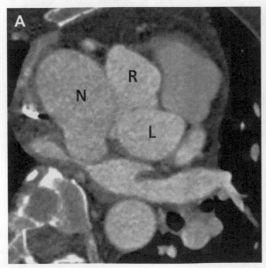
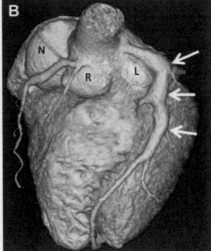

Fig. 13. Sinus of Valsalva aneurysm on contrast-enhanced CT. (*A*) Short axis view through the aortic root shows asymmetric dilation of all sinuses of Valsalva, most severe in the noncoronary sinus, in this patient with underlying connective tissue disorder. (*B*) Three-dimensional reconstruction of the heart shows asymmetric dilation of the sinuses of Valsalva. There is also aneurysmal dilation of the left anterior descending artery (*arrows*). N, noncoronary sinus; R, right coronary sinus; L, left coronary sinus.

AORTIC COARCTATION

Aortic coarctation is focal narrowing of the thoracic aorta, which can occur anywhere in the aorta, although it is most common at the isthmus. Aortic coarctation is a common malformation, affecting men 2 to 5 times more often than women.[65] Aortic coarctation has three major subtypes: focal (aortic coarctation), diffuse (hypoplastic isthmus), and complete (aortic arch interruption). The narrowing in aortic coarctation is caused by a fibrous ridge, arising from abnormal hyperplasia of the tunica media. Hemodynamic compromise leads to the development of collaterals to bypass the narrowed aorta (Fig. 14). The extent of collaterals depends on the severity of stenosis. Collaterals may compress the spinal cord or may rupture.[66]

Most aortic coarctation classifications are based on anatomy. Aortic coarctations have been traditionally divided into preductal (infantile) and postductal (adult) subtypes; however, this classification system can be misleading. The contemporary approach is to use left subclavian artery as a landmark for distinguishing between the more common distal (juxtaductal) and less common proximal subtypes.[65]

Aortic coarctations are associated with multiple other abnormalities. Among patients with aortic coarctation, 30% to 40% will also have a bicuspid aortic valve, although most of these will not have a coarctation.[67]

Patients with Turner syndrome have a higher prevalence of aortic coarctation. Other abnormalities associated with aortic coarctation include ventricular septal defect, patent ductus arteriosus, aortic stenosis, and mitral stenosis.[68] Patients with aortic coarctation must also be evaluated for intracerebral berry aneurysms. Intracerebral aneurysms can rupture, leading to subarachnoid or intracerebral hemorrhage, even long after successful coarctation repair.[69]

Rare cases of acquired aortic narrowing have also been reported. Inflammatory aortitis (Takayasu aortitis) is a well-described cause of acquired aortic stenosis and usually involves the midthoracic or abdominal aorta.[70] Takayasu aortitis predominantly affects young women of Asian descent, with a mean age of 35 years at diagnosis.[71] Imaging findings suggesting Takayasu aortitis include thickening of the walls of the aorta and its branches (Fig. 15), stenosis of the aorta and arch vessels, aneurysmal dilation of the aorta and its major branches, and aortic regurgitation from aortic root dilation.

Treatment of congenital aortic coarctation is largely dependent on age, clinical presentation, and severity. Early repair is important to prevent long-standing hypertension. Indications for repair include arterial hypertension, congestive heart

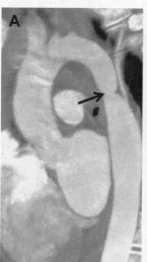
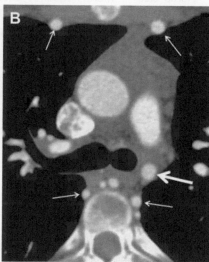
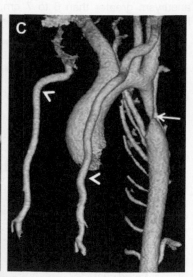

Fig. 14. Aortic coarctation on contrast-enhanced CT. (*A*) Oblique sagittal (candy cane) view of the thoracic aorta shows narrowing (*arrow*) of the proximal descending aorta. (*B*) Axial view through the mid chest shows high-grade stenosis of the descending thoracic aorta (*thick arrow*); multiple enlarged collateral arteries are present (*thin arrows*), including internal mammary arteries, which bypass the stenotic portion of the aorta and provide blood flow to the lower body. (*C*) Three-dimensional reconstruction shows multiple dilated collateral arteries and severe narrowing of the proximal descending aorta (*arrow*). The internal mammary arteries (*arrowheads*) are markedly enlarged.

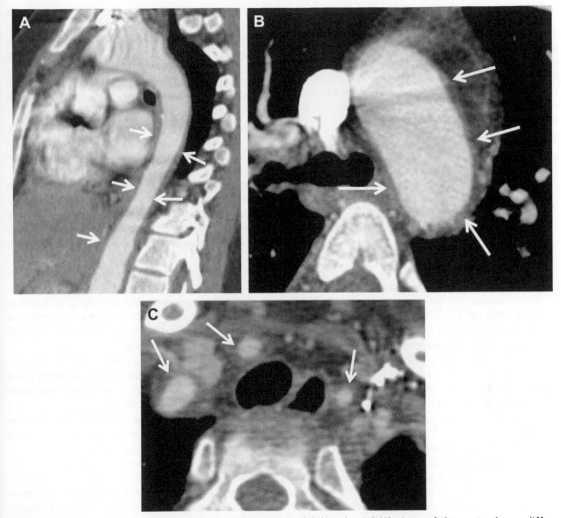

Fig. 15. Takayasu aortitis on contrast enhanced CT. Sagittal (*A*) and axial (*B*) views of the aorta shows diffuse thickening of the aortic wall (*arrows*) with smooth narrowing of the mid descending thoracic aorta. As opposed to cases of atherosclerosis, the aortic wall shows a general paucity of calcification. (*C*) Axial view through the upper thorax shows circumferential thickening of the innominate, carotid, and subclavian arteries (*arrows*).

failure, and pressure gradient greater than 30 mmHg (though resting pressure gradient in isolation is an unreliable indicator of severity in the presence of extensive collaterals).[72] Multiple surgical techniques are available, including resection with end-to-end anastomosis, subclavian flap aortoplasty in infants with long-segment coarctation, prosthetic patch (now rarely used because of increased risk for postoperative aneurysms and ruptures), and bypass grafting across the coarctation.[73] Balloon angioplasty is a viable alternative to surgery and can be used in patients with native coarctation or those who develop restenosis after surgery.[74,75] Postprocedural surveillance of these patients is mandatory to monitor for

residual coarctation (most common with resection and end-to-end anastomosis), aortic arch hypoplasia, aneurysm formation at the site of repair, restenosis, aortic dissection, and pseudoaneurysm formation (most common with balloon angioplasty).[76]

Pseudocoarctation should not be misdiagnosed as true aortic coarctation. In pseudocoarctation, the aortic arch is elongated and has a kinked appearance from fixation of the proximal descending aorta by the ligamentum arteriosum. Chest wall collaterals, fibrous ridge, and pressure gradient are absent. Over time, progressive dilation and aortic dissection may complicate pseudocoarctations (see **Fig. 5**).[77,78]

SUMMARY

This article reviews the MDCT imaging appearance of common entities that are part of the wide spectrum of diseases involving the thoracic aorta. ECG-gated MDCT is poised to become the reference standard method in assessing the thoracic aorta. Reproducible images of the aorta can be acquired independent of operator skill.

REFERENCES

1. Kaatee R, Van Leeuwen M, De Lange E, et al. Spiral CT angiography of the renal arteries: should a scan delay based on a test bolus injection or a fixed scan delay be used to obtain maximum enhancement of the vessels? J Comput Assist Tomogr 1998;22: 541–7.

2. Van Hoe L, Baert A, Gryspeerdt S, et al. Supra- and juxtarenal aneurysms of the abdominal aorta: preoperative assessment with thin-section spiral CT. Radiology 1996;198:443–8.

3. Armerding M, Rubin G, Beaulieu C, et al. Aortic aneurysmal disease: assessment of stent-graft treatment-CT versus conventional angiography. Radiology 2000;215:138–46.

4. Katz D, Jorgensen M, Rubin G. Detection and follow-up of important extra-arterial lesions with helical CT angiography. Clin Radiol 1999;54:294–300.

5. Rubin G. MDCT imaging of the aorta and peripheral vessels. Eur J Radiol 2003;45(Suppl 1):S42–9.

6. Lee C, Goo J, Ye H, et al. Radiation dose modulation techniques in the multidetector CT era: from basics to practice. Radiographics 2008;28:1451–9.

7. Abbara S, Kalva S, Cury R, et al. Thoracic aortic disease: spectrum of multidetector computed tomography imaging findings. J Cardiovasc Comput Tomogr 2007;1:40–54.

8. Mao S, Ahmadi N, Shah B, et al. Normal thoracic aorta diameter on cardiac computed tomography in healthy asymptomatic adults: impact of age and gender. Acad Radiol 2008;15:827–34.

9. Berko N, Jain V, Godelman A, et al. Variants and anomalies of thoracic vasculature on computed tomographic angiography in adults. J Comput Assist Tomogr 2009;33:523–8.

10. Layton K, Kallmes D, Cloft H, et al. Bovine aortic arch variant in humans: clarification of a common misnomer. AJNR Am J Neuroradiol 2006;27:1541–2.

11. Roos J, Willmann J, Weishaupt D, et al. Thoracic aorta: motion artifact reduction with retrospective and prospective electrocardiography-assisted multi-detector row CT. Radiology 2002;222:271–7.

12. Mészáros I, Mórocz J, Szlávi J, et al. Epidemiology and clinicopathology of aortic dissection. Chest 2000;117:1271–8.

13. Isselbacher EM, Eagle KA, Desanctis RW. Diseases of the aorta: aortic dissection. In: Braunwald E, Zipes DP, Libby P, et al, editors. Braunwald's heart disease: a textbook of cardiovascular medicine. 7th edition. Philadelphia: Saunders; 2005. p. 1415–31.

14. Rojas C, Restrepo C. Mediastinal hematomas: aortic injury and beyond. J Comput Assist Tomogr 2009; 33:218–24.

15. DeSanctis R, Doroghazi R, Austen W, et al. Aortic dissection. N Engl J Med 1987;317:1060–7.

16. Coady M, Rizzo J, Goldstein L, et al. Natural history, pathogenesis, and etiology of thoracic aortic aneurysms and dissections. Cardiol Clin 1999;17:615–35, vii.

17. Hagan P, Nienaber C, Isselbacher E, et al. The International Registry of Acute Aortic Dissection (IRAD): new insights into an old disease. JAMA 2000;283: 897–903.

18. Moore A, Eagle K, Bruckman D, et al. Choice of computed tomography, transesophageal echocardiography, magnetic resonance imaging, and aortography in acute aortic dissection: International Registry of Acute Aortic Dissection (IRAD). Am J Cardiol 2002;89:1235–8.

19. Cigarroa J, Isselbacher E, DeSanctis R, et al. Diagnostic imaging in the evaluation of suspected aortic dissection. Old standards and new directions. N Engl J Med 1993;328:35–43.

20. Nienaber C, von Kodolitsch Y, Nicolas V, et al. The diagnosis of thoracic aortic dissection by noninvasive imaging procedures. N Engl J Med 1993;328:1–9.

21. Bansal R, Chandrasekaran K, Ayala K, et al. Frequency and explanation of false negative diagnosis of aortic dissection by aortography and transesophageal echocardiography. J Am Coll Cardiol 1995;25:1393–401.

22. Mammen L, Yucel EK, Khan A, et al. Expert Panel on Cardiac Imaging. ACR appropriateness criteria® acute chest pain–suspected aortic dissection. Reston (VA): American College of Radiology (ACR); 2008. online publication.

23. Morgan-Hughes G, Marshall A, Roobottom C. Refined computed tomography of the thoracic aorta: the impact of electrocardiographic assistance. Clin Radiol 2003;58:581–8.

24. Greenberg R, Secor J, Painter T. Computed tomography assessment of thoracic aortic pathology. Semin Vasc Surg 2004;17:166–72.

25. Batra P, Bigoni B, Manning J, et al. Pitfalls in the diagnosis of thoracic aortic dissection at CT angiography. Radiographics 2000;20:309–20.

26. LePage M, Quint L, Sonnad S, et al. Aortic dissection: CT features that distinguish true lumen from false lumen. AJR Am J Roentgenol 2001;177:207–11.

27. Williams M, Farrow R. Atypical patterns in the CT diagnosis of aortic dissection. Clin Radiol 1994;49: 686–9.

28. Nelsen K, Spizarny D, Kastan D. Intimointimal intussusception in aortic dissection: CT diagnosis. AJR Am J Roentgenol 1994;162:813–4.

29. Fan Z, Zhang Z, Ma X, et al. Acute aortic dissection with intimal intussusception: MRI appearances. AJR Am J Roentgenol 2006;186:841–3.

30. Heinemann M, Laas J, Karck M, et al. Thoracic aortic aneurysms after acute type A aortic dissection: necessity for follow-up. Ann Thorac Surg 1990;49:580–4.

31. Fattori R, Bertaccini P, Celletti F, et al. Intramural posttraumatic hematoma of the ascending aorta in a patient with a double aortic arch. Eur Radiol 1997;7:51–3.

32. Nienaber C, von Kodolitsch Y, Petersen B, et al. Intramural hemorrhage of the thoracic aorta. Diagnostic and therapeutic implications. Circulation 1995;92:1465–72.

33. von Kodolitsch Y, Nienaber C. [Intramural hemorrhage of the thoracic aorta: diagnosis, therapy and prognosis of 209 in vivo diagnosed cases]. Z Kardiol 1998;87:797–807 [in German].

34. von Kodolitsch Y, Csösz S, Koschyk D, et al. Intramural hematoma of the aorta: predictors of progression to dissection and rupture. Circulation 2003;107:1158–63.

35. Kaji S, Nishigami K, Akasaka T, et al. Prediction of progression or regression of type A aortic intramural hematoma by computed tomography. Circulation 1999;100:II281–6.

36. Quint L, Williams D, Francis I, et al. Ulcerlike lesions of the aorta: imaging features and natural history. Radiology 2001;218:719–23.

37. Hayashi H, Matsuoka Y, Sakamoto I, et al. Penetrating atherosclerotic ulcer of the aorta: imaging features and disease concept. Radiographics 2000;20:995–1005.

38. Kazerooni E, Bree R, Williams D. Penetrating atherosclerotic ulcers of the descending thoracic aorta: evaluation with CT and distinction from aortic dissection. Radiology 1992;183:759–65.

39. Stanson A, Kazmier F, Hollier L, et al. Penetrating atherosclerotic ulcers of the thoracic aorta: natural history and clinicopathologic correlations. Ann Vasc Surg 1986;1:15–23.

40. Feczko J, Lynch L, Pless J, et al. An autopsy case review of 142 nonpenetrating (blunt) injuries of the aorta. J Trauma 1992;33:846–9.

41. Burkhart H, Gomez G, Jacobson L, et al. Fatal blunt aortic injuries: a review of 242 autopsy cases. J Trauma 2001;50:113–5.

42. Steenburg S, Ravenel J, Ikonomidis J, et al. Acute traumatic aortic injury: imaging evaluation and management. Radiology 2008;248:748–62.

43. Johnston K, Rutherford R, Tilson M, et al. Suggested standards for reporting on arterial aneurysms. Subcommittee on Reporting Standards for Arterial Aneurysms, Ad Hoc Committee on Reporting Standards, Society for Vascular Surgery and North American Chapter, International Society for Cardiovascular Surgery. J Vasc Surg 1991;13:452–8.

44. Clouse W, Hallett JJ, Schaff H, et al. Improved prognosis of thoracic aortic aneurysms: a population-based study. JAMA 1998;280:1926–9.

45. Crawford E, Cohen E. Aortic aneurysm: a multifocal disease. Presidential address. Arch Surg 1982;117:1393–400.

46. Isselbacher E. Thoracic and abdominal aortic aneurysms. Circulation 2005;111:816–28.

47. Quint L, Francis I, Williams D, et al. Evaluation of thoracic aortic disease with the use of helical CT and multiplanar reconstructions: comparison with surgical findings. Radiology 1996;201:37–41.

48. Svensson L, Crawford E, Hess K, et al. Experience with 1509 patients undergoing thoracoabdominal aortic operations. J Vasc Surg 1993;17:357–68 [discussion: 368–70].

49. Bonser R, Pagano D, Lewis M, et al. Clinical and patho-anatomical factors affecting expansion of thoracic aortic aneurysms. Heart 2000;84:277–83.

50. Dapunt O, Galla J, Sadeghi A, et al. The natural history of thoracic aortic aneurysms. J Thorac Cardiovasc Surg 1994;107:1323–32 [discussion: 1332–3].

51. Davies R, Goldstein L, Coady M, et al. Yearly rupture or dissection rates for thoracic aortic aneurysms: simple prediction based on size. Ann Thorac Surg 2002;73:17–27 [discussion: 27–8].

52. Adams J, Trent R. Aortic complications of Marfan's syndrome. Lancet 1998;352:1722–3.

53. Nistri S, Sorbo M, Marin M, et al. Aortic root dilatation in young men with normally functioning bicuspid aortic valves. Heart 1999;82:19–22.

54. von Kodolitsch Y, Aydin M, Koschyk D, et al. Predictors of aneurysmal formation after surgical correction of aortic coarctation. J Am Coll Cardiol 2002;39:617–24.

55. Coady M, Davies R, Roberts M, et al. Familial patterns of thoracic aortic aneurysms. Arch Surg 1999;134:361–7.

56. Nuenninghoff D, Hunder G, Christianson T, et al. Incidence and predictors of large-artery complication (aortic aneurysm, aortic dissection, and/or large-artery stenosis) in patients with giant cell arteritis: a population-based study over 50 years. Arthritis Rheum 2003;48:3522–31.

57. Coady M, Rizzo J, Hammond G, et al. Surgical intervention criteria for thoracic aortic aneurysms: a study of growth rates and complications. Ann Thorac Surg 1999;67:1922–6 [discussion: 1953–8].

58. Davies R, Gallo A, Coady M, et al. Novel measurement of relative aortic size predicts rupture of thoracic aortic aneurysms. Ann Thorac Surg 2006;81:169–77.

59. Lobato A, Puech-Leão P. Predictive factors for rupture of thoracoabdominal aortic aneurysm. J Vasc Surg 1998;27:446–53.

60. Bonow R, Carabello B, Chatterjee K, et al. ACC/AHA 2006 guidelines for the management of patients with valvular heart disease: a report of the American College of Cardiology/American Heart Association Task Force on Practice Guidelines (writing Committee to Revise the 1998 guidelines for the management of patients with valvular heart disease) developed in collaboration with the Society of Cardiovascular Anesthesiologists endorsed by the Society for Cardiovascular Angiography and Interventions and the Society of Thoracic Surgeons. J Am Coll Cardiol 2006;48:e1–148.

61. Gott V, Pyeritz R, Magovern GJ, et al. Surgical treatment of aneurysms of the ascending aorta in the Marfan syndrome. Results of composite-graft repair in 50 patients. N Engl J Med 1986;314:1070–4.

62. Meier J, Seward J, Miller FJ, et al. Aneurysms in the left ventricular outflow tract: clinical presentation, causes, and echocardiographic features. J Am Soc Echocardiogr 1998;11:729–45.

63. Takach T, Reul G, Duncan J, et al. Sinus of Valsalva aneurysm or fistula: management and outcome. Ann Thorac Surg 1999;68:1573–7.

64. Webb GDSJ, Therrier J. Congenital heart disease: sinus of Valsalva aneurysm and fistula. In: Braunwald E, Zipes DP, Libby P, et al, editors. Braunwald's heart disease: a textbook of cardiovascular medicine. 7th edition. Philadelphia: Saunders; 2005. p. 1535–6.

65. Brickner M, Hillis L, Lange R. Congenital heart disease in adults. First of two parts. N Engl J Med 2000;342:256–63.

66. Watson A. Spinal subarachnoid haemorrhage in patient with coarctation of aorta. Br Med J 1967;4:278–9.

67. Nihoyannopoulos P, Karas S, Sapsford R, et al. Accuracy of two-dimensional echocardiography in the diagnosis of aortic arch obstruction. J Am Coll Cardiol 1987;10:1072–7.

68. Levine J, Sanders S, Colan S, et al. The risk of having additional obstructive lesions in neonatal coarctation of the aorta. Cardiol Young 2001;11:44–53.

69. Hodes H, Steinfeld L, Blumenthal S. Congenital cerebral aneurysms and coarctation of the aorta. Arch Pediatr 1959;76:28–43.

70. Pagni S, Denatale R, Boltax R. Takayasu's arteritis: the middle aortic syndrome. Am Surg 1996;62:409–12.

71. Maksimowicz-McKinnon K, Hoffman GS. Takayasu arteritis: what is the long-term prognosis? Rheum Dis Clin North Am 2007;33:777–86, vi.

72. Attenhofer Jost C, Schaff H, Connolly H, et al. Spectrum of reoperations after repair of aortic coarctation: importance of an individualized approach because of coexistent cardiovascular disease. Mayo Clin Proc 2002;77:646–53.

73. Parikh S, Hurwitz R, Hubbard J, et al. Preoperative and postoperative "aneurysm" associated with coarctation of the aorta. J Am Coll Cardiol 1991;17:1367–72.

74. Fawzy M, Awad M, Hassan W, et al. Long-term outcome (up to 15 years) of balloon angioplasty of discrete native coarctation of the aorta in adolescents and adults. J Am Coll Cardiol 2004;43:1062–7.

75. Hellenbrand W, Allen H, Golinko R, et al. Balloon angioplasty for aortic recoarctation: results of Valvuloplasty and Angioplasty of Congenital Anomalies Registry. Am J Cardiol 1990;65:793–7.

76. Therrien J, Thorne S, Wright A, et al. Repaired coarctation: a "cost-effective" approach to identify complications in adults. J Am Coll Cardiol 2000;35:997–1002.

77. Safir J, Kerr A, Morehouse H, et al. Magnetic resonance imaging of dissection in pseudocoarctation of the aorta. Cardiovasc Intervent Radiol 1993;16:180–2.

78. Sebastià C, Quiroga S, Boyé R, et al. Aortic stenosis: spectrum of diseases depicted at multisection CT. Radiographics 2003;23(Spec No):S79–91.

79. Lu T, Huber C, Rizzo E, et al. Ascending aorta measurements as assessed by ECG-gated multidetector computed tomography: a pilot study to establish normative values for transcatheter therapies. Eur Radiol 2009;19:664–9.

80. Lin F, Devereux R, Roman M, et al. Assessment of the thoracic aorta by multidetector computed tomography: age- and sex-specific reference values in adults without evident cardiovascular disease. J Cardiovasc Comput Tomogr 2008;2:298–308.

81. Tops L, Wood D, Delgado V, et al. Noninvasive evaluation of the aortic root with multislice computed tomography implications for transcatheter aortic valve replacement. JACC Cardiovasc Imaging 2008;1:321–30.

82. Ocak I, Lacomis J, Deible C, et al. The aortic root: comparison of measurements from ECG-gated CT angiography with transthoracic echocardiography. J Thorac Imaging 2009;24:223–6.

Computed Tomography Angiography of the Carotid and Cerebral Circulation

Josser E. Delgado Almandoz, MD[a,b,*],
Javier M. Romero, MD[a], Stuart R. Pomerantz, MD[a],
Michael H. Lev, MD[a]

KEYWORDS

- CT angiography • Neuroradiology
- Multidetector row CT • Acute stroke

Several important advances in computed tomography (CT) technology in the last decade have allowed CT angiography (CTA) to become the first-line imaging study for an increasing number of neurovascular applications, including the evaluation of patients with steno-occlusive carotid disease, acute ischemic and hemorrhagic stroke, subarachnoid hemorrhage (SAH), and craniocervical trauma. At many medical centers around the world, including the authors' own, CTA has replaced catheter angiography as the initial examination for most neurovascular indications.

The growing clinical applications of CTA in the past decade can be attributed to the development of helical multidetector row CT (MDCT) scanners with increasing numbers of detector rows, which enable the acquisition of CTA with greatly increased speed and quality. However, because of the increase in the number of image slices per study and the difficulty of depicting the complex neurovascular tree with multidetector CTA (MDCTA), three-dimensional (3D) postprocessing has become increasingly important for the interpretation of MDCTA examinations.

Hence, to attain prompt and accurate diagnoses for the different neurovascular conditions to be evaluated, the MDCTA acquisition parameters and standardized 3D views must be specifically tailored to clearly show the relevant pathologic conditions for the various MDCTA indications. Table 1 describes sample MDCTA protocols used at the authors' institution in common clinical scenarios in which examination of the neurovascular tree is pivotal.

INTRAVENOUS CONTRAST CONSIDERATIONS IN CTA OF THE CAROTID AND CEREBRAL CIRCULATION

The use of nonionic iodinated contrast material has been shown to be safe in the setting of cerebral ischemia in animal models[1] and clinical studies.[2] However, patients who have diabetes, preexisting renal dysfunction, or both at baseline are at an increased risk for contrast-induced nephropathy (CIN). Nevertheless, several recent studies with large numbers of patients with acute ischemic and hemorrhagic stroke evaluated with MDCTA on admission have found that the incidence of acute CIN in this patient

[a] Division of Neuroradiology, Massachusetts General Hospital, Harvard Medical School, Gray 2, Room 273A, 55 Fruit Street, Boston, MA 02114, USA
[b] Division of Neuroradiology, Mallinckrodt Institute of Radiology, Washington University School of Medicine, Campus Box 8131, 510 South Kingshighway Boulevard, Saint Louis, MO 63110, USA
* Corresponding author. Division of Neuroradiology, Mallinckrodt Institute of Radiology, Washington University School of Medicine, Campus Box 8131, 510 South Kingshighway Boulevard, Saint Louis, MO 63110.
E-mail address: delgadoj@mir.wustl.edu

Radiol Clin N Am 48 (2010) 265–281
doi:10.1016/j.rcl.2010.02.007

Table 1
Common neurovascular MDCTA examinations and indications

MDCTA Examination	Indications
CT angiogram of the neck	1. Carotid and vertebral steno-occlusive disease 2. Acute craniocervical trauma 3. Spontaneous dissection
CT angiogram of the head	1. Subarachnoid hemorrhage 2. Acute hemorrhagic stroke 3. Cerebral vasospasm 4. Follow-up of unruptured and clipped aneurysms 5. Follow-up of arteriovenous malformations and fistulae not embolized with onyx
CT angiogram of the head and neck	1. Acute ischemic stroke 2. Acute craniocervical trauma
CT perfusion	1. Acute ischemic stroke 2. Cerebral vasospasm

population is low (ranging from 2% to 7%), and that this risk is not higher in patients whose baseline creatinine value is unknown at the time of scanning.[3–7]

In addition, the risk of CIN can be reduced by adopting several strategies. First, adequate pre- and postprocedure hydration is considered by most experts to be the most important factor in preventing CIN. Second, because nephrotoxicity from contrast material is dose-dependent,[8] MDCTA protocols are designed to use the smallest amount of contrast possible. The availability of denser contrast agents and innovative strategies enabled by the latest generation of MDCT scanners and power injectors have increasingly resulted in reduced contrast loads. At our institution, a routine MDCTA/CT perfusion (CTP) evaluation for acute ischemic stroke is performed by administering a total volume of 110 mL of nonionic low-osmolar iodinated contrast material with a concentration of 370 mgI/mL. This combined MDCTA/CTP contrast dose is similar to or slightly lower than the typical contrast load of a 3-vessel catheter angiogram and does not hinder pursuing intra-arterial thrombolysis or mechanical thrombectomy in eligible patients.

Thomsen and Morcos[9] recently conducted a pooled analysis of 2 randomized trials that evaluated the incidence of CIN in patients with moderate or severe renal impairment who received either low-osmolar or iso-osmolar contrast material for MDCT. In their analysis, they found that the overall incidence of CIN in this patient population was low (2.3%), and was directly related to the patient's baseline glomerular filtration rate (GFR): 0.6% in patients with GFR greater than 40 mL/min, 4.6% in patients with GFR less than 40 mL/min, and 7.8% in patients with GFR less than 30 mL/min. Furthermore, whereas 4.7% of patients who received iso-osmolar contrast material developed CIN, no patients who received low-osmolar contrast material developed CIN, although the differences in osmolality between these contrast agents did not seem to play a role in the pathogenesis of CIN.

Hence, in patients with neurologic emergencies requiring rapid evaluation of the neurovascular tree, emergent MDCTA evaluation with adequate pre- and postexamination hydration and administration of the lowest possible dose of a low-osmolar iodinated contrast agent is safe with respect to the nephrotoxicity related to the iodinated contrast material, even in the setting of preexisting renal dysfunction.

For patients who have experienced mild allergic reactions to iodinated contrast material, premedication with antihistamines and steroids can blunt the anaphylactoid response. However, in the setting of an acute stroke there is not enough time to complete a course of steroid administration. In this difficult situation, a gadolinium contrast agent may be used as an alternative to iodinated contrast for MDCTA evaluation.[10] Nevertheless, although these scans are usually diagnostic, peak vessel opacification is less than with iodinated contrast agents. Furthermore, in light of the recently described risk of nephrogenic systemic fibrosis in patients with renal dysfunction who receive gadolinium contrast material,[11] documentation of a GFR 30 mL/min or greater and minimization of the gadolinium contrast dose are imperative before administering this alternative contrast agent for MDCTA evaluation.

CTA IN THE EVALUATION OF CAROTID ARTERY STENO-OCCLUSIVE DISEASE

Several recent studies have shown that measurements of residual carotid luminal diameter obtained with MDCTA are comparable with those obtained with digital subtraction angiography (DSA).[12–19] However, careful attention must be paid to applying appropriate window settings because differences in luminal contrast density in serial examinations can produce significant differences in the measured residual lumen, and beam-hardening artifact from heavy plaque calcifications can result in overestimation of the degree of stenosis. To avoid this potential pitfall, Saba and Mallarini[20] have recently proposed a practical formula to calculate the optimal window settings for the evaluation of carotid stenosis with MDCTA: window width, intraluminal Hounsfield unit (HU) $\times$ 2.07; window level, intraluminal HU $\times$ 0.72. Software applications for semi-automated detection of cross-sectional area and luminal diameters orthogonal to a computer-generated centerline have been developed, which may reduce interobserver variability in the measurement of residual luminal diameter (RLD).[12,16,19] However, these techniques perform best when coupled with direct inspection of the axial CT angiogram source images (CTA-SIs) by the reader and should not be relied on as the primary means of diagnosis.

The degree of carotid stenosis can be reported in terms of percent stenosis, residual luminal area, or RLD. Percent stenosis, defined as the ratio of maximal luminal narrowing to the normal internal carotid artery distal to the bulb, was the measurement used in the North American Symptomatic Carotid Endarterectomy Trial (NASCET) and is the most commonly used measure in North America. However, the reference diameter of the distal internal carotid artery can range from 5 to 8 mm, which can alter the calculated percent stenosis for a given RLD. To avert this potential pitfall, several research groups have advocated using RLD instead of percent stenosis in the assessment of the severity of carotid steno-occlusive disease,[15,21–24] and Waaijer and colleagues[18] have recently advocated using simple visual estimation of the degree of stenosis rather than caliper measurements. At the authors' institution, in addition to the now standard percent stenosis measurements based on NASCET, we also report the degree of carotid stenosis based on the RLD, using 1.5 mm as the cutoff for hemodynamically

significant stenosis, which correlates approximately to an ultrasound peak systolic velocity of more than 250 cm/s and a NASCET measurement of more than 70% stenosis.[25]

Before performing MDCTA of the neck for evaluation of carotid steno-occlusive disease, any available ultrasound or magnetic resonance (MR) angiography studies should be reviewed to determine what clinical questions are to be answered. If the clinical question is whether there is a complete internal carotid artery occlusion versus a hairline residual lumen, an immediate delayed acquisition through the neck is helpful in the detection of the slow opacification of a hairline residual lumen and aids in distinguishing it from a complete internal carotid artery occlusion. An important potential pitfall to be cognizant of when making this crucial determination is that, on occasion, the ascending pharyngeal artery may mimic an internal carotid artery hairline residual lumen. However, the ascending pharyngeal artery should not reach the skull base, and a hairline internal carotid artery residual lumen should. Accurately making this differentiation is critically important because those patients with a hairline residual lumen are at risk for embolic stroke and are candidates for carotid endarterectomy or stenting, whereas those patients with complete internal carotid occlusions are usually treated medically. Several studies have shown that MDCTA is an excellent tool in making this critical distinction.[26–28] **Fig. 1** illustrates the usefulness of MDCTA in the evaluation of carotid artery steno-occlusive disease.

Plaque characteristics such as ulceration, amount of calcification, thin fibrous cap, lipid core, and hemorrhage are potential predictors of stroke risk. Although early studies evaluating the usefulness of CTA for carotid plaque characterization yielded inconsistent results,[29–31] more recent studies with MDCTA and dual-source CT have shown excellent sensitivity and specificity of this technique for the detection of plaque ulcerations, thin fibrous caps, and large lipid cores.[32–35] Furthermore, a recent study from our institution showed that arterial wall enhancement overlying carotid plaque in patients with high-grade carotid stenosis (likely a proxy for inflammatory changes within the plaque) correlated well with patient symptomatology such as transient ischemic attacks and strokes (**Fig. 2**).[36]

Hence, MDCTA is an accurate examination for the determination of carotid stenosis and shows promise as a valuable diagnostic test for plaque characterization and the identification of vulnerable plaque.

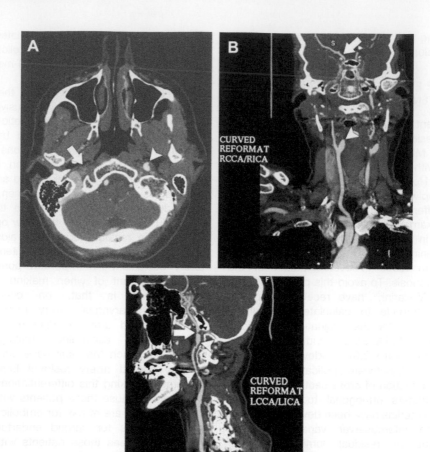

Fig. 1. A 52-year-old woman presented with intermittent tinnitus and mild neck pain after being hit by a wave while swimming. (*A*) Axial CTA-SI shows occlusion of the right internal carotid artery (*arrow*) and dissection with pseudoaneurysm formation of the left internal carotid artery (*arrowhead*). (*B*) Curved reformat of the right common and internal carotid arteries shows occlusion of the proximal right internal carotid artery (*arrowhead*) with reconstitution of flow within the supraclinoid segment of this vessel (*arrow*). (*C*) Curved reformat of the left common and internal carotid arteries shows a dissection with pseudoaneurysm formation of the left cervical internal carotid artery (*arrowheads*) with a superimposed focal severe stenosis of this vessel at the skull base (*arrow*).

CTA IN THE EVALUATION OF ACUTE ISCHEMIC STROKE

According to the National Stroke Association 2009 Fact Sheet, nearly 800,000 people in the United States were expected to suffer a stroke in 2009, with an estimated cost of nearly $69 billion. Stroke will continue to be the third leading cause of death in the United States, with more than 140,000 Americans expected to die from a stroke in 2009. There are 2 types of stroke: ischemic and hemorrhagic. Ischemic stroke is more common, accounting for approximately 85% of cases. Although the severity of brain damage from ischemic stroke increases as time passes, death

or severe disability can be prevented or diminished if thrombolytic treatment is administered within a short time after the onset of symptoms.

Because of its accuracy in the identification of intravascular thrombus, vascular stenosis, and parenchymal ischemia, as well as the widespread availability of MDCT scanners in emergency departments, MDCTA and CTP have become integral components of the early management of patients presenting with acute ischemic stroke at many institutions in North America and around the world. At our institution, the acute ischemic stroke protocol consists of (1) unenhanced head CT, (2) MDCTA of the head and neck, and (3) CTP of the head at 1 to 2 nonoverlapping levels with 4 to 8 cm of brain

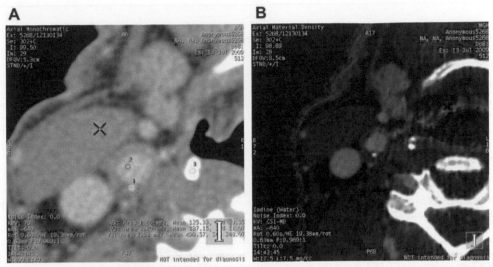

Fig. 2. A 45-year-old woman presented with intermittent episodes of transient left-sided weakness. (*A*) Axial CTA-SI acquired with a spectral source CT shows luminal irregularity within the proximal right internal carotid artery, consistent with mild atherosclerotic changes. In addition, there is associated circumferential carotid wall enhancement (region of interest 1). (*B*) CTA iodine image better shows the circumferential carotid wall enhancement in the region of the atherosclerotic plaque.

coverage with a 64-slice detector. The total estimated effective radiation dose to the head of this imaging protocol is 8.3 to 11.6 mSv (unenhanced CT of the head, 2.5 mSv; CTA of the head, 2.5 mSv; 1–2 slab CTP of the head, 3.3–6.7 mSv), and to the neck is 7.1 mSv (neck CTA).[37] Thus, the total effective radiation dose for our comprehensive acute ischemic stroke protocol is 15.4 to 18.7 mSv, which is similar to that reported by Mnyusiwalla and colleagues[38] (16.4 mSv), and is approximately 5 to 6 times the estimated annual background effective radiation dose for a person in the United States (3 mSv). Hence, it is of utmost importance that the comprehensive protocol (and especially the CTP of the head) only be performed in patients who may be eligible for intra-arterial thrombolysis or mechanical thrombectomy. Furthermore, although CTP is generally indicated for acute ischemic stroke management, serial CTP examinations are typically unnecessary and discouraged because of cumulative radiation dose considerations. Although serial CTP examinations may be of greater value in the evaluation of symptomatic vasospasm following aneurysmal SAH, similar radiation dose considerations exist.

Given the large number of images that are generated by this imaging protocol, adhering to a systematic algorithm for review of the MDCTA/CTP examination is imperative to ensure that the 4 cardinal questions of acute stroke imaging are answered in a timely and accurate manner (Table 2). To ensure that this protocol is performed seamlessly, at our institution a neuroradiologist

reviews all acute stroke MDCTA/CTP examinations directly at the CT scanner console in conjunction with the Acute Stroke Team.

The first question (Is there intracranial hemorrhage?) is easily answered through a rapid review of the unenhanced CT examination. The second question (Is there intravascular thrombus that can be targeted for thrombolysis?) is answered in 2 steps. First, patency of the cervical and proximal intracranial vasculature is determined through direct review of the CTA-SIs as soon as they are reconstructed by the CT scanner. Second, patency of the more distal intracranial vasculature is determined through careful review of 3 sets of orthogonal thick-slab maximum intensity projection (MIP) angiographic images generated by the CT technologist at the scanner console in less than 1 minute. The third question (Is there a core of irreversibly infarcted tissue?) is answered in 3 steps. First, the unenhanced CT examination is reviewed to determine the location and extent of parenchymal hypodensity and regions with loss of gray-white matter differentiation. Second, the CTA-SIs are reviewed in narrow perfusion windows to determine the extent of the parenchymal hypodensity within the affected vascular territory, which has been shown to correlate well with final infarct size.[39–42] Third, after the CTP examination has been processed by the neuroradiologist at a 3D workstation, the CTP cerebral blood volume (CBV) maps are reviewed to determine the extent of brain parenchyma with decreased CBV, which also correlates well with

Table 2
The 4 cardinal questions of acute stroke imaging

Acute Stroke Imaging Question	MDCT Examination(s) Used to Provide Answer
Is there intracranial hemorrhage?	Unenhanced CT
Is there intravascular thrombus that can be targeted for thrombolysis?	1. CTA-SI for the proximal intracranial and cervical vasculature 2. Thick-slab angiographic MIP images for the distal intracranial vasculature
Is there a core of irreversibly infarcted tissue?	1. Unenhanced CT 2. CTA-SI in narrow perfusion windows 3. CTP CBV map
Is there a penumbra of severely ischemic but potentially salvageable tissue?	CTP CBF and MTT maps compared directly with unenhanced CT, CTA-SI in narrow perfusion windows and CTP CBV map

Abbreviations: CBF, cerebral blood flow; CBV, cerebral blood volume; CTA-SI, CT angiogram source image; CTP, CT perfusion; MDCT, multidetector CT; MIP, maximum intensity projection; MTT, mean transit time.

final infarct size.[43–47] Finally, the fourth question (Is there a penumbra of severely ischemic but potentially salvageable tissue?) is answered by directly comparing the CTP cerebral blood flow and mean transit time (MTT) maps with the unenhanced CT, CTA-SI, and CBV maps. This direct comparison is done to determine if (1) there is abnormally perfused tissue surrounding a core of infarcted tissue, the ischemic penumbra, which although viable is believed to be at risk for imminent infarction and may benefit from immediate reperfusion; or (2) all or most of the abnormally perfused tissue has already progressed to infarction, in which case initiating thrombolytic treatment could worsen the outcome by precipitating intracranial hemorrhage. Typically, these 4 questions can be answered within 20 to 25 minutes from the time that the patient is brought to the CT scanner suite, thus allowing for the rapid identification of those patients who are most likely to benefit from intravenous and/or intra-arterial thrombolysis, or mechanical thrombectomy.

In addition, the CTA-SIs can be helpful in the risk stratification and prognosis of patients with acute stroke. Several studies have found a significant correlation between (1) the extent of parenchymal hypoattenuation,[41,48–51] (2) intravascular thrombus burden,[52–54] and (3) degree of collateral circulation to the affected vascular territory[54,55] in the initial CTA-SIs and patient outcome. Because MDCTA of the neck is included in the routine acute stroke evaluation, when the source of the embolic infarct is atherosclerotic disease at the carotid bifurcation, it can depict the causative lesion rapidly and accurately. Furthermore, recent research suggests that adding a cardiac CTA to the routine acute stroke evaluation may be useful in the

identification of cardiac lesions responsible for the embolic stroke such as left atrial thrombus or a patent foramen ovale.[56] Fig. 3 illustrates the usefulness of MDCTA in the evaluation of acute ischemic stroke.

MDCTA and CTP have become integral components of the emergent diagnostic work-up of patients with acute ischemic stroke, yielding accurate and timely answers to the 4 cardinal questions of acute stroke imaging and enabling the rapid triage of patients to thrombolytic therapy.

CTA IN THE EVALUATION OF ACUTE HEMORRHAGIC STROKE

Hemorrhagic stroke accounts for approximately 15% of cases of acute stroke in the United States and has a worse prognosis than ischemic stroke, with up to 50% mortality and high rates of severe neurologic disability among survivors.[57] There are 2 types of hemorrhagic stroke: (1) those that are caused by an underlying vascular lesion such as an arteriovenous malformation (AVM), aneurysm, or dural venous sinus thrombosis (DVST), which are potentially treatable (secondary intracerebral hemorrhage [ICH]); and (2) those that are not caused by an underlying vascular lesion (primary ICH). The total volume of extravasated intracranial blood is the most potent predictor of mortality and poor outcome in patients with primary ICH, and those who develop hematoma expansion after admission have a worse prognosis than those who do not.[58] Although current treatment options for primary ICH are limited, emerging hemostatic therapies aiming to limit the extent of hematoma expansion such as recombinant activated factor VII or intensive blood pressure reduction may be

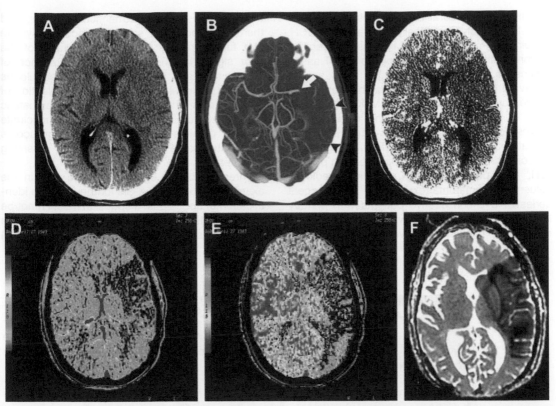

Fig. 3. A 64-year-old woman presented after the acute onset of right hemiparesis and expressive aphasia 4 hours before presentation. (*A*) Unenhanced CT examination shows hypodensity and loss of gray-white matter differentiation within the left basal ganglia and frontal operculum, consistent with ischemia in the left middle cerebral artery territory. (*B*) Axial CTA MIP image shows a proximal left M1 cutoff (*arrow*) with poor collaterals within the left middle cerebral artery territory (*arrowheads*). (*C*) Axial CTA-SI in narrow perfusion windows shows hypoattenuation within the left middle cerebral artery territory consistent with ischemia, larger in extent than the unenhanced CT hypodensity. (*D* and *E*) CTP CBV and MTT maps show decreased CBV and increased MTT within the left middle cerebral artery territory. The MTT defect is slightly larger than the CBV defect and approximately the same size as the CTA-SI hypoattenuation, consistent with a small penumbra. Based on these findings, no intervention was undertaken. (*F*) Follow-up apparent diffusion coefficient (ADC) map 24 hours after presentation shows the final infarct volume, which closely approximates the MTT and CTA-SI defects and was slightly larger than the initial CBV defect.

able to reduce the morbidity and mortality of this disease.[59,60] However, accurate patient selection to target hemostatic therapy only to those patients who are actively bleeding at the time of presentation (and hence are most likely to benefit from hemostatic therapy) is imperative.

MDCTA is becoming an increasingly important diagnostic tool in the evaluation of patients with hemorrhagic stroke. Several recent studies have shown that MDCTA can accurately and promptly diagnose those patients with hemorrhagic stroke who have secondary ICH,[61–64] allowing for the prompt institution of endovascular or surgical treatment to prevent rebleeding from the causative vascular lesion. These studies have shown that, depending on the population examined, the incidence of underlying vascular causes for ICH can

range from 15% in adults[64] to 65% in patients younger than 40 years.[62] A recent series of 623 consecutive patients presenting with hemorrhagic stroke at our institution identified independent predictors of a higher yield of MDCTA for the identification of causative vascular lesions in ICH: age younger than 46 years, lobar or infratentorial ICH location, female sex, and absence of known hypertension or impaired coagulation at presentation (Fig. 4).[64] There is an important potential pitfall to be aware of when making the diagnosis of DVST as the ICH cause. Since the introduction of 64-slice CT scanners, the time delay from contrast injection to scanning has decreased and, as a result, the normal dural venous sinuses may or may not be opacified at the time of scanning. Hence, if in the first-pass CTA there is inadequate opacification of a dural venous sinus in a distribution that could potentially explain the ICH, acquiring immediate delayed images is imperative to confidently make the diagnosis of DVST as the ICH cause.

Several studies have shown that the presence of active contrast extravasation at MDCTA, the spot sign, is an indicator of ongoing bleeding and serves as an accurate and powerful predictor of hematoma expansion, mortality, and poor outcome among survivors in patients with primary ICH, with particularly high negative predictive values for hematoma expansion.[65–72] A recent series of 573 consecutive patients with primary ICH from our institution showed that all spot signs do not have the same positive predictive value for

the outcome measures mentioned earlier, and thereby proposed a spot sign scoring system that further refines the predictive value of the spot sign (Fig. 5).[71,72] Thus, the presence of a spot sign and the spot sign score could be used as powerful triage tools in the selection of patients with primary ICH for early hemostatic therapy. Future research may also elucidate whether patients with different spot sign scores derive the same benefit from these emerging treatments.

Three important criteria must be met in the examination of the CTA-SIs for the accurate identification of spot signs: a spot sign must (1) not be present in the unenhanced CT, (2) be separate from the vasculature adjacent to the ICH, and (3)

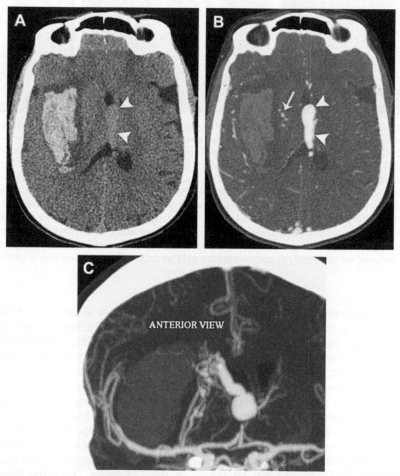

Fig. 4. A 59-year-old woman without known hypertension or impaired coagulation presented with sudden onset of left-sided weakness and increasing unresponsiveness. (A) Unenhanced CT shows a large right basal ganglia hemorrhage with an enlarged vessel in the region of the third ventricle (arrowheads). (B) Axial CTA-SI shows abnormal vascularity in the right basal ganglia (arrow) with an enlarged right internal cerebral draining vein (arrowheads), consistent with an AVM. (C) Coronal CTA MIP image shows the AVM nidus in the right basal ganglia and the enlarged right internal cerebral draining vein.

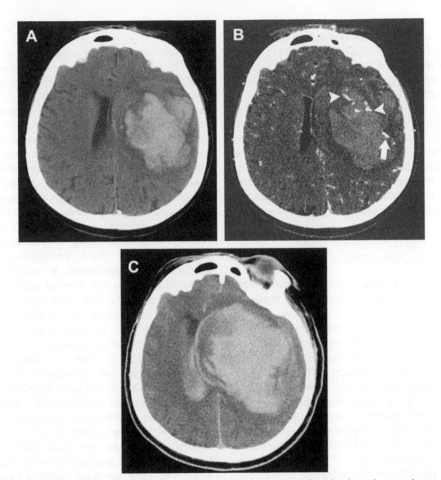

Fig. 5. An 81-year-old woman with a history of hypertension presented with altered mental status 2.5 hours before presentation. (*A*) Unenhanced CT shows a left basal ganglia hemorrhage (93 mL) with minimal intraventricular extension. (*B*) Axial CTA-SI shows at least 6 foci of contrast pooling within the ICH, separate from the vasculature adjacent to the ICH and with an attenuation 120 HU or greater, consistent with spot signs (*arrowheads*). The largest spot sign measures 7 mm in axial dimension and has an attenuation of 362 HU (*arrow*, spot sign score: 4). (*C*) Follow-up unenhanced CT examination 2 hours after the CTA shows marked interval enlargement of the intracerebral (229 mL) and intraventricular hemorrhage (39 mL). The patient died shortly after the follow-up unenhanced CT examination.

have an attenuation of at least 120 HU. The first 2 criteria allow the reader to make the important differentiation between spot signs and spot sign mimics such as choroidal calcifications, aneurysms, and AVMs,[73] whereas the third criterion minimizes the likelihood that hematoma heterogeneity and inherent CTA-SI noise may be misdiagnosed as a spot sign.

Several studies have found that a significant minority of spot signs are found on the delayed MDCTA acquisitions only (typically performed 2–3 minutes after the first-pass CTA), ranging from 8% to 23% of all spot signs identified in different series.[68,69,71,72] These delayed spot signs carry the same predictive value as the spot signs

identified in the first-pass CTAs and increase the sensitivity of this finding for hematoma expansion. In addition, delayed MDCTA acquisitions are of utmost usefulness in cases in which the distinction between a spot sign and an aneurysm or small AVM is challenging. Given that, by definition, spot signs are extravascular collections of contrast and aneurysms or AVMs are intravascular, it follows that on a delayed MDCTA acquisition a spot sign should change in configuration and attenuation relative to the vasculature adjacent to the hematoma as it mixes with the unopacified blood within the hematoma (often layering in the dependent portions of the hematoma). However, being intravascular, an aneurysm or small AVM should maintain its morphology and have the same attenuation as the vasculature adjacent to the hematoma on the delayed MDCTA acquisition. Distinguishing spot signs from aneurysms or small AVMs is of great clinical importance because the treatment implications are vastly different.

MDCTA is rapidly becoming a central examination in the initial evaluation of patients with acute hemorrhagic stroke, allowing for the prompt and accurate diagnosis of a potentially treatable underlying vascular cause in an important minority of patients, and serving as a key triage tool in the selection of patients for emerging early hemostatic therapies or early surgery.

CTA IN THE EVALUATION OF SAH AND CEREBRAL VASOSPASM

Several recent studies have shown that, compared with DSA and intraoperative findings, MDCTA has excellent overall sensitivity for the detection of intracranial aneurysms, ranging from 93% to 99%.[74–84] Although a few of these studies have reported a lower sensitivity of MDCTA for the detection of aneurysms measuring less than 3 mm (70%–76%),[75,77] most have reported excellent sensitivity for the detection of aneurysms measuring less than 3 to 4 mm (85%–100%), particularly when systematic review of the axial CTA-SIs is coupled with standard 3D reformations.[76,79,80,82–84] However, the use of MDCTA for the detection of intracranial aneurysms in patients with SAH continues to be a controversial topic in the literature, with some investigators arguing that the lower sensitivity of MDCTA for the detection of intracranial aneurysms compared with DSA is unacceptable and poses a danger to patients if DSA is not subsequently performed in all patients with CTA-negative SAH.[85] At our institution, MDCTA is used as the primary diagnostic examination in the evaluation of patients with SAH, showing efficacy in the detection and characterization of ruptured and unruptured intracranial aneurysms, and allowing for the decision whether to undertake endovascular or surgical treatment to be made promptly.[86] Nevertheless, we routinely perform DSA in patients with CTA-negative SAH if the hemorrhage is not clearly posttraumatic or does not conform to the classic pattern of a benign perimesencephalic hemorrhage. Although the presence of extensive streak artifact renders MDCTA evaluation of coiled aneurysms nondiagnostic, there is growing evidence that MDCTA is useful in the follow-up of aneurysms that have undergone surgical clipping, with reported sensitivities for the detection of residual/recurrent aneurysms ranging from 83% to 100%.[87–89]

Several studies have shown that in the evaluation of cerebral vasospasm secondary to SAH, MDCTA provides an accurate depiction of the anatomic location and severity of luminal narrowing of the intracranial vasculature using DSA as the reference standard,[90–93] whereas CTP provides important additional information regarding the resulting changes in cerebrovascular flow within the affected vascular bed and predicts the development of delayed cerebral ischemia.[90,92,94–103] Although diagnosing severe vasospasm is straightforward, detecting mild or moderate vasospasm can be difficult at times. Hence, when evaluating a vascular structure for vasospasm, direct comparison with the admission CT angiogram is crucial to detect slight changes in the luminal caliber or subtle luminal irregularity that may represent mild or moderate vasospasm. In addition, taking into account the CTP findings when assessing the CT angiogram for vasospasm is also useful, as brain perfusion changes correlate well with moderate or severe vasospasm and denote an increased risk of delayed cerebral ischemia. Thus, a combined MDCTA/CTP examination is useful in the noninvasive evaluation of patients with SAH for the detection of cerebral vasospasm, allowing for the rapid triage of patients to either medical therapy or endovascular treatment. However, because cerebral vasospasm is a dynamic disease process, if there is a long time interval between the MDCTA/CTP and DSA examinations, there is a possibility of discordant findings, which may be a result of the dynamic nature of this disease process rather than the accuracy of MDCTA/CTP. Fig. 6 illustrates the usefulness of MDCTA and CTP in the evaluation of patients with SAH and cerebral vasospasm.

MDCTA is becoming the preferred diagnostic examination for the initial evaluation of patients with SAH at an increasing number of medical centers around the world, allowing for the rapid and accurate detection and characterization of cerebral aneurysms and, in combination with CTP, is also playing an increasingly important role in the detection and treatment triage of vasospasm. Nevertheless, this continues to be a controversial topic in the literature.

FUTURE DEVELOPMENTS IN CTA OF THE CAROTID AND CEREBRAL CIRCULATION

In the early 1990s CT technology was revolutionized by the introduction of helical CT, in which

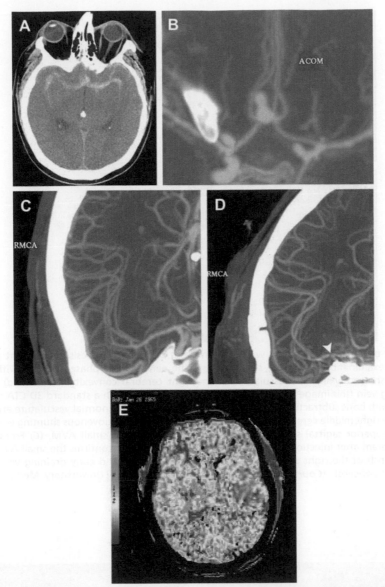

Fig. 6. A 44-year-old man presented after the "worst headache of his life". (*A*) Unenhanced CT shows diffuse SAH in the basal cisterns. (*B*) Curved reformat of the anterior communicating artery shows a wide-neck aneurysm. (*C*) Coronal MIP image of the right middle cerebral artery shows a normal caliber of the right M1 segment. (*D*) Coronal MIP image of a follow-up CTA examination 7 days after the hemorrhage shows diffusely decreased caliber of the right M1 segment with a focal short segment of severe stenosis (*arrowhead*), consistent with vasospasm. (*E*) CTP MTT map shows increased MTT in the right middle cerebral artery territory secondary to the vasospasm. The patient was successfully treated with intra-arterial nicardipine and did not develop an infarct.

data were continuously acquired as an x-ray source and detector combination spun continuously around the patient.[104] The subsequent introduction of scanners with progressively more detector rows in this decade has enabled significantly larger coverage in a shorter amount of time and 3D isotropic voxel resolution.[105] The latest 64-slice CT scanner units can scan the entire craniocervical neurovascular tree in 12 to 15 seconds.

With the recent introduction of the 320-detector row CT units, featuring a detector width of 16 cm, whole-brain imaging can be accomplished during peak arterial phase of contrast administration with a single gantry rotation in 1 second and the entire neurovascular tree (arch to vertex) can be imaged

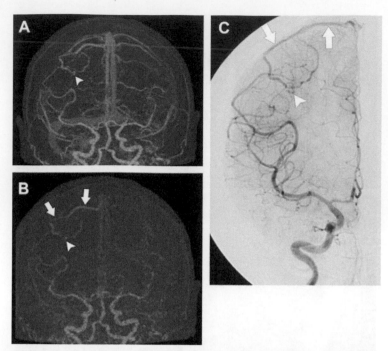

Fig. 7. A 64-year-old woman presented with sudden onset of left hemiparesis and a right parietal ICH. (*A*) Coronal 4D CTA examination with bone subtraction in the early venous phase acquired with a 320-detector row CT scanner shows asymmetric vasculature in the right cerebral convexity (*arrowhead*) but no definite enlarged draining vein (this image is comparable with that obtained with a standard 3D CTA examination). (*B*) Coronal 4D CTA with bone subtraction in the early arterial phase shows abnormal vasculature arising from a parietal branch of the right middle cerebral artery (*arrowhead*) as well as arteriovenous shunting with an early draining vein to the superior sagittal sinus (*arrowheads*), consistent with a small AVM. (*C*) Frontal projection of a catheter angiogram after injection of the right internal carotid artery confirms the small AVM nidus supplied by a parietal branch of the right middle cerebral artery (*arrowhead*) and early draining vein to the superior sagittal sinus (*arrowheads*). (*Courtesy of* Dr Eberhard Siebert, Charité Universitary Medicine Berlin, Berlin, Germany.)

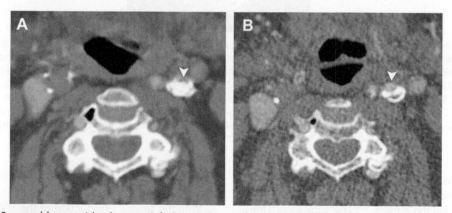

Fig. 8. A 76-year-old man with a known right internal carotid artery occlusion presented for evaluation of the left internal carotid artery. (*A*) Axial CTA source image at 120 kVp shows the known right internal carotid artery occlusion as well as heavily calcified plaque at the origin of the left internal carotid artery, which makes evaluation of the RLD difficult because of calcium blooming (*arrowhead*). (*B*) Axial CTA source image at 140 kVp decreases the amount of calcium blooming and allows for more accurate determination of the RLD of the left internal carotid artery (mild stenosis, *arrowhead*).

in 4 to 5 seconds. Hence, with the current development of time-resolved four-dimensional (4D) MDCTA and whole-brain CTP, this technique is addressing some of the current disadvantages of MDCTA compared with DSA (temporal resolution, **Fig. 7**) and MR perfusion (whole-brain coverage).[106–108] Moreover, the recent development of dual and spectral energy source CT scanner technology has allowed for significant improvements to be made on another disadvantage of MDCTA compared with DSA: automated bone and heavily calcified plaque removal.[109–114] This innovation enables the creation of MDCTA images that effortlessly depict neurovascular pathology in the internal carotid arteries at the skull base, the vertebral arteries in the neck, and within carotid arteries affected by heavily calcified plaque (**Fig. 8**).

Thus, future MDCT technology will perhaps develop scanners in which a dual or spectral energy source is coupled with a detector row wide enough to provide whole-brain coverage in 1 gantry rotation, which will allow for time-resolved cerebral 4D MDCTA with automated bone removal, whole-brain CTP, as well as accurate depiction and characterization of steno-occlusive carotid disease, even in patients with heavily calcified carotid plaque.

ACKNOWLEDGMENTS

The authors would like to thank M. Shervin Kamalian, MD (Massachusetts General Hospital, Boston, MA, USA), Seyedmehdi Payabvash, MD (Massachusetts General Hospital, Boston, MA, USA), Michael J. Stone, MD (Massachusetts General Hospital, Boston, MA, USA) and Eberhard Siebert, MD (Charité Universitary Medicine Berlin, Berlin, Germany) for their assistance in the image collection, and Eleni K. Balasalle, BA (Massachusetts General Hospital Radiology Educational Media Services, Boston, MA) for her assistance in the artwork for this manuscript.

REFERENCES

1. Doerfler A, Engelhorn T, von Kummer R, et al. Are iodinated contrast agents detrimental in acute cerebral ischemia? An experimental study in rats. Radiology 1998;206:211–7.

2. Palomäki H, Muuronen A, Raininko R, et al. Administration of nonionic iodinated contrast medium does not influence the outcome of patients with ischemic brain infarction. Cerebrovasc Dis 2003; 15:45–50.

3. Krol AL, Dzialowski I, Roy J, et al. Incidence of radiocontrast nephropathy in patients undergoing acute stroke computed tomography angiography. Stroke 2007;38:2364–6 [Erratum in: Stroke 2007; 38: e97].

4. Dittrich R, Akdeniz S, Kloska SP, et al. Low rate of contrast-induced nephropathy after CT perfusion and CT angiography in acute stroke patients. J Neurol 2007;254:1491–7.

5. Langner S, Stumpe S, Kirsch M, et al. No increased risk for contrast-induced nephropathy after multiple CT perfusion studies of the brain with a nonionic, dimeric, iso-osmolal contrast medium. AJNR Am J Neuroradiol 2008;29:1525–9.

6. Hopyan JJ, Gladstone DJ, Mallia G, et al. Renal safety of CT angiography and perfusion imaging in the emergency evaluation of acute stroke. AJNR Am J Neuroradiol 2008;29:1826–30.

7. Oleinik A, Romero JM, Schwab K, et al. CT angiography for intracerebral hemorrhage does not increase risk of acute nephropathy. Stroke 2009; 40:2393–7.

8. Thomsen HS, Morcos SK, Barrett BJ. Contrast-induced nephropathy: the wheel has turned 360 degrees. Acta Radiol 2008;49:646–57.

9. Thomsen HS, Morcos SK. Risk of contrast-medium-induced nephropathy in high-risk patients undergoing MDCT–a pooled analysis of two randomized trials. Eur Radiol 2009;19:891–7.

10. Henson JW, Nogueira RG, Covarrubias DJ, et al. Gadolinium-enhanced CT angiography of the circle of Willis and neck. AJNR Am J Neuroradiol 2004; 25:969–72.

11. Morcos SK, Thomsen HS. Nephrogenic systemic fibrosis: more questions and some answers. Nephron Clin Pract 2008;110:c24–31.

12. Zhang Z, Berg MH, Ikonen AE, et al. Carotid artery stenosis: reproducibility of automated 3D CT angiography analysis method. Eur Radiol 2004;14: 665–72.

13. Josephson SA, Bryant SO, Mak HK, et al. Evaluation of carotid stenosis using CT angiography in the initial evaluation of stroke and TIA. Neurology 2004;63:457–60.

14. Berg M, Zhang Z, Ikonen A, et al. Multi-detector row CT angiography in the assessment of carotid artery disease in symptomatic patients: comparison with rotational angiography and digital subtraction angiography. AJNR Am J Neuroradiol 2005;26:1022–34.

15. Zhang Z, Berg M, Ikonen A, et al. Carotid stenosis degree in CT angiography: assessment based on luminal area versus luminal diameter measurements. Eur Radiol 2005;15:2359–65.

16. Silvennoinen HM, Ikonen S, Soinne L, et al. CT angiographic analysis of carotid artery stenosis: comparison of manual assessment, semiautomatic vessel analysis, and digital subtraction angiography. AJNR Am J Neuroradiol 2007;28: 97–103.

17. Bucek RA, Puchner S, Haumer M, et al. CTA quantification of internal carotid artery stenosis: application of luminal area vs. luminal diameter measurements and assessment of inter-observer variability. J Neuroimaging 2007;17:219–26.

18. Waaijer A, Weber M, van Leeuwen MS, et al. Grading of carotid artery stenosis with multidetector-row CT angiography: visual estimation or caliper measurements? Eur Radiol 2009;19:2809–18.

19. Puchner S, Popovic M, Wolf F, et al. Multidetector CTA in the quantification of internal carotid artery stenosis: value of different reformation techniques and axial source images compared with selective carotid arteriography. J Endovasc Ther 2009;16:336–42.

20. Saba L, Mallarini G. Window settings for the study of calcified carotid plaques with multidetector CT angiography. AJNR Am J Neuroradiol 2009;30:1445–50.

21. Bartlett ES, Walters TD, Symons SP, et al. Quantification of carotid stenosis on CT angiography. AJNR Am J Neuroradiol 2006;27:13–9.

22. Bartlett ES, Symons SP, Fox AJ. Correlation of carotid stenosis diameter and cross-sectional areas with CT angiography. AJNR Am J Neuroradiol 2006;27:638–42.

23. Bartlett ES, Walters TD, Symons SP, et al. Carotid stenosis index revisited with direct CT angiography measurement of carotid arteries to quantify carotid stenosis. Stroke 2007;38:286–91.

24. Bartlett ES, Walters TD, Symons SP, et al. Classification of carotid stenosis by millimeter CT angiography measures: effects of prevalence and gender. AJNR Am J Neuroradiol 2008;29:1677–83.

25. Suwanwela N, Can U, Furie KL, et al. Carotid Doppler ultrasound criteria for internal carotid artery stenosis based on residual lumen diameter calculated from en bloc carotid endarterectomy specimens. Stroke 1996;27:1965–9.

26. Lev MH, Romero JM, Goodman DN, et al. Total occlusion versus hairline residual lumen of the internal carotid arteries: accuracy of single section helical CT angiography. AJNR Am J Neuroradiol 2003;24:1123–9.

27. Chen CJ, Lee TH, Hsu HL, et al. Multi-slice CT angiography in diagnosing total versus near occlusions of the internal carotid artery: comparison with catheter angiography. Stroke 2004;35:83–5.

28. Bartlett ES, Walters TD, Symons SP, et al. Diagnosing carotid stenosis near-occlusion by using CT angiography. AJNR Am J Neuroradiol 2006;27:632–7.

29. Oliver TB, Lammie GA, Wright AR, et al. Atherosclerotic plaque at the carotid bifurcation: CT angiographic appearance with histopathologic correlation. AJNR Am J Neuroradiol 1999;20:897–901.

30. Walker LJ, Ismail A, McMeekin W, et al. Computed tomography angiography for the evaluation of carotid atherosclerotic plaque: correlation with histopathology of endarterectomy specimens. Stroke 2002;33:977–81.

31. Debernardi S, Martincich L, Lazzaro D, et al. CT angiography in the assessment of carotid atherosclerotic disease: results of more than two years' experience. Radiol Med 2004;108:116–27.

32. Saba L, Caddeo G, Sanfilippo R, et al. Efficacy and sensitivity of axial scans and different reconstruction methods in the study of the ulcerated carotid plaque using multidetector-row CT angiography: comparison with surgical results. AJNR Am J Neuroradiol 2007;28:716–23.

33. Saba L, Caddeo G, Sanfilippo R, et al. CT and ultrasound in the study of ulcerated carotid plaque compared with surgical results: potentialities and advantages of multidetector row CT angiography. AJNR Am J Neuroradiol 2007;28:1061–6.

34. Wintermark M, Jawadi SS, Rapp JH, et al. High-resolution CT imaging of carotid artery atherosclerotic plaques. AJNR Am J Neuroradiol 2008;29:875–82.

35. Das M, Braunschweig T, Mühlenbruch G, et al. Carotid plaque analysis: comparison of dual-source computed tomography (CT) findings and histopathological correlation. Eur J Vasc Endovasc Surg 2009;38:14–9.

36. Romero JM, Babiarz LS, Forero NP, et al. Arterial wall enhancement overlying carotid plaque on CT angiography correlates with symptoms in patients with high grade stenosis. Stroke 2009;40:1894–6.

37. Jessen KA, Shrimpton PC, Geleijns J, et al. Dosimetry for optimization of patient protection in computed tomography. Appl Radiat Isot 1999;50:165–72.

38. Mnyusiwalla A, Aviv RI, Symons SP. Radiation dose from multidetector row CT imaging for acute stroke. Neuroradiology 2009;51:635–40.

39. Schramm P, Schellinger PD, Fiebach JB, et al. Comparison of CT and CT angiography source images with diffusion-weighted imaging in patients with acute stroke within 6 hours after onset. Stroke 2002;33:2426–32.

40. Schramm P, Schellinger PD, Klotz E, et al. Comparison of perfusion computed tomography and computed tomography angiography source images with perfusion-weighted imaging and diffusion-weighted imaging in patients with acute stroke of less than 6 hours' duration. Stroke 2004;35:1652–8.

41. Coutts SB, Lev MH, Eliasziw M, et al. ASPECTS on CTA source images versus unenhanced CT: added value in predicting final infarct extent and clinical outcome. Stroke 2004;35:2472–6.

42. Puetz V, Sylaja PN, Hill MD, et al. CT angiography source images predict final infarct extent in

patients with basilar artery occlusion. AJNR Am J Neuroradiol 2009;30:1877–83.

43. Wintermark M, Reichhart M, Cuisenaire O, et al. Comparison of admission perfusion computed tomography and qualitative diffusion- and perfusion-weighted magnetic resonance imaging in acute stroke patients. Stroke 2002;33:2025–31.

44. Wintermark M, Fischbein NJ, Smith WS, et al. Accuracy of dynamic perfusion CT with deconvolution in detecting acute hemispheric stroke. AJNR Am J Neuroradiol 2005;26:104–12.

45. Wintermark M, Meuli R, Browaeys P, et al. Comparison of CT perfusion and angiography and MRI in selecting stroke patients for acute treatment. Neurology 2007;68:694–7.

46. Tan JC, Dillon WP, Liu S, et al. Systematic comparison of perfusion-CT and CT-angiography in acute stroke patients. Ann Neurol 2007;61:533–43.

47. Schaefer PW, Barak ER, Kamalian S, et al. Quantitative assessment of core/penumbra mismatch in acute stroke: CT and MR perfusion imaging are strongly correlated when sufficient brain volume is imaged. Stroke 2008;39:2986–92.

48. Schwamm LH, Rosenthal ES, Swap CJ, et al. Hypoattenuation on CT angiographic source images predicts risk of intracerebral hemorrhage and outcome after intra-arterial reperfusion therapy. AJNR Am J Neuroradiol 2005;26:1798–803.

49. Puetz V, Sylaja PN, Coutts SB, et al. Extent of hypoattenuation on CT angiography source images predicts functional outcome in patients with basilar artery occlusion. Stroke 2008;39:2485–90.

50. Schaefer PW, Yoo AJ, Bell D, et al. CT angiography-source image hypoattenuation predicts clinical outcome in posterior circulation strokes treated with intra-arterial therapy. Stroke 2008; 39:3107–9.

51. Rosenthal ES, Schwamm LH, Roccatagliata L, et al. Role of recanalization in acute stroke outcome: rationale for a CT angiogram-based "benefit of recanalization" model. AJNR Am J Neuroradiol 2008;29:1471–5.

52. Puetz V, Dzialowski I, Hill MD, et al. Intracranial thrombus extent predicts clinical outcome, final infarct size and hemorrhagic transformation in ischemic stroke: the clot burden score. Int J Stroke 2008;3:230–6.

53. Barreto AD, Albright KC, Hallevi H, et al. Thrombus burden is associated with clinical outcome after intra-arterial therapy for acute ischemic stroke. Stroke 2008;39:3231–5.

54. Tan IY, Demchuk AM, Hopyan J, et al. CT angiography clot burden score and collateral score: correlation with clinical and radiologic outcomes in acute middle cerebral artery infarct. AJNR Am J Neuroradiol 2009;30:525–31.

55. Maas MB, Lev MH, Ay H, et al. Collateral vessels on CT angiography predict outcome in acute ischemic stroke. Stroke 2009;40:3001–5.

56. Hur J, Kim YJ, Lee HJ, et al. Cardiac computed tomographic angiography for detection of cardiac sources of embolism in stroke patients. Stroke 2009;40:2073–8.

57. Qureshi AI, Tuhrim S, Broderick JP, et al. Spontaneous intracerebral hemorrhage. N Engl J Med 2001;344:1450–60.

58. Davis SM, Broderick J, Hennerici M, et al. Hematoma growth is a determinant of mortality and poor outcome after intracerebral hemorrhage. Neurology 2006;66:1175–81.

59. Mayer SA, Brun NC, Begtrup K, et al. Efficacy and safety of recombinant activated factor VII for acute intracerebral hemorrhage. N Engl J Med 2008;358: 2127–37.

60. Anderson CS, Huang Y, Wang JG, et al. Intensive blood pressure reduction in acute cerebral haemorrhage trial (INTERACT): a randomised pilot trial. Lancet Neurol 2008;7:391–9.

61. Yeung R, Ahmad T, Aviv RI, et al. Comparison of CTA to DSA in determining the etiology of spontaneous ICH. Can J Neurol Sci 2009;36(2): 176–80.

62. Romero JM, Artunduaga M, Forero NP, et al. Accuracy of CT angiography for the diagnosis of vascular abnormalities causing intraparenchymal hemorrhage in young patients. Emerg Radiol 2009;16:195–201.

63. Yoon DY, Chang SK, Choi CS, et al. Multidetector row CT angiography in spontaneous lobar intracerebral hemorrhage: a prospective comparison with conventional angiography. AJNR Am J Neuroradiol 2009;30:962–7.

64. Delgado Almandoz JE, Schaefer PW, Forero NP, et al. Diagnostic accuracy and yield of multidetector CT angiography in the evaluation of spontaneous intraparenchymal cerebral hemorrhage. AJNR Am J Neuroradiol 2009;30:1213–21.

65. Becker KJ, Baxter AB, Bybee HM, et al. Extravasation of radiographic contrast is an independent predictor of death in primary intracerebral hemorrhage. Stroke 1999;30:2025–32.

66. Wada R, Aviv RI, Fox AJ, et al. CT angiography "spot sign" predicts hematoma expansion in acute intracerebral hemorrhage. Stroke 2007;38: 1257–62.

67. Goldstein JN, Fazen LE, Snider R, et al. Contrast extravasation on CT angiography predicts hematoma expansion in intracerebral hemorrhage. Neurology 2007;68:889–94.

68. Kim J, Smith A, Hemphill JC III, et al. Contrast extravasation on CT predicts mortality in primary intracerebral hemorrhage. AJNR Am J Neuroradiol 2008;29:520–5.

69. Ederies A, Demchuk A, Chia T, et al. Postcontrast CT extravasation is associated with hematoma expansion in CTA spot negative patients. Stroke 2009;40:1672–6.

70. Thompson AL, Kosior JC, Gladstone DJ, et al. PREDICTS/Sunnybrook ICH CTA Study Group. Defining the CT angiography 'spot sign' in primary intracerebral hemorrhage. Can J Neurol Sci 2009; 36:456–61.

71. Delgado Almandoz JE, Yoo AJ, Stone MJ, et al. Systematic characterization of the computed tomography angiography spot sign in primary intracerebral hemorrhage identifies patients at highest risk for hematoma expansion. The spot sign score. Stroke 2009;40:2994–3000.

72. Delgado Almandoz JE, Yoo AJ, Stone MJ, et al. The spot sign score in primary intra-cerebral hemorrhage identifies patients at highest risk of in-hospital mortality and poor outcome among survivors. Stroke 2010;41:54–60.

73. Gazzola S, Aviv RI, Gladstone DJ, et al. Vascular and nonvascular mimics of the CT angiography "spot sign" in patients with secondary intracerebral hemorrhage. Stroke 2008;39:1177–83.

74. Agid R, Lee SK, Willinsky RA, et al. Acute subarachnoid hemorrhage: using 64-slice multidetector CT angiography to "triage" patients' treatment. Neuroradiology 2006;48:787–94.

75. Yoon DY, Lim KJ, Choi CS, et al. Detection and characterization of intracranial aneurysms with 16-channel multidetector row CT angiography: a prospective comparison of volume-rendered images and digital subtraction angiography. AJNR Am J Neuroradiol 2007;28:60–7.

76. El Khaldi M, Pernter P, Ferro F, et al. Detection of cerebral aneurysms in nontraumatic subarachnoid haemorrhage: role of multislice CT angiography in 130 consecutive patients. Radiol Med 2007;112: 123–37.

77. Lubicz B, Levivier M, François O, et al. Sixty-four-row multisection CT angiography for detection and evaluation of ruptured intracranial aneurysms: interobserver and intertechnique reproducibility. AJNR Am J Neuroradiol 2007;28:1949–55.

78. Westerlaan HE, Gravendeel J, Fiore D, et al. Multislice CT angiography in the selection of patients with ruptured intracranial aneurysms suitable for clipping or coiling. Neuroradiology 2007;49:997–1007.

79. McKinney AM, Palmer CS, Truwit CL, et al. Detection of aneurysms by 64-section multidetector CT angiography in patients acutely suspected of having an intracranial aneurysm and comparison with digital subtraction and 3D rotational angiography. AJNR Am J Neuroradiol 2008;29:594–602.

80. Uysal E, Oztora F, Ozel A, et al. Detection and evaluation of intracranial aneurysms with 16-row multislice CT angiography: comparison with conventional angiography. Emerg Radiol 2008;15:311–6.

81. Chen W, Yang Y, Xing W, et al. Sixteen-row multislice computed tomography angiography in the diagnosis and characterization of intracranial aneurysms: comparison with conventional angiography and intraoperative findings. J Neurosurg 2008;108:1184–91.

82. Chen W, Wang J, Xing W, et al. Accuracy of 16-row multislice computerized tomography angiography for assessment of intracranial aneurysms. Surg Neurol 2009;71:32–42.

83. Li Q, Lv F, Li Y, et al. Evaluation of 64-section CT angiography for detection and treatment planning of intracranial aneurysms by using DSA and surgical findings. Radiology 2009;252:808–15.

84. Gerardin E, Daumas-Duport B, Tollard E, et al. Usefulness of multislice computerized tomography angiography in preoperative diagnosis of ruptured cerebral aneurysms. J Neuroradiol 2009;36:278–84.

85. Kallmes DF, Layton K, Marx WF, et al. Death by nondiagnosis: why emergent CT angiography should not be done for patients with subarachnoid hemorrhage. AJNR Am J Neuroradiol 2007;28: 1837–8.

86. Hoh BL, Cheung AC, Rabinov JD, et al. Results of a prospective protocol of computed tomographic angiography in place of catheter angiography as the only diagnostic and pretreatment planning study for cerebral aneurysms by a combined neurovascular team. Neurosurgery 2004;54:1329–40.

87. Dehdashti AR, Binaghi S, Uske A, et al. Comparison of multislice computerized tomography angiography and digital subtraction angiography in the postoperative evaluation of patients with clipped aneurysms. J Neurosurg 2006;104:395–403.

88. Uysal E, Ozel A, Erturk SM, et al. Comparison of multislice computed tomography angiography and digital subtraction angiography in the detection of residual or recurrent aneurysm after surgical clipping with titanium clips. Acta Neurochir (Wien) 2009;151:131–5.

89. Gerardin E, Tollard E, Derrey S, et al. Usefulness of multislice computerized tomographic angiography in the postoperative evaluation of patients with clipped aneurysms. Acta Neurochir (Wien) 2009. [Epub ahead of print].

90. Wintermark M, Ko NU, Smith WS, et al. Vasospasm after subarachnoid hemorrhage: utility of perfusion CT and CT angiography on diagnosis and management. AJNR Am J Neuroradiol 2006;27:26–34.

91. Yoon DY, Choi CS, Kim KH, et al. Multidetector-row CT angiography of cerebral vasospasm after aneurysmal subarachnoid hemorrhage: comparison of volume-

rendered images and digital subtraction angiography. AJNR Am J Neuroradiol 2006;27:370–7.

92. Binaghi S, Colleoni ML, Maeder P, et al. CT angiography and perfusion CT in cerebral vasospasm after subarachnoid hemorrhage. AJNR Am J Neuroradiol 2007;28:750–8.

93. Chaudhary SR, Ko N, Dillon WP, et al. Prospective evaluation of multidetector-row CT angiography for the diagnosis of vasospasm following subarachnoid hemorrhage: a comparison with digital subtraction angiography. Cerebrovasc Dis 2008; 25:144–50.

94. van der Schaaf I, Wermer MJ, van der Graaf Y, et al. Prognostic value of cerebral perfusion-computed tomography in the acute stage after subarachnoid hemorrhage for the development of delayed cerebral ischemia. Stroke 2006;37:409–13.

95. Sviri GE, Mesiwala AH, Lewis DH, et al. Dynamic perfusion computerized tomography in cerebral vasospasm following aneurysmal subarachnoid hemorrhage: a comparison with technetium-99m-labeled ethyl cysteinate dimer-single-photon emission computerized tomography. J Neurosurg 2006; 104:404–10.

96. van der Schaaf I, Wermer MJ, van der Graaf Y, et al. CT after subarachnoid hemorrhage: relation of cerebral perfusion to delayed cerebral ischemia. Neurology 2006;66:1533–8.

97. Sviri GE, Britz GW, Lewis DH, et al. Dynamic perfusion computed tomography in the diagnosis of cerebral vasospasm. Neurosurgery 2006;59:319–25.

98. Pham M, Johnson A, Bartsch AJ, et al. CT perfusion predicts secondary cerebral infarction after aneurysmal subarachnoid hemorrhage. Neurology 2007;69:762–5.

99. Wintermark M, Dillon WP, Smith WS, et al. Visual grading system for vasospasm based on perfusion CT imaging: comparisons with conventional angiography and quantitative perfusion CT. Cerebrovasc Dis 2008;26:163–70.

100. Rijsdijk M, van der Schaaf IC, Velthuis BK, et al. Global and focal cerebral perfusion after aneurysmal subarachnoid hemorrhage in relation with delayed cerebral ischemia. Neuroradiology 2008; 50:813–20.

101. Aralasmak A, Akyuz M, Ozkaynak C, et al. CT angiography and perfusion imaging in patients with subarachnoid hemorrhage: correlation of vasospasm to perfusion abnormality. Neuroradiology 2009;51:85–93.

102. Dankbaar JW, Rijsdijk M, van der Schaaf IC, et al. Relationship between vasospasm, cerebral perfusion, and delayed cerebral ischemia after aneurysmal subarachnoid hemorrhage. Neuroradiology 2009;51:813–9.

103. Dankbaar JW, de Rooij NK, Velthuis BK, et al. Diagnosing delayed cerebral ischemia with different CT modalities in patients with subarachnoid hemorrhage with clinical deterioration. Diagnosing delayed cerebral ischemia with different CT modalities in patients with subarachnoid hemorrhage with clinical deterioration. Stroke 2009;40:3493–8.

104. Flohr TG, Schaller S, Stierstorfer K, et al. Multidetector row CT systems and image-reconstruction techniques. Radiology 2005;235:756–73.

105. Hu H, He HD, Foley WD, et al. Four multidetector-row helical CT: image quality and volume coverage speed. Radiology 2000;215:55–62.

106. Klingebiel R, Siebert E, Diekmann S, et al. 4-D imaging in cerebrovascular disorders by using 320-slice CT: feasibility and preliminary clinical experience. Acad Radiol 2009;16:123–9.

107. Siebert E, Bohner G, Dewey M, et al. 320-slice CT neuroimaging: initial clinical experience and image quality evaluation. Br J Radiol 2009;82: 561–70.

108. Siebert E, Bohner G, Dewey M, et al. Letter to the editor concerning "320-slice CT neuroimaging: initial clinical experience and image quality evaluation" (Siebert E et al: Br J Radiol 2009; 82: 561–70). Br J Radiol 2009;82:615.

109. Watanabe Y, Uotani K, Nakazawa T, et al. Dual-energy direct bone removal CT angiography for evaluation of intracranial aneurysm or stenosis: comparison with conventional digital subtraction angiography. Eur Radiol 2009;19:1019–24.

110. Deng K, Liu C, Ma R, et al. Clinical evaluation of dual-energy bone removal in CT angiography of the head and neck: comparison with conventional bone-subtraction CT angiography. Clin Radiol 2009;64:534–41.

111. Lell MM, Kramer M, Klotz E, et al. Carotid computed tomography angiography with automated bone suppression: a comparative study between dual energy and bone subtraction techniques. Invest Radiol 2009;44:322–8.

112. Uotani K, Watanabe Y, Higashi M, et al. Dual-energy CT head bone and hard plaque removal for quantification of calcified carotid stenosis: utility and comparison with digital subtraction angiography. Eur Radiol 2009;19: 2060–5.

113. Buerke B, Wittkamp G, Seifarth H, et al. Dual-energy CTA with bone removal for transcranial arteries intraindividual comparison with standard CTA without bone removal and TOF-MRA. Acad Radiol 2009;16:1348–55.

114. Mühlenbruch G, Das M, Mommertz G, et al. Comparison of dual-source CT angiography and MR angiography in preoperative evaluation of intra- and extracranial vessels: a pilot study. Eur Radiol 2010;20:469–76.

Update on Multidetector Computed Tomography Angiography of the Abdominal Aorta

Joseph J. Budovec, MD[a],*, Matthew Pollema, MD[b], Michael Grogan, MD, JD[b]

KEYWORDS

- Multidetector computed tomography • Aorta
- Vascular disease

The development of 16-slice multidetector computed tomography angiography (MDCTA) and beyond allows high spatial resolution, including nearly isotropic submillimeter resolution in the X, Y, and Z planes, and rapid image acquisition in a single breath hold, with greatly enhanced diagnostic capabilities over conventional CT. MDCTA has inherent advantages over digital subtraction angiography (DSA), including being a less invasive technique and facilitating the evaluation of the aortic wall and lining mural thrombus, detection of unsuspected extraluminal abnormalities, and multiplanar postprocessing for interventional planning. Because of these advantages and its widespread availability, MDCTA of the abdominal aorta and iliac arteries has largely replaced DSA in many practices for the evaluation of abdominal aortic aneurysm (AAA), surveillance of known AAA, and follow-up postsurgical or endovascular treatment of AAA. Other diseases affecting the aortoiliac system, including intramural hematoma and aortic dissection, atherosclerotic disease and penetrating aortic ulcer, posttraumatic vascular injury, and vasculitis, may be evaluated by MDCTA. This article discusses the technical components and optimization of MDCTA of the abdominal aorta and iliac arteries (aortoiliac system), as well as diseases of the aortoiliac system evaluated by MDCTA.

TECHNICAL PARAMETERS AND OPTIMIZATION

Important issues to consider before performing an MDCTA of the aortoiliac system relate to scanner type, contrast factors, postprocessing, and patient radiation dose.

Scanner

MDCTA allows for the acquisition of a volumetric data set, which was not achievable with single-detector, incremental, or helical CT. More importantly for CTA, 16-slice or greater MDCTA allowed for the rapid acquisition of a large volumetric data set with submillimeter isotropic spatial resolution. The higher table speed and increased number of detectors available on the current MDCTA platforms allows for faster acquisition and greater coverage during a single breath hold.

Contrast

Contrast bolus shaping for MDCTA is determined by the rate and duration of injection, type and

[a] Body and Digital Imaging Section, Department of Radiology, Medical College of Wisconsin, 9200 West Wisconsin Avenue, Milwaukee, WI 53226, USA
[b] Department of Radiology, Medical College of Wisconsin, 9200 West Wisconsin Avenue, Milwaukee, WI 53226, USA
* Corresponding author.
E-mail address: jbudovec@mcw.edu

Radiol Clin N Am 48 (2010) 283–309
doi:10.1016/j.rcl.2010.02.009

concentration of contrast material, and use of a saline flush technique. The shape of the contrast bolus influences the contrast arrival time, time to aortoiliac peak enhancement, and the duration of acceptable enhancement (generally more than 250 Hounsfield units [HU]) for image acquisition.

Contrast arrival time is most commonly evaluated by 1 of 2 methods. Bolus-tracking software with automatic triggering of the CT scanner allows the initiation of image acquisition once attenuation at a specified location (such as the celiac axis) reaches a threshold value. Arrival time can also be assessed by performing a test bolus injection of 10 to 15 mL at a high rate used during MDCTA acquisition, such as 5 to 6 mL/s. Arrival time at the authors' institution is evaluated by performing 2 separate test bolus injections of 15 mL of contrast at 5 to 6 mL/s. The time to peak enhancement after the test bolus injection is calculated at the celiac axis, as well as 30 cm below the celiac axis. Performing 2 rather than 1 test bolus injection allows calculation of flow velocity within the abdominal aorta, which varies from patient to patient. Common conditions that may alter circulation time include congestive heart failure and cardiac arrhythmias with associated delay in aortic contrast arrival and decreased peak enhancement, or an AAA with prolonged contrast transit time through the aneurysmal segment. Aligning the flow velocity and table speed using modern MDCTA scanners can minimize the risk of outrunning the contrast bolus.[1,2]

For identical injection durations, higher concentrations of contrast medium are associated with earlier and greater peak aortic enhancement[1,3–5] and greater attenuation and conspicuity of smaller vessels.[6]

Injection duration determines the time to peak aortic enhancement and attenuation of the contrast column over time. A short injection duration may lead to insufficient arterial enhancement, whereas prolonged injection duration may result in venous contamination. Decreased duration of injection is more important for angiographic MDCT applications than for parenchymal applications. Higher rates of injection at a fixed volume of contrast are associated with significantly increased enhancement of the aorta compared with that of abdominal parenchymal organs such as the liver.[1]

In the authors' practice, duration of contrast injection equals a delay time from aortic arrival to the beginning of acquisition plus the acquisition interval. The delay time after aortic arrival allows for continued upslope of enhancement to produce a relatively homogeneous plateau of enhancement during acquisition.[1,7] The acquisition interval depends on the imaging distance (generally 30–40 cm) and table speed, with the table speed set to equal the arterial flow velocity. Arterial flow velocity, determined by aortoiliac transit time, is usually less than the routine table speed of 8 to 11 cm/s. The table speed can be decelerated by changing the scan rotation speed, pitch, or, if necessary, beam width. Adequate intravenous access, preferably with 18-gauge plastic venous cannulas in an antecubital vein, is required for injection rates of 5 to 6 cm/s.

The administered contrast volume, which is determined by injection duration multiplied by rate of injection, will be increased with longer acquisition times determined by slower flow velocities. However, this is kept within the bounds of contrast volume related to patient weight. Patients of larger size have larger circulating blood volumes and thus require larger doses of contrast for MDCTA, which is achieved by increasing contrast volume and/or concentration. At the authors' institution, 60 mL of 370 mg iodine/mL contrast medium followed by saline flush is administered to patients weighing up to 68 kg, with incremental increases of 20 mL of contrast volume for every additional 22.68-kg increase in patient weight for aortoiliac MDCTA (maximum 140 mL of contrast for patients >136 kg). Adequate aortic attenuation in MDCTA is at least 250 HU and preferably 300 to 350 HU. Using patient weight and flow velocity in determining contrast load has resulted in an average contrast volume of 100 mL of 370 mg iodine/mL contrast medium across a broad representative range of patients with peripheral arterial disease. Lower volumes of contrast without degradation of image quality or diagnostic performance are advantageous, because chronic kidney disease has been reported in up to 7% to 25% of patients undergoing evaluation for endovascular aneurysm repair (EVAR) of AAA.[6]

Performing a saline flush with 20 to 30 mL of saline at the same rate of injection as that of the contrast bolus with use of a dual-head injector pushes the tail of the contrast bolus from the upper extremity venous system into the central circulating blood volume. This procedure also increases length of peak aortic enhancement and decreases the amount of total injected contrast required for adequate aortic enhancement by 10 to 15 mL.[1] Elevating the patient's arm during acquisition is important, because this position avoids venous constriction at the thoracic inlet and allows more contrast to enter the central circulating blood volume than to remain within the upper extremity venous system. Sample abdominal and aortoiliac CTA protocols using a 64-channel MDCTA system (LightSpeed VCT

[General Electric Healthcare, Little Chalfont, Buckinghamshire, UK]) are provided.

Postprocessing

Postprocessing of acquired data includes volume rendering (VR), maximum intensity projection (MIP), and curved planar reformations. VR provides a topographic display of aortoiliac vessels and abdominal visceral arterial branches, and can be performed with and without bone segmentation. MIP techniques, which display the maximum attenuation within a voxel of data, are 2-dimensional representations of 3-dimensional data and require viewing from different angles for a 3-dimensional perspective. A subvolume MIP without superimposition of celiac and mesenteric branches is useful in displaying lining mural thrombus in the aortorenal and aortoiliac circulation (Fig. 1). MIP is limited in the evaluation of vascular stenoses because of the high attenuation and superimposition of vascular calcifications over the vessel lumen. In these circumstances, curved plane reformations can display inner lumen and outer mural calcification and accurately portray the degree of arterial stenosis.

Dose Reduction

Patient dose considerations are important in any MDCTA protocol, particularly with increased public attention to radiation dose recently raised by medical and popular literature.[8] Although radiation dose should follow the as low as reasonably achievable principle, certain factors, such as thin collimation allowing for adequate multiplanar reconstructions, are essential in providing high-quality MDCTA images. Multiple strategies for patient dose reduction—including, but not limited to, low peak tube voltage (kVp), automatic tube current modulation, and virtual noncontrast imaging provided by dual-energy CT techniques—have been introduced in an attempt to reduce radiation dose without degradation of image quality in MDCTA, and may have applications in MDCTA.[7]

For MDCTA, increased peak aortic attenuation and decreased radiation dose without significant change in image quality has been demonstrated at 100 kVp compared with 120 kVp.[9] A recent phantom study tailored to patient body habitus suggested adequate capability of detecting endoleaks measuring 6 mm or larger at 80 kVp in patients of small to intermediate size and 100 kVp in patients of larger size. For endoleaks as small as 4 mm, 80 kVp MDCTA could be applied to small patients, 100 kVp in intermediate-sized patients, and 120 kVp in larger patients, with dose reduction of greater than 50% for 80 kVp versus 120 kVp in smaller patients.[10]

Automatic tube current modulation allows adjustment of tube current in the x-y plane (angular modulation) or the z-axis (z-axis modulation), based on the weight or cross-sectional dimensions of the patient or size and attenuation of the

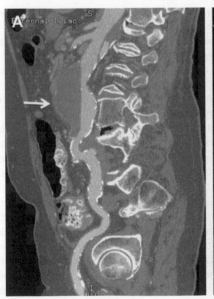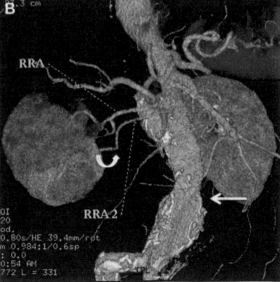

Fig. 1. Curved plane reformatted image. (A) The inner lumen, lining mural thrombus, and mural calcifications within a fusiform aneurysm (*arrow*). The lining mural thrombus is not appreciated on the volume-rendered image (*B, arrow*) An accessory right renal artery (RRA) is observed.

imaged body part, without significant degradation in image quality.[7] Automated tube current modulation has been associated with 40% to 60% reduction in CT dose index, and is now routinely implemented on most scanners.[11]

Dual-energy CTA may allow decreased amounts of administered iodinated contrast medium because of the improved contrast resolution with the low kVp data set. The dual-energy technique is also useful in differentiating iodinated contrast material from calcified plaque or bone. Postprocessing of high and low kVp data sets allows production of "virtual unenhanced" and "iodine only" data sets, which may have future applications in the evaluation for endoleak in patients who have undergone EVAR of AAA.[12–14]

ABDOMINAL AORTA
Anatomy

The thoracic aorta becomes the abdominal aorta after passing through the diaphragmatic hiatus, the most caudal and posterior of all the large openings in the diaphragm. The abdominal aorta begins immediately before the superior adrenal arteries arise, approximately at the level of the T12 vertebral body. The juxtarenal abdominal aorta diameter normally measures less than 3 cm. The abdominal aorta supplies visceral and parietal arteries that arise in 3 vascular planes before it bifurcates to form the common iliac arteries at the level of the L4. The bifurcation tends to migrate and increase in tortuosity with age. The unpaired visceral arteries to the gastrointestinal tract include the celiac artery, and superior and inferior mesenteric arteries. These arteries arise in the midline anterior plane. The paired visceral arteries include the renal, adrenal, and gonadal (testicular or ovarian) arteries, which run through the lateral plane to supply the urogenital and endocrine organs. The subcostal, inferior phrenic, and lumbar arteries are paired parietal arteries to the diaphragm and body wall, arising in the posterior oblique plane. The only unpaired parietal artery, the middle sacral, arises posteriorly.

The common iliac artery bifurcates at the pelvic brim, where the ureter crosses ventrally, to yield the hypogastric arteries. The hypogastric arteries subsequently divide into anterior and posterior divisions. The posterior division provides the branches of the lateral sacral, iliolumbar, and superior gluteal arteries. The anterior division branches into the inferior gluteal, obturator, vesicular, middle hemorrhoidal, internal pudendal, uterine (female), and deferential (male) arteries. Variations in the branching patterns of the posterior and anterior division vessels are common.

The pelvic arteries form an important potential collateral network in patients with aortoiliac occlusive disease. Major potential connections include those from the lumbar to iliolumbar, medial to lateral sacral, and superior to middle hemorrhoidal (the superior hemorrhoidal is a branch of the inferior mesenteric artery [IMA]) arteries.

Three important arterial branches arise from the distal external iliac artery immediately proximal to the common femoral artery. These arteries are the circumflex iliac, inferior epigastric, and external pudendal arteries. The circumflex iliac and inferior epigastric arteries also make important contributions to arterial collateral networks, the circumflex artery communicating with the parietal branches of the lumbar arteries, and the inferior epigastric with the superior epigastric branches, in turn deriving inflow from the internal mammary arteries (Fig. 2).

Variant Anatomy

Multiple configurations of the origin and branching pattern of abdominal aortic visceral arterial branches occur commonly. Up to 30% of patients have more than one renal artery, the accessory artery most commonly supplying the lower pole. Lower pole accessory arteries usually arise from the mid-abdominal aorta but may also arise from the distal aorta or common iliac arteries (Fig. 3). Accessory renal arteries may arise from an abdominal aortic or iliac aneurysm, and may require vessel sacrifice during endovascular stent graft placement or reimplantation during open aneurysm repair.

The number of accessory renal arteries varies and is usually not more than 4. Multiple renal arteries are typical in patients with horseshoe kidney. In patients with horseshoe kidney and AAA, a major renal arterial branch may arise from the aortic midline to supply both lower-pole moieties, and poses a technical challenge in an open aneurysm repair procedure.

The celiac axis is usually a single trunk, but separate aortic origins of the hepatic, left gastric, and splenic arteries do occur. A combined origin for the celiac and superior mesenteric artery is unusual.

An important but rare congenital anomaly is the absence of the common and external iliac and femoral arteries with replacement by a persistent sciatic artery. The sciatic artery usually regresses during development, with the residual vessel forming the superior gluteal artery. A persistent sciatic artery runs adjacent to the nerve, exiting the pelvis via the sciatic notch and continuing superficial to the adductor magnus muscle. A sciatic artery is associated with the clinical conundrum of absent

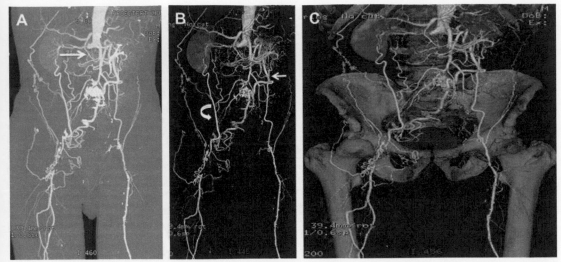

Fig. 2. A 66-year-old man with infrarenal aortic occlusion and lower extremity claudication. Coronal MIP image (*A*) demonstrates occlusion of the infrarenal abdominal aorta (*arrow*) with reconstitution of the IMA via a Riolan arch, circumflex iliac, and inferior epigastric arteries. Segmented and nonsegmented coronal volume-rendered images (*B*) and (*C*), respectively, demonstrate the extensive infrarenal collaterals with reconstitution of the superficial femoral arteries distally. The common and external iliac arteries are completely occluded. The straight and curved arrows in *B* demonstrate the prominent Riolan arch and inferior epigastric collateral to the RRA.

femoral pulse and normal pulse pressures in the distal extremity arteries. Importance relates to recognition of a congenital variation and avoidance of attempted femoral catheterization.

ABDOMINAL AORTIC ANEURYSM
Epidemiology and Etiology

An AAA is defined as a structural failure of the vessel wall resulting in segmental dilatation, which increases the normal vessel diameter by 50% or results in an anteroposterior (AP) diameter greater than 3 cm.[15] Dilatation of the aorta by less than 50% of its original diameter is called ectasia.[16] AAAs are now the 13th leading cause of death in the United States.[17] Unlike coronary artery disease and stroke, AAA has increased in incidence in the last 40 years.[18] AAA occurs in 4% to 8% of men and in 1% of women older than 50 years.[15] Approximately 80% of AAAs occur between the renal arteries and the bifurcation.[19] The principal risk factors include smoking, male sex, white race, and family history.[20]

Among the major risk factors, smoking has the strongest correlation with AAA, with a prevalence of 5.1% in smokers versus 1.5% in nonsmokers.[21] In addition, an AAA grows faster[22] and ruptures more often in current smokers.[23] The risk of AAA associated with the male sex may be related to genetic predisposition, hormonal environment, and anatomic factors such as the larger caliber

of the male aorta compared with that of the female aorta.[24] A few examples of pertinent risk factors are vasculitis such as Takayasu or giant cell arteritis, metabolic syndromes such as homocysteinuria[25] or pseudoxanthoma elasticum,[26] and connective tissue disorders such as Marfan syndrome.

AAA formation is most likely a polygenomic disease under the influence of multiple environmental factors.[24] Diabetes, black race, and female sex have a reduced risk of AAA unless other significant risk factors, such as family history or multiple risk factors for atherosclerotic disease, are present.[20] Atherosclerosis has been postulated as an environmental factor. The connection, however, between atherosclerosis and aneurysm formation remains obscure. The association between diabetes mellitus and atherosclerosis remains firm, but diabetes mellitus negatively correlates with the development and progression of AAA.[27]

Current research on the pathogenesis of AAA focuses on the extracellular matrix, which provides mechanical strength and integrity to the aortic wall. Because autopsy specimens demonstrate disruption of the ordered layering of collagen and early disappearance of the elastin fibers in AAAs, it is thought that proinflammatory mediators trigger an intricate network of enzymes that digest the extracellular matrix and impair its subsequent repair, leading to aneurysm formation. Vascular inflammation traditionally occurs within the intima

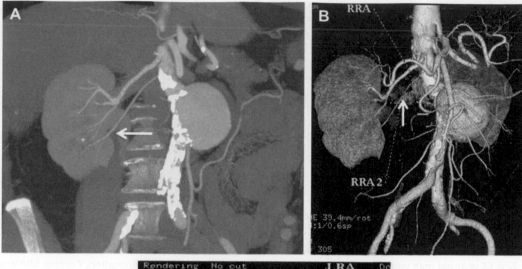

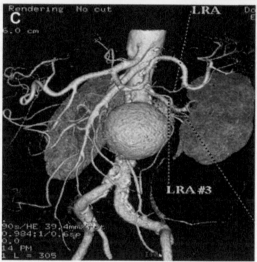

Fig. 3. A 70-year-old woman with a saccular infrarenal AAA. Coronal MIP image (*A*) demonstrates an accessory renal artery to the right inferior pole (*arrow*). Volume-rendered image (*B*) demonstrates the RRA (*arrow*). Three renal arteries are present on the left, as seen on the volume-rendered image (*C*).

and eventually involves the adventitia. More recent evidence suggests that the inflammatory process starts in the adventitia and works inward to the intima.[28] Oxidative stress plays a role in this inflammatory cascade,[29] because perpetuation of this inflammatory process by matrix metalloproteinases (MMPs), MMP-9 and MMP-2 in particular, leads to aneurysm.

The detection of an increased incidence of AAA in World War II veterans with above-the-knee amputation (5.8%) versus nonamputees (1.1%) elevated the suspicion for turbulent flow as a cause for AAA formation.[30] Turbulent flow results in kinetic energy creating shear forces, leading to aneurysmal dilatation and eventual rupture.[31] The systolic pulsatile wave results in the highest pressure load occurring within the infrarenal aorta. This infrarenal localization of hemodynamic stress occurs secondary to the distal tapering of the aorta, progressive senile stiffening of the aortic wall secondary to changes in the collagen/elastin ratio, and the synergistic effects of retrograde pressure waves that reflect from the iliac bifurcation with the incoming antegrade systolic pressure waves.[32] Further support for the turbulent flow hypothesis comes from the protective nature of lower extremity exercise and promotion of aneurysm by sedentary lifestyles, such as those of patients with spinal cord injuries.[33]

Screening

Palpation is moderately sensitive for larger aneurysms, but it cannot reliably rule out the disease.[19]

Ultrasound is the preferred screening modality, but recommendations for the population that should be screened vary among organizations.[15] The recent study of the Cochrane Collaboration on ultrasound screening for AAA in men aged between 65 and 74 years found that it significantly reduces the risk of death from AAA rupture, with an odds ratio of 0.60, but fails to reduce the all-cause mortality.[34] However, when considering several newer studies not included in the Cochrane meta-analysis and having a longer follow-up (ranging from 7.1 to 15 years), the all-cause mortality was significantly reduced.[35] Thus, the centers for Medicare and Medicaid services in the United States will pay for a one-time screening duplex ultrasound, if performed within 6 months of Medicare eligibility, in 2 patient populations. These populations are men aged between 65 and 75 years with a history of smoking more than 100 cigarettes in their lifetime and anyone older than 60 years with a family history of AAA.[15]

Ultrasound is reportedly 95% sensitive and 100% specific for diagnosing AAAs larger than 3 cm.[36] Ultrasound is an inexpensive way to detect abdominal aneurysms and, if present, the location of the aneurysm in relation to aortic branch vessels and presence of lining mural thrombus. Ultrasound has no inherent contraindications.[37]

Ultrasound has several limitations. This technique is unreliable in determining whether an aneurysm may be juxtarenal or suprarenal, and whether an aneurysm involves the common iliac artery or extends to the iliac artery bifurcation. Furthermore, additional aneurysmal disease or stenotic disease of abdominal visceral vessels is not generally evaluated. Ultrasound interrogation is limited when the aorta is tortuous or the aneurysm is eccentric, and it can be imprecise by up to 5 mm, which may result in misclassification of patients.[38] In addition, ultrasound would be limited in the 26.5% of Americans[39] who, in 2008, met the definition of obesity.

When screening with ultrasound, if the abdominal aorta is less than 3 cm in maximum AP dimension, no further imaging is recommended.[40] If the abdominal aorta measures between 3 and 4 cm, annual follow-up is suggested.[15] Ultrasound screening should be performed every 6 months if the aneurysm measures between 4 and 5 cm.[15] If the AP diameter is greater than 5.5 cm or the growth exceeds 1 cm in a year, these patients should be referred to a vascular surgeon or interventional radiologist.[15] Once the patient is 75 years old, most recommendations suggest that no further screening is necessary, given the increasing comorbidities and decreased life expectancy.[41] Recent evidence shows, however, the mortality rate after endovascular or open repair

for selected octogenarians, although higher than younger patients, seems acceptable.[41]

Although magnetic resonance (MR) imaging and CT provide excellent characterization of AAAs, they are not recommended for screening because of their cost, use of ionizing radiation, and contrast. Radiologists should encourage clinicians to reserve these modalities for patients in whom intervention is planned. Plain radiographs are insensitive for AAA and fail to provide essential aneurysm measurements, although intramural calcium deposits may herald aneurysm.[19]

Clinical Features

AAA rupture classically (50%) presents with hypotension, back pain, and a pulsatile abdominal mass.[42] Rupture may also present as constipation, urinary retention, urge to defecate, or syncope, as the expanding hematoma compresses the bowel, ureters, or their supplying blood vessels.[19] Contained rupture can present with a normal hematocrit and blood pressure.[19] Misdiagnosis of ruptured AAA remains distressingly common despite the awareness of the disease for more than a century.[19] Vague AAA syndrome symptoms of the back, groin, flank, or abdominal pain may be attributed to more common entities such as urinary tract infections, renal stones, lumbago, or gastroesophageal reflux disease.

Natural History

Aneurysm formation leads to progressive aortic wall degeneration over many years culminating with rupture. Aneurysms smaller than 5.5 cm on average grow by 2.6 to 3.2 mm per year.[43] Annual growth rate increases with aneurysm size, accelerating the time to rupture, and 70% of aneurysms 4 to 5.5 cm will surpass the 5.5-cm intervening point within 10 years.[43] Risk of rupture correlates with the amount of hemodynamic stress placed on the weakened aortic wall, because tensile strength is largely a function of aneurysm size and geometry (Laplace's law).[16] The cumulative incidence of rupture over 6 years for AAAs that are 4 cm or smaller is only 1%.[42] The annual risk of rupture increases to as much as 3% for aneurysms of 4 to 5 cm, 11% for aneurysms of 5 to 7 cm, and 20% for those larger than 7 cm.[17]

Most AAAs are asymptomatic until rupture, which carries a poor prognosis with a community-based mortality of 79% and a 50% 30-day perioperative mortality risk.[36] For patients with a rupture who make it to the hospital, surgery carries a 40% mortality risk.[44] When the AAA reaches 5.5 cm, the risk of rupture (approximately 27.8%)[15] and the associated overwhelming morbidity and mortality that rupture brings (79%)[36] are thought to exceed the risk of elective surgery (5%)[36] or EVAR.

Once the AAA surpasses 5.5 cm in AP diameter, referral to a specialist is recommended. Additional concern is required in 2 important circumstances. First, rapid expansion of a saccular aneurysm should raise suspicion for infection of the aneurysm, because mycotic aneurysms tend to increase in size more rapidly than aneurysm from other causes.[45] Second, if significant perianeurysmal fibrosis and adhesions are present, an inflammatory aneurysm should be suspected. Inflammatory aneurysms are often symptomatic and have a much higher rate of rupture independent of their size.[46]

CT Imaging and Classification of AAA

Ninety percent of AAAs are found before they reach the threshold for intervention (5.5 cm).[47,48] Regardless of the indication for CTA, either automated software measurement or manual technique using curved planar reformation and subsequent length measurement should be used to determine the axial length of the aneurysm neck (the distance between the lowermost renal artery to the start of the aneurysm), the shape and angulation of the neck, the maximum AP

diameter of the aneurysm sac, the diameter of the iliac arteries (for access through the groin), and the potential length and condition of the distal iliac arteries (**Fig. 4**). Aneurysmal mural thrombus and calcifications are common. Noting the amount of or change in mural thrombus and calcification within an aneurysm is important.

This information should be provided in the radiology report because certain findings will improve or limit technical success, particularly with EVAR. The angle between the superior neck and the long axis of the aneurysm should be detailed because most stent grafts work better when this angle measures less than 60°. The shape and wall characteristics of the superior neck are also important because stent graft devices fixate better when the neck is straight (**Fig. 5**). Fixation within a conical or flared aneurysm neck has a higher incidence of stent migration. In addition, fixation with either friction devices or barb devices into a superior neck or the iliac arteries with significant atherosclerotic plaque or ulceration may lead to distal embolization during procedure, poor fixation, and/or possible endoleak.

Approximately 5% of AAAs are juxtarenal or suprarenal. A juxtarenal aneurysm has a short superior neck unsuitable for operative clamping, and a suprarenal aneurysm extends to the level of the superior mesenteric artery or above.[49] There

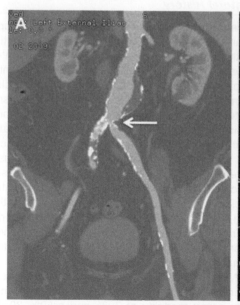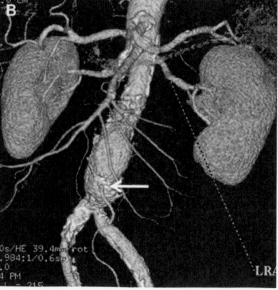

Fig. 4. A 73-year-old man with a fusiform infrarenal AAA extending to the aortic bifurcation. Curved planar reformatted image (*A*) demonstrates a moderately high-grade stenosis at the origin of the left common internal iliac artery (*arrow*) and extensive calcification within the origin of the right common iliac artery. Although the volume-rendered image (*B*) demonstrates the moderately extensive calcification at the aortoiliac bifurcation, it does not demonstrate the high degree of stenosis within the origin of the left common iliac artery. A patent IMA is also noted arising from the aneurysm (*arrow*).

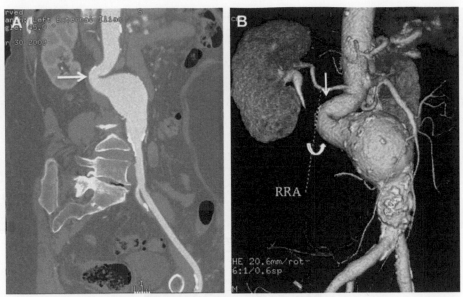

Fig. 5. A 72-year-old woman with a fusiform infrarenal AAA extending to the aortic bifurcation. The curved planar image along with the left external iliac artery axis (A) demonstrates marked angulation of the neck with reference to the long axis of the aneurysm, measuring approximately 90° (arrow). The volume-rendered image (B) demonstrates the marked angulation of the neck in reference to the long axis of the aneurysm (straight arrow). There is marked kinking of the aneurysm sac in relationship to the neck, measuring approximately 70° to 90° (curved arrow). A patent IMA arises from the aneurysm.

is no commonly accepted definition for juxtarenal aneurysm, although the term is used often (Fig. 6). Crawford's initial definition of juxtarenal aneurysm actually was "juxtarenal infrarenal" and referred to infrarenal AAAs that came close enough to or involved the renal arteries such that suprarenal cross-clamping during open repair was needed. Crawford's term was modified by Qvarfordt and colleagues,[50] who used the term "pararenal aneurysm." The Ad Hoc Committee on Reporting Standards on Arterial Aneurysms chose not to use the term pararenal.[51] Because all these terms result in increased surgical risk, some have proposed a classification system, in which type A refers to AAAs of the infrarenal aorta, which involve the suprarenal aorta; type B, which extend to and involve the renal arteries but not the suprarenal aorta; and type C, which extend to the renal arteries without involving them.[52]

Identifying the number and location of renal arteries as well as the presence of a retroaortic left renal vein is important for operative planning.[53] An accessory renal artery arising from the aneurysm may be sacrificed by an endoluminal stent graft procedure if the artery supplies a small portion of the kidney, the patient has normal renal function, and the main renal arteries are not stenotic.

As in all potential stent grafting, careful assessment of patency of the mesenteric and hypogastric arteries should be performed. Discussing the arterial communication between the middle colic branch of the superior mesenteric artery and the superior left colic branch of the IMA is important because these connections maintain left colon perfusion in patients when the IMA is occluded or sacrificed (Fig. 7). This arterial communication between the 2 colic arterial branches at the splenic flexure has been labeled as the Griffith point. Integrity of this communication maintains left colon perfusion when the IMA is occluded by plaque, deliberately occluded (as when an AAA is excluded by an endovascular stent graft), or ligated (at open repair). Collateral communication between the middle hemorrhoidal branch of the hypogastric artery and the superior hemorrhoidal branch of the IMA also contributes to left colon perfusion.

A comment on the iliofemoral vessel tortuosity, plaque burden, and vessel caliber is also essential. In addition to determining the route of endovascular access,[54] they affect the planned intervention, especially if the aneurysm extends into the iliac arteries, which occurs 5% to 46% of the time.[55] Such aneurysms usually involve the proximal common iliac arteries with normal-caliber distal common iliac arteries and hypogastric arteries. As with aortic aneurysms, lining mural thrombus and mural calcification are common with iliac aneurysms. Although most iliac aneurysms are

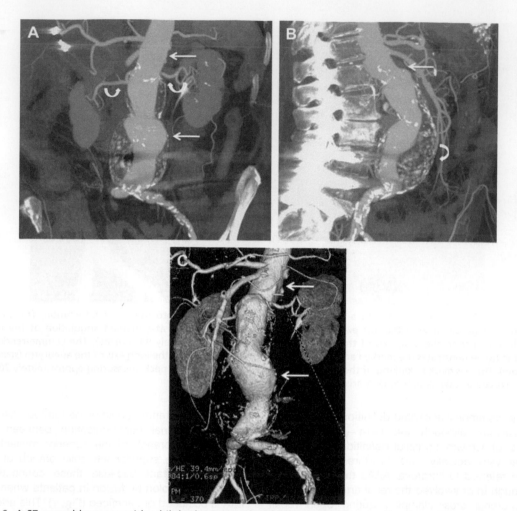

Fig. 6. A 67-year-old woman with a bilobed suprarenal and infrarenal AAA extending from the superior mesenteric artery origin to the aortic bifurcation. Coronal curved planar reformatted image (*A*) demonstrates a suprarenal and infrarenal aneurysm (*straight arrows*) with single bilateral renal arteries arising from the aneurysm (*curved arrows*). Sagittal curved planar reformatted image (*B*) demonstrates the ectatic nature of the suprarenal infrarenal AAA (*arrow*). Calcification is seen lining the walls of the aneurysm (*curved arrow*). Volume-rendered reformatted image in the coronal plane (*C*) demonstrates the extent of the suprarenal infrarenal aneurysm (*arrow*).

fusiform, saccular aneurysms also occur. Saccular aneurysms are more likely in instances of isolated common iliac artery aneurysms or hypogastric artery aneurysms.[56]

Diagnosis of Rupture

CT, pre- and postcontrast, should be performed in all conscious, hemodynamically stable patients with suspected AAA rupture.[57,58] MDCTA provides essential information for urgent preoperative or pre–stent graft planning and can be performed expeditiously. DSA cannot diagnose contained rupture or provide all appropriate information to determine appropriate stent graft selection.[59]

Ultrasound is relatively insensitive to rupture,[60] and MR imaging has issues in relation to availability, length of scan, and monitoring or resuscitating a hemodynamically unstable patient in an intense magnetic field. Contained AAA ruptures may be noted on MR imaging examinations of the lumbar spine,[61] and ultrasound may still have a role in the diagnosis of AAA at the bedside of a patient too unstable for a CT scan.[47] CT is 80% to 90% sensitive for detection of aortic aneurysm rupture.[62] The slightly low sensitivity is caused by interobserver variability with small ruptures.[61,63]

AAA rupture most commonly occurs through the posterior lateral wall into the retroperitoneum.[61]

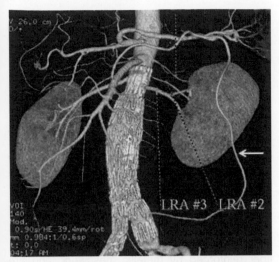

Fig. 7. Volume-rendered image of a 72-year-old man with an aortobiiliac endovascular stent graft with right external iliac extender and coil occlusion of the right internal iliac artery. The IMA is reconstituted by a middle colic to left colic arterial anastomosis (*arrow*).

Periaortic blood may extend into the perirenal space, pararenal space, or both (Fig. 8).[47] The blood may also extend into the psoas muscle. When intraperitoneal rupture occurs, the anterior or anterolateral aortic wall is usually the source. Less commonly, rupture may occur into the bowel, most often the duodenum, resulting in exsanguination.[42] Occasionally, rupture into bowel can

result in slow leaks mimicking peptic ulcer disease.[42] Rarely, AAA rupture into the inferior vena cava causes high-output cardiac failure, lower extremity swelling, and engorgement of the leg veins (aortocaval fistula).[42]

Prompt diagnosis of frank or impending rupture of AAA is essential. Ruptured aneurysms tend to have more thrombus, less calcification within thrombus, and crescents of high attenuation within the thrombus compared with nonruptured aneurysms.[64] Focal discontinuity of an otherwise circumferential calcification is specific for rupture.[64] Most mural calcifications have multifocal areas of discontinuity, but if the discontinuity has changed since an old examination, rupture is likely.[64]

One of the most specific signs for frank or impending rupture is the "crescent sign," which is best seen on a non–contrast-enhanced image. This sign is most specific for rupture when a well-defined area of higher attenuation than the psoas muscle on a contrast study or an area of the aortic lumen on a noncontrast study is noted within the aneurysm wall.[64] A crescent represents acute dissection into the thrombus or aneurysm wall, thereby weakening it, and signifies penetration of the protective shield supplied by the mural thrombus.[65] Hemorrhage into the retroperitoneum after initial intrathrombus or intramural hemorrhage usually takes several hours.

The "drape sign" is also specific for rupture. The posterior aortic wall should be sharp, and a distinct fat plane should be present between the adjacent

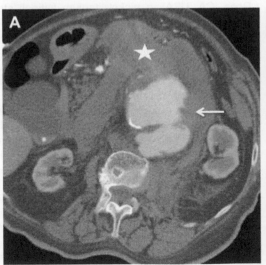
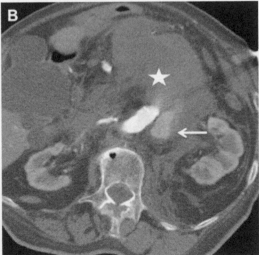

Fig. 8. A 95-year-old woman with syncope and an AAA. Axial CT image (*A*) demonstrates a large infrarenal AAA (*arrow*) with surrounding hematoma (*star*). Axial CT image just below the level of the renal arteries (*B*) demonstrates active contrast extravasation from the posterior lateral aspect of the aneurysm (*arrow*) with a large retroperitoneal and intraperitoneal hematoma (*star*).

vertebral bodies. A drape sign should be questioned when the posterior aneurysm wall lacks sharpness or closely conforms to the vertebral body (ie, it drapes over the vertebral body),[47] especially if there is erosion of the vertebral body (Fig. 9).[66] Occasionally, the drape sign may be confused with the duodenum, periaortic aneurysm fibrosis, or lymph nodes.[47] Likewise, a thrombus-filled saccular aortic aneurysm compressing a vertebral body should not be confused with a periaortic malignant mass such as multiple myeloma or plasmacytoma. Chronic ruptures do occur. The diagnosis requires the patient to have an AAA, a previous pain syndrome, a CT scan showing retroperitoneal hemorrhage, and pathologic confirmation of organizing hematoma.[67]

Treatment of AAA

Pharmacotherapy is an intense focus of current research. Cardiovascular risk factor reduction is beneficial to patients with AAAs. Some studies assert that statins decrease the risk of rupture by as much as 50%.[57] Most current research focuses on inhibiting metalloproteinase activity.[16]

Open surgical repair has been the gold standard for treatment of AAAs. Surgical repair was initially performed with homografts in the 1950s.[68] Nowadays the surgeon performs open repair by approaching the aneurysm from the retroperitoneum or peritoneal cavity and subsequently obtains proximal and distal control of the aorta.

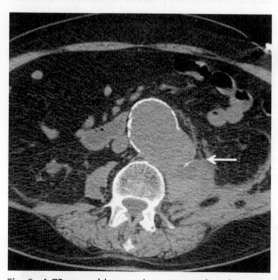

Fig. 9. A 72-year-old man who presented to the emergency department with severe back pain. Noncontrast axial CT image demonstrates an infrarenal AAA with posterior lateral displacement of mural calcification and soft tissue "draping" over the vertebral body (arrow).

Next, the surgeon opens the aneurysm, ligates any back feeding vessels, and sews a graft from the normal proximal aorta to normal distal aorta/iliac vessels. Surgery, compared with EVAR, is associated with a longer hospital stay, greater use of critical or intensive care, more pain, more blood products, and a higher 30-day mortality risk (4.7%), and requires general anesthesia.[69] Surgical risk may be prohibitive in some patients with certain comorbidities.

EVAR was first reported in 1991, and likely reflects the growing trend toward minimally invasive procedures and concern about excessive risks of open repair.[60] The surgeon performs bilateral incisions over the common femoral arteries, allowing direct access using the Seldinger technique. These devices are composed of synthetic fiber reinforced by metallic meshwork, and are thus capable of preventing pressure transmission of the systolic pulse through the endograft into the native AAA wall. The less tortuous and/or larger iliofemoral arteries are used for delivering the main stent graft, whereas the contralateral side is used to deliver the contralateral limb. An extension limb is available to ensure accurate placement. At the proximal neck of the aneurysm, angiographic balloons are used to deploy the main graft, which uses barbs or hooks to avoid migration through satisfactory fixation. The ipsilateral and contralateral iliac limbs are deployed in a similar fashion, albeit through their respective common femoral arteries.

The Food and Drug Administration (FDA) has approved the use of 5 different devices for EVAR of AAAs.[70] The AneuRx (Medtronic AVE, Santa Rosa, CA, USA), a nickel-titanium (nitinol) stent graft with friction seal but no barbs, was the first device approved (in 1999). As of 2 years previously, more than 55,000 devices had been placed worldwide. The device is compatible with an MR imaging field strength of less than 3 T. Because of its lack of proximal barb fixation, there is concern about device migration. The Talent (Medtronic AVE, Santa Rosa, CA, USA) device is also a modular, self-expanding nitinol stent, covered with a woven polyester fabric. The Talent device seals by friction, similar to the Zenith graft (Cook Vascular Inc, Vandergrift, PA, USA) system. The proximal end of the stent is uncovered, permitting suprarenal fixation. The Talent device was approved by the FDA in 2008. The Excluder (WL Gore & Associates Inc, Flagstaff, AZ, USA) is a nitinol device with friction seal, but it has staggered barbs, and was approved in 2002. During the first 5 years after approval, approximately 42,200 devices were placed, likely because of its ease of deployment. The Excluder is MR imaging–compatible up to a field strength of 1.5 T. The Zenith Flex endoprosthesis (Cook Vascular Inc, Vandergrift, PA, USA), first approved by the FDA in 2003, is made of self-expanding stainless steel stents and polyester fabric. The Zenith Flex is, therefore, not MR imaging–compatible. Deployment of this device is thought to be less intuitive and takes more steps than the other delivery systems. The device is gaining rapid acceptance, however, for its ability to achieve suprarenal fixation with barbs and permit endograft placement in wider-necked or more angulated aneurysms. The Powerlink (Endologix Inc, Irvine, CA, USA) is a unibody cobalt-chromium device with an expanding polytetrafluoroethylene graft, which has been available in Europe since 1999 but received FDA approval only in 2004. The unibody construction requires only a single femoral artery cutdown, facilitating delivery in a patient with difficult access. Deployment requires some manipulation and is more complex than other systems. The Powerlink device is MR imaging–compatible up to a field strength of 0.5 T.

Anatomic factors that facilitate technical success for EVAR vary with the device being used. For the AneuRx and Excluder devices, the following measurements are recommended. The proximal neck should be 28 mm in maximum external AP and transverse diameter and 15 mm in length, with a 60° or less angulation in relation to the long axis of the aneurysm. The aneurysm neck should not be excessively conical or flared and should be free of excessive atherothrombosis (<25% of neck circumference and <2 mm thrombus thickness is suggested as suitable for stent grafting). The distal placement zone in the iliac arteries should be 13 to 15 mm in maximal external AP diameter and 20 mm in length, and proximal to iliac artery bifurcation. The external and common iliac arteries should allow access, have no focally significant stenosis (particularly calcific stenosis), and have a maximum allowable angle of tortuosity of less than 120°. The constant evolution of device design has allowed successful EVAR of most AAAs.

Aortoiliac aneurysms, where the common iliac aneurysms extend to the iliac artery bifurcation, require the use of a bifurcated endovascular stent graft with extenders into the external iliac artery on the involved side.[71] Concomitantly, occlusion of the ipsilateral hypogastric artery must be performed to prevent a reflow endoleak into the distal graft (Fig. 10). In this circumstance, arterial inflow into the pelvis should be maintained by a patent contralateral hypogastric artery, thus requiring any contralateral common iliac artery aneurysm to have a distal margin proximal to the iliac artery bifurcation. An isolated common iliac artery aneurysm that is not in continuity with an aortic aneurysm can be treated by a separate iliac endovascular stent graft.[72] An isolated hypogastric artery aneurysm with a normal diameter patent hypogastric artery of the opposite side can be treated with coil embolization.

Some aneurysms may be juxtarenal and suprarenal. Juxtarenal aneurysms were previously

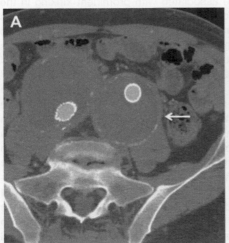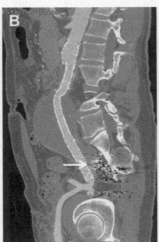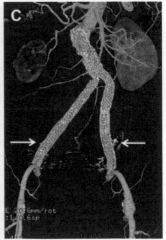

Fig. 10. A 64-year-old man with an endovascular stent graft for treatment of an abdominal aortic, bilateral common iliac, and proximal external iliac artery aneurysms. Axial CT image at the level of the common iliac arteries (A) demonstrates large common iliac artery aneurysms with iliac extenders (arrow). Curved planar reformatted image at the right external iliac artery (B) demonstrates the iliac extender with occlusion of the hypogastric artery via the graft limb and coil occlusion (arrow). Coronal volume-rendered image (C) demonstrates the iliac extenders with occlusion of hypogastric artery (arrows).

considered unsuitable for conventional endovascular stent grafting because of the need for unfenestrated stent grafts to occupy an infrarenal location in order to avoid encroaching on the pararenal aorta and thus compromising renal perfusion. The shorter the nondilated segment between the aneurysm and the renal arteries (neck), the higher was the likelihood of a type I endoleak or stent graft migration.

Fenestration allows the stent graft to overlay the renal artery ostia while providing for transgraft flow to the renal artery, which improves sealing everywhere except the area immediately around the fenestration. The risk of endoleak is minimized by orienting a small fenestration precisely so that the margin of the fenestration impinges on the arterial ostia. The key advance in fenestrated stent graft implantation was the development of a method of staged stent graft deployment, using bridging catheters to align the fenestration with the renal artery and a flared bridging stent to maintain alignment.[73]

EVAR for suprarenal AAAs using fenestrated grafts is gaining acceptance, and early results are promising, especially in patients too ill to tolerate open repair.[74] At present, most suprarenal aneurysms are treated by surgical tube-graft replacement with implantation of the abdominal visceral branches.

A patent IMA arising from an aneurysm may be implanted into an aortic graft during surgery, or it may be ligated if there is adequate collateral circulation from the middle colic to the left colic artery via the marginal colonic circulation. Such assessments can be made intraoperatively by evaluating pulse pressure in the stump of an IMA after separation from the aorta. In patients treated with endovascular stent grafting and in whom the IMA is patent and arises from the aneurysm, a preintervention display of the middle colic and superior left colic arteries is important to determine the likelihood of adequate left colon perfusion after aneurysm exclusion. In addition to evaluating colic artery patency, stenosis of the superior mesenteric artery and/or hypogastric artery is also important. A stenosed superior mesenteric artery may not provide adequate pulse pressure through the mesenteric arterial collateral circulation to facilitate sufficient left colon perfusion following aneurysm exclusion. The hypogastric artery, through its middle hemorrhoidal to superior hemorrhoidal anastomoses, also contributes to sigmoid and left colonic arterial perfusion. Stenosis of the hypogastric arteries in the presence of a patent IMA arising from the aneurysm introduces a relative risk of postendograft colonic ischemia. Postintervention colonic ischemia may also result from periprocedural cholesterol embolization of the superior and inferior mesenteric arteries and the hypogastric artery.

Immediate Complications Post EVAR

EVAR of abdominal aortic rupture involves performing a complex procedure on a high-risk patient. Risk of aneurysm rupture during the procedure is less than 1%.[75] Ischemic complications to the spinal cord, buttocks, genitalia, colon, and lower extremity have been reported to be as high as 10%, although the number is likely lower, given advancements in endograft device design.[76] The cause of renal complications post EVAR is likely multifactorial and associated with placement of the device, contrast load, and embolization. Suprarenal fixation, although still uncertain, likely has a higher associated rate of renal complications. The renal deterioration post EVAR is lower than in open repair (2%–10%) and tends to occur more slowly over time.[77] However, hemodialysis requirements are comparable between EVAR and open repair (2%).[78]

Infrarenal aortic enlargement develops in healthy individuals as they age and in patients after surgical or endovascular therapy.[79–81] Following surgical aortobiiliac or aortobifemoral tube grafting, a pseudoaneurysm may develop at the proximal anastomotic site, or a true aneurysm may develop either in the infrarenal, juxtarenal, or suprarenal aorta (Fig. 11).[82] This dilatation has been shown to be present in 35.3%[83] of patients with endograft migration and tends to result in late type I endoleaks.[84] This late type I endoleak may be associated with prominent kinking in the aortic or iliac limb, and this type of migration is the primary cause of postoperative conversion to open repair.[85] Some studies suggest EVAR is protective of infrarenal aortic enlargement.[86]

Graft limb thrombosis is uncommon (2.2%–3.9%), and may be secondary to kinking of the aortic component of the stent graft within the aneurysm sac or kinking of the iliac limbs within the iliac arteries.[87] Kinking of the iliac limb is most often associated with use of the iliac limb extenders, and is thought to be related to poor distal fixation. Iliac artery dissection by the catheter or delivery system during initial placement of the endovascular graft may result in ipsilateral iliac artery thrombosis distal to the graft. Iliac graft limb thrombosis may require use of a femorofemoral bypass graft to provide ipsilateral lower limb perfusion (Fig. 12). Aortic thrombosis requires urgent conversion to open repair.

Major branch vessel occlusion should not occur if there is proper preprocedural patient selection and appropriate placement of a suitable

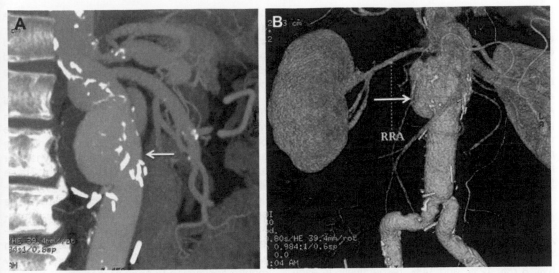

Fig. 11. A 72-year-old man with an abdominal aortic tube graft and infrarenal AAA arising from the margin of the tube graft. Curved planar image (*A*) demonstrates the bilobed aneurysm arising at the junction of the aorta and aortic tube graft (*arrow*). A coronal volume-rendered image (*B*) better depicts the relationship of the aneurysm to the tube graft (*arrow*). The renal arteries arise superior to the cranial extent of the aneurysm.

endovascular stent graft. If the proximal margin of a covered stent graft overlays a renal artery, renal artery occlusion and infarction can occur. More commonly, inferior accessory renal arteries are overlain by the covered portion of the stent graft, and are occluded if they supply a small proportion of kidney parenchyma in a patient with normal renal function and without main renal artery stenosis.

According to a recent meta-analysis, EVAR offers faster recovery, less pain, less blood product replacement (1022–1900 mL), and

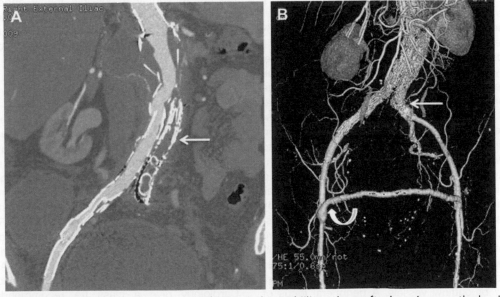

Fig. 12. A 78-year-old woman with a history of a surgical aortobiiliac tube graft who subsequently developed a supra-anastomotic juxtarenal aortic aneurysm. The patient was treated with an aortoiliac endovascular stent graft with an occluder device placed in the left limb, as seen (*arrow*) on the curved planar reformatted image (*A*). The endograft was extended into the right external iliac artery and a femoral-femoral bypass graft was performed, as depicted on the coronal volume-rendered image (*B*). The straight arrow denotes the occlusion within the left iliac limb. The curved arrow denotes the right femoral to left femoral bypass graft.

significantly lower 30-day mortality risk (1.2%–1.7%), and can be performed without general anesthesia.[88,89] Although EVAR offers significant decreases in perioperative adverse events and aneurysm-related mortality, it fails to reduce the all-cause mortality over open repair.[89] Interim analysis from the Open versus EVAR Veterans Affairs Cooperative Study Group suggests that perioperative mortality was low for both procedures and lower for endovascular than open repair, and that the early advantage of EVAR was not offset by increased morbidity or mortality in the first 2 years after repair.[90]

Endoleaks

According to data from patients with EVAR from 1999 to 2004, reintervention was necessary in 6%, 8.7%, 12%, and 14%, respectively, in each subsequent year after placement of the device.[91] Reintervention was as high as 20% in patients fitted with older devices and followed for 15 months.[92] The typical reason for reintervention is endoleak, which has 5 categories based on the site of leakage. All endoleaks cause increased pressurization of the aneurysm sac and thus potential for continued aneurysm growth and rupture.

A type I endoleak is an attachment site endoleak, either proximal or distal, usually recognized at stent graft placement. Type I endoleaks maintain arterial pressure inside the sac and, if untreated, can eventually result in aortic rupture.[93] These endoleaks require treatment either by placement of aortic cuffs at the proximal or distal attachment site or by open surgical suture closure. Delayed development of a type I endoleak may be related to changes in tortuosity of the aorta secondary to aneurysm shrinkage or enlargement.[94] On CT, a type I endoleak should be suspected when acute hemorrhage or contrast pooling is found in the aneurysm sac adjacent to a device attachment site (Fig. 13).

A type II endoleak is caused by continued blood flow into the repaired aneurysm sac through small arterial branches of the aorta that are excluded by the stent graft. Type II endoleaks are the most common (40% of all endoleaks), and often resolve spontaneously.[95] A type II endoleak requires an inflow and outflow vessel, and the lumbar and inferior mesenteric arteries may function as either inflow or outflow vessels. A peripheral focus of acute hemorrhage or contrast is often seen within the aneurysm sac when this type of leak is present (Fig. 14). These leaks are treated with expectant management to assess for sac growth over 6 months. If interval growth is noted, embolization

of lumbar or mesenteric vessels or translumbar injection of hemostatic agent into the nonthrombosed component of the aneurysm sac should be considered. Contrast opacification of excluded aortic branches does not always implicate the correct vessel.[96]

A type III endoleak is caused by mechanical disruption involving either the fabric of an endograft or mechanical separation of an iliac module or extender from the main graft. Type III endoleaks are considered high pressure and high risk for rupture, necessitating immediate treatment. These leaks are suggested to occur when large collections of pooling contrast or acute hemorrhage are seen centrally at a distance from the attachment sites of the native vessels.[97] Type III endoleaks may be treated by placement of an additional endograft to seal the local leak, or may require conversion to open procedure.

A type IV endoleak is secondary to graft porosity, a condition that usually occurs immediately after placement before the graft fabric has been sealed by incorporation of fibrin. A type IV endoleak is self-healing by nature and often resolves with cessation of anticoagulation.[93]

A type V endoleak is described as endotension and occurs when arterial pressure is recorded in the aneurysm sac or the sac enlarges over time, but there is no identifiable cause. Endotension is a diagnosis of exclusion in that MDCTA and catheter angiography (with injection of all potential feeders to supply a possible reflow endoleak) have been performed before diagnosis. Endotension associated with expansion of the aneurysm sac is low risk but may require conversion to open repair.[94]

Late Complications

The long-term comparison of aneurysm-related mortality between EVAR and open surgery remains uncertain.[98] The long-term follow-up available is based on devices that have been reengineered multiple times since their initial placement, and several of these devices have been taken off the market. EVAR trials suggest the patients most likely to benefit from EVAR are younger, healthier patients, who could undergo open surgery with an acceptable operative risk.[54] However, the 2005 guidelines issued by the American Heart Association and American College of Cardiology give a class IIA recommendation (evidence favors usefulness or efficacy) for EVAR in patients with high surgical risk and a class IIB (evidence is less well established) recommendation for EVAR in patients with low or average surgical risk.[99]

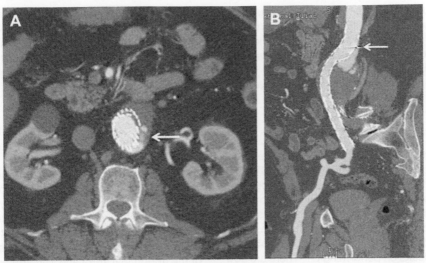

Fig. 13. An 83-year-old man with an aortoiliac stent graft, left common iliac artery occlusion, and femoral-femoral bypass graft. Axial CT image (A) demonstrates contrast in the aneurysm sac at the superior margin of the stent graft (arrow), consistent with a type I endoleak, with inflow between the first uncovered and second covered segments of the endograft. A curved planar reformatted image along the external iliac artery access (B) demonstrates the extent of the type I endoleak (arrow).

Infection of the endograft is rare[100] but devastating, with mortality approaching 75%.[101] Infected endograft presents in a typical fashion with fever, leukocytosis, and elevated erythrocyte sedimentation rate. Nonspecific presentations also occur, in which gastrointestinal bleeding, hydronephrosis, osteomyelitis, or ischemia from a clotted graft is present. The pathogen is usually *Staphylococcus epidermidis*, but there are reports of *Clostridium sodelli*[102] and *Aspergillus*.[103] Some fluid is expected around the aorta immediately after the procedure or surgery. Persistent or expanding soft tissue, fluid, and/or gas adjacent to the graft suggest graft infection, with or without aortoenteric fistula.

Indium-111–tagged white blood cell scans, gallium, or ultrasound may help diagnose graft infection. An MR image has not been studied for diagnosing graft infection. An infected anastomotic aneurysm or an infected aortic graft usually requires antibiotic therapy and surgical correction. The latter most frequently necessitates graft

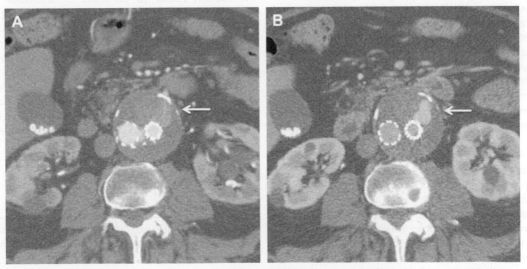

Fig. 14. An 85-year-old man with a Zenith aortobiiliac endovascular stent graft. Axial CT image (A) during the arterial phase demonstrates a faint blush within the aneurysm sac (arrow). On delayed phase imaging (B), contrast is noted within the aneurysm sac consistent with a type II endoleak supplied by the IMA (arrow).

removal and extra-anatomic surgical bypass using an axillofemoral and femorofemoral bypass graft in combination with subrenal aortic graft removal. It is suggested that surgery is safer if perigraft fluid aspiration is performed percutaneously before operative repair.[104] The infection results in a pseudoaneurysm about 25% of the time.[100]

Surveillance

MDCTA is the modality of choice for surveillance post EVAR.[105] The superiority of MDCTA for detection of endoleaks compared with conventional angiography is well known.[106] However, every modality has its disadvantages. For example, beam-hardening artifact from stent material and aortic wall calcifications can obscure subtle endoleaks on performing CT. There are now reported cases where MR imaging has been more sensitive than CT for the detection of aortic endoleak.[107] The disadvantages of MR imaging are the potential susceptibility artifacts (especially in stainless steel and some nitinol devices), which may obscure crucial detail so that the MR imaging might miss significant findings. Radiographs are limited to evaluating stent graft position and integrity. Sonography has limited sensitivity, although recent studies suggest that contrast-enhanced ultrasound has significantly improved sensitivity for endoleak detection.

Follow-up imaging after EVAR is usually performed with CT at 1, 6, and 12 months, and then annually. In MDCTA, a post–stent graft imaging examination uses precontrast, dynamic first circulation imaging and "immediate delayed" postcontrast imaging. The precontrast images allow one to distinguish calcifications or high attenuation foci from true endoleaks. The delayed images help detect less conspicuous slow-flow endoleaks.[108,109] The precontrast and immediate delayed postcontrast imaging can be performed with a relatively thick image (of thickness 2–3 mm). The dynamic first circulation study is performed with maximum z-axis resolution which, depending on the MDCTA system used, may vary from 0.5 mm to 1.25 mm detector collimation.

As with preoperative imaging, a first circulation study requires accurate circulation timing, equivalence of injection and acquisition intervals, and sufficiently rapidly injected contrast bolus to elevate aortic CT attenuation to 250 to 300 HU throughout acquisition. Images are evaluated in stacked axial cine mode, full volume and subvolume MIP, VR, and multiplanar and curved planar reformations. In addition to measuring the maximum external AP and transverse dimensions of the aneurysm sac and the endoluminal measurements of the aortic stent graft and its 2 limbs, the distance between the proximal margin of the stent graft and the inferior margin of the most inferior renal artery, and the lower margin of the stent graft and the iliac artery bifurcation of each side are measured.

AORTIC DISSECTION

Dissection is a disruption of the aortic wall, with separation of the intima and inner medial layer of the aorta from the outer medial layer and serosa. Focal dissection of the abdominal aorta is rare, occurring in 1.3% of all aortic dissections.[110] Focal dissection is associated most strongly with hypertension and also with smoking, diabetes, previous aneurysm surgery, and hypercholesterolemia.[111] The most common cause for nonfocal dissection of the abdominal aorta and iliac arteries is a thoracoabdominal dissection, either type A or B. On occasion, patients may have a coexistent thoracoabdominal aortic dissection, and a separate subrenal AAA (Fig. 15). Connective tissue disorders, including Marfan and Ehlers-Danlos syndromes and fibrodysplasia, may all result in a focal aortoiliac dissection.

Patients typically present with chest, back, or abdominal pain. Focal abdominal aortic dissections most often occur spontaneously, but trauma and iatrogenic causes (such as cardiac catheterization) also contribute. Proximally, the abdominal aortic dissection tends to occur either between the renal arteries and the IMA (33%) or the celiac trunk and the renal arteries (23%). The distal extent almost always terminates before the common iliac artery.[111] Clinical manifestations of aortoiliac dissection relate to stenoses or occlusion of abdominal visceral branch vessels resulting in mesenteric ischemia, renovascular hypertension, or iliac dissection and extremity ischemia. On occasion, aortoiliac dissection will result in focal aneurysmal disease.

Focal abdominal aortic dissection is most commonly treated with open repair, although medical management/observation and EVAR are also used.[111] The risk of in-hospital mortality is 4% and the complication rate is 9%.[111]

AORTOILIAC OCCLUSIVE DISEASE AND ATHEROMATOUS ULCER
Aortoiliac Stenosis

Aortoiliac stenosis occurs in the setting of chronic atherosclerotic disease. The infrarenal aorta and the iliac arteries are the most common locations where symptomatic aortoiliac disease occurs. Hemodynamically significant aortoiliac arterial occlusive disease (≥50% stenosis), or inflow

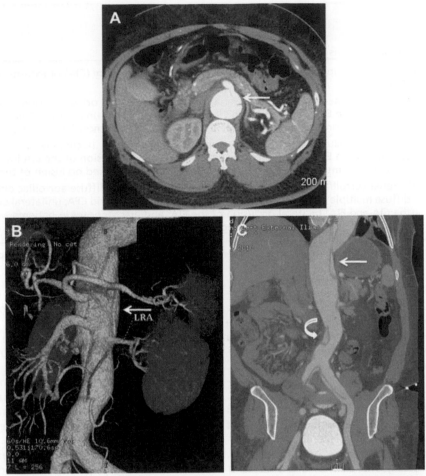

Fig. 15. A 45-year-old man with a type B dissection extending to the iliac artery bifurcation and a suprarenal and infrarenal fusiform AAA. Axial CT image (*A*) shows a dissection flap and a suprarenal aortic aneurysm at the level of the superior mesenteric artery. The superior mesenteric artery is supplied by the true lumen (*arrow*). A volume-rendered image (*B*) demonstrates the fusiform suprarenal and infrarenal AAA. A curved planar reformatted image (*C*) along the axis of the left external iliac artery demonstrates the dissection flaps and the aneurysm (*straight arrow and curved arrow*).

disease, tends to occur at arterial bifurcation points. Proximal common iliac artery stenosis is common, and may be bilateral or isolated. Patient presentation is dependent on acuity of findings, typically intermittent thigh or hip/buttock claudication symptoms, but symptoms vary with extent of collateral flow and coexistent disease. Among men with aortoiliac occlusive disease, 30% to 50% will have complaints of impotence.[112]

Aortoiliac lesion morphology is categorized according to the TransAtlantic InterSociety Consensus (TASC II) classification, which also provides a therapeutic framework for the decision regarding appropriateness of either percutaneous treatment or surgery.[113] Aortoiliac lesions are divided into 4 types depending on location, length, multiplicity, unilateral or bilateral involvement, and degree of stenosis or occlusion (Table 1).[113] MDCTA is most often extended through the lower extremity runoff to evaluate for coexistent femoral-popliteal or below-knee runoff arterial disease. MDCTA of the lower extremities is discussed elsewhere in this issue.

Very high interobserver agreement between MDCTA and DSA has been demonstrated in evaluation of aortoiliac arterial disease.[114,115] Reconstitution of flow distal to occlusion is better demonstrated with MDCTA than with DSA.[114] A recent meta-analysis demonstrated pooled sensitivity of 96% and pooled specificity of 97% in MDCTA evaluation of aortoiliac arterial disease (≥50% stenosis).[116] No significant difference between magnetic resonance angiography (MRA) and MDCTA has been demonstrated in the

Table 1
TransAtlantic InterSociety Consensus (TASC II) classification[113]

Type	Aortoiliac Lesions Morphology
Type A	Single stenoses up to 3 cm in length in the common iliac artery (CIA) or external iliac artery (EIA)
Type B	Less than 3-cm stenosis of the infrarenal aorta, unilateral CIA occlusion, single or multiple stenosis of the EIA between 3 and 10 cm in total length or unilateral EIA occlusion not involving the origins of the internal iliac artery or the common femoral artery (CFA)
Type C	Bilateral CIA occlusions, bilateral EIA stenoses between 3 and 10 cm in length, unilateral stenosis of the EIA extending into the CFA, unilateral occlusion of the EIA involving the origin of the internal iliac artery and/or the CFA, and calcified occlusion of the EIA
Type D	Infrarenal aortoiliac occlusion; hemodynamically significant diffuse aortoiliac disease; diffuse multiple stenoses involving the unilateral CIA, EIA, and CFA; unilateral occlusion of the CIA and EIA; bilateral occlusion of the EIA; and iliac stenoses in patients with an infrarenal aortic aneurysm requiring treatment

(*Data from* Norgren L, Hiatt WR, Dormandy JA, et al. Inter-society consensus for the management for peripheral arterial disease (TASC II). J Vasc Surg 2007;45(Suppl 5):S5–67.

evaluation of hemodynamically significant aortoiliac stenosis.[116,117]

Surgical or endovascular treatment options are available and, as with aneurysmal disease, data acquired from MDCTA can guide definitive treatment of aortoiliac occlusive arterial disease. Advantages of MDCTA and MRA in the preoperative or preendovascular workup of focal aortoiliac occlusive disease include evaluation of length and multiplicity of involved segments, degree of stenosis, development of collaterals, and evaluation of coexistent femoral-popliteal disease. Balloon angioplasty, with or without endovascular stent placement, is best for concentric, noncalcified stenosis less than 3 cm (type A and B lesions). Bilateral proximal common iliac artery stenoses are often treated with the "kissing" stent technique. Surgery, either aortobifemoral or axillofemoral with femoral-femoral bypass, is often performed in the setting of chronic aortoiliac occlusion. As with the treatment of AAA, a collaborative surgical/interventional approach tailored to each individual patient is optimal. For example, patients who may otherwise undergo surgery may be poor operative candidates and are best served by endovascular treatment, if possible. MDCTA or MRA guides therapeutic decision making for definitive surgical, endovascular, or combined repair, and guides access route in the case of EVAR.

Aortoiliac Atheromatous Ulceration

Atheromatous ulcerations confined to the intima of the aortic wall occur in patients with advanced atherosclerosis. Although usually asymptomatic, atheromatous aortoiliac ulceration may result in peripheral embolism or "blue toe" syndrome, with the infrarenal abdominal aorta or proximal iliac artery as common source sites for distal embolism. A penetrating atherosclerotic ulcer refers to an ulcerating atherosclerotic lesion penetrating through the intima into the media of the aortic wall with associated hematoma.[118] Penetrating atheromatous ulcerations most commonly occur in the descending thoracic aorta but may also occur in the abdominal aorta. Penetrating ulcers may uncommonly lead to pseudoaneurysm formation, dissection, aortocaval fistula, or rupture (Fig. 16). Surgical or endovascular treatment may be performed in symptomatic cases, on enlarging ulceration, or on signs of impending rupture. Short-term follow-up is recommended in nontreated cases.

TRAUMA

Acute traumatic aortic injury (ATAI) occurs much more commonly in the thorax, with traumatic injury to the abdominal aorta occurring in 0.08% to 0.62% of nonpenetrating trauma and accounting for only 4% to 6% of ATAI cases. Nevertheless, life-threatening injury to the abdominal aorta may also occur in the setting of trauma. Imaging findings in ATAI include intimal disruption with focal flap, propagation of dissection, formation of pseudoaneurysm, or rarely, frank disruption with active extravasation (Fig. 17).[119] CT angiographic images of the thorax of the patient experiencing trauma are routinely obtained at the authors' institution to evaluate for ATAI, and images of the abdomen are obtained in the parenchymal phase.[120] An abdominal aortic pseudoaneurysm may be subtle, and careful evaluation of the aorta should be performed in every trauma patient. Generally, patients

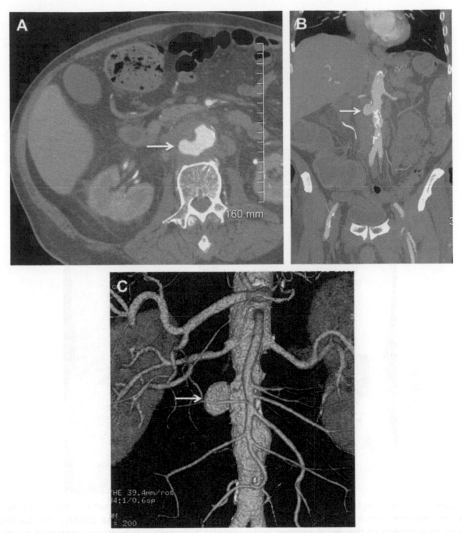

Fig. 16. A 73-year-old man with a penetrating atheromatous ulcer. Axial CT image of the infrarenal aorta (*A*) demonstrates a penetrating atherosclerotic ulcer in the lateral wall of the aorta (*arrow*). Coronal MIP image (*B*) demonstrates the focal outpouching and pseudoaneurysm formation (*arrow*). The volume-rendered image (*C*) demonstrates the saccular nature of the penetrating atherosclerotic ulcer and pseudoaneurysm formation (*arrow*).

with definitive or suspected traumatic pseudoaneurysm of the abdominal aorta are evaluated further by DSA to confirm the diagnosis and provide definitive management. MDCTA of the abdominal aorta may also be obtained as a follow-up examination post-endograft placement.

Aortocaval fistula may occur after penetrating trauma or penetrating aortic ulcer with focal aneurysm formation. Patients with aortocaval fistula have a hyperdynamic state secondary to high-flow arteriovenous communication, which may lead to heart failure.

VASCULITIS

Takayasu arteritis is a large-vessel vasculitis found most often in young Asian women, and is the most common vasculitis involving the thoracoabdominal aorta and primary branches as well as the pulmonary artery. Four subtypes have been described, with type 1 confined to the aortic arch and branches, type 2 involving the descending

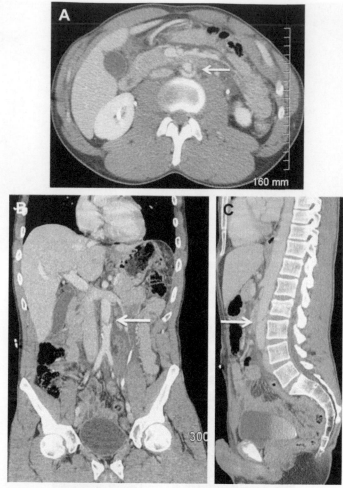

Fig. 17. Traumatic focal dissection in a 43-year-old man involved in a high-speed motor vehicle collision. Axial (*A*) CT angiogram demonstrates a focal dissection in the infrarenal abdominal aorta (*arrow*). The location of the dissection in relationship to the renal arteries and aortoiliac bifurcation is best demonstrated on the coronal (*B*) and sagittal (*C*) CT angiographic images (*arrow*).

thoracic and abdominal aortas, and visceral branches of the latter, type 3 involving type 1 and 2 components, and type 4 combining types 1, 2, or 3 with concomitant pulmonary arterial vasculitis. Early imaging findings may include thickening and enhancement of the vessel wall, whereas more chronic disease may demonstrate arterial stenosis, occlusion, or aneurysm formation.[121] Although early diagnosis and treatment with corticosteroids are associated with improved prognosis, contrast-enhanced CT or MDCTA may not be ordered by the referring clinician in the acute phase because symptoms are often nonspecific early in the disease. MDCTA and MRA are well suited to demonstrate early and late imaging findings.[121] Most patients present

with the late form of the disease and often require intervention depending on whether stenosis, occlusion, or aneurysm is present. Rarely, aneurysm enlargement may occur despite corticosteroid therapy, particularly in aneurysms with wall thickening.[122]

SUMMARY

MDCTA provides the radiologist with the information needed to diagnosis life-threatening diseases of the aortoiliac system, offers critical information for the vascular surgeon or interventional radiologist to treat that disease, and identifies subsequent complications related to therapy. As the population continues to age, the prevalence of aortic disease will continue to increase, requiring radiologists to be familiar with optimization of MDCTA of the aortoiliac system, evaluation and treatment of abdominal aortic and aortoiliac artery aneurysms, dissection, and atherosclerotic disease, and follow-up evaluations of endovascular and surgical therapies designed to treat these diseases.

REFERENCES

1. Bae KT, Heiken JP. Scan and contrast administration principles of MDCT. Eur Radiol 2005;15(Suppl 5):E46–59.

2. Lin PH, Huynh TT, Kougias P, et al. Descending thoracic aortic dissection: evaluation and management in the era of endovascular technology. Vasc Endovascular Surg 2009;43(1):5–24.

3. Yanaga Y, Awai K, Nakaura T, et al. Effect of contrast injection protocols with dose adjusted to the estimated lean patient body weight on aortic enhancement at CT angiography. AJR Am J Roentgenol 2009;192(4):1071–8.

4. Rist C, Nikolaou K, Kirchin MA, et al. Contrast bolus optimization for cardiac 16-slice computed tomography: comparison of contrast medium formulations containing 300 and 400 milligrams of iodine per milliliter. Invest Radiol 2006;41(5):460–7.

5. Bae KT. Test-bolus versus bolus-tracking techniques for CT angiographic timing. Radiology 2005;236(1):369–70 [author reply: 370].

6. Diehm N, Pena C, Benenati JF, et al. Adequacy of an early arterial phase low-volume contrast protocol in 64-detector computed tomography angiography for aortoiliac aneurysms. J Vasc Surg 2008;47(3):492–8.

7. Kalra MK, Maher MM, Toth TL, et al. Strategies for CT radiation dose optimization. Radiology 2004; 230(3):619–28.

8. Brenner DJ, Hall EJ. Computed tomography—an increasing source of radiation exposure. N Engl J Med 2007;357(22):2277–84.

9. Wintersperger B, Jakobs T, Herzog P, et al. Aortoiliac multidetector-row CT angiography with low kV settings: improved vessel enhancement and simultaneous reduction of radiation dose. Eur Radiol 2005;15(2):334–41.

10. Szucs-Farkas Z, Semadeni M, Bensler S, et al. Endoleak detection with CT angiography in an abdominal aortic aneurysm phantom: effect of tube energy, simulated patient size, and physical properties of endoleaks. Radiology 2009;251(2): 590–8.

11. Hara AK, Paden RG, Silva AC, et al. Iterative reconstruction technique for reducing body radiation dose at CT: feasibility study. AJR Am J Roentgenol 2009;193(3):764–71.

12. Yeh BM, Shepherd JA, Wang ZJ, et al. Dual-energy and low-kVp CT in the abdomen. AJR Am J Roentgenol 2009;193(1):47–54.

13. Chandarana H, Godoy MC, Vlahos I, et al. Abdominal aorta: evaluation with dual-source dual-energy multidetector CT after endovascular repair of aneurysms—initial observations. Radiology 2008; 249(2):692–700.

14. Stolzmann P, Leschka S, Scheffel H, et al. Dual-source CT in step-and-shoot mode: noninvasive coronary angiography with low radiation dose. Radiology 2008;249(1):71–80.

15. Pande RL, Beckman JA. Abdominal aortic aneurysm: populations at risk and how to screen. J Vasc Interv Radiol 2008;19(Suppl 6):S2–8.

16. Annambhotla S, Bourgeois S, Wang X, et al. Recent advances in molecular mechanisms of abdominal aortic aneurysm formation. World J Surg 2008;32(6):976–86.

17. Gloviczki P, Ricotta JJ II. Sabiston Textbook of surgery. In: Townsend CM, Beauchamp RD, Evers BM, et al, editors. Aneurysmal vascular disease. 18th edition. Philadelphia: Saunders; 2007.

18. Jemal A, Ward E, Hao Y, et al. Trends in the leading causes of death in the United States, 1970–2002. [comment]. JAMA 2005;294(10): 1255–9.

19. Lederle FA. In the clinic. Abdominal aortic aneurysm. Ann Intern Med 2009;150(9):ITC5-1–15 [quiz: ITC15–6].

20. Lederle FA, Johnson GR, Wilson SE, et al. The aneurysm detection and management study screening program: validation cohort and final results. Aneurysm Detection and Management Veterans Affairs Cooperative Study Investigators. Arch Intern Med 2000;160(10):1425–30.

21. Fleming C, Whitlock EP, Beil TL, et al. Screening for abdominal aortic aneurysm: a best-evidence systematic review for the U.S. Preventive Services Task Force. Ann Intern Med 2005;142(3):203–11.

22. Brady AR, Thompson SG, Fowkes FG, et al. Abdominal aortic aneurysm expansion: risk factors and time intervals for surveillance. Circulation 2004;110(1):16–21.

23. Smoking, lung function and the prognosis of abdominal aortic aneurysm. The UK Small Aneurysm Trial Participants. Eur J Vasc Endovasc Surg 2000;19(6):636–42.

24. Aoki H, Yoshimura K, Matsuzaki M. Turning back the clock: regression of abdominal aortic aneurysms via pharmacotherapy. J Mol Med 2007;85(10):1077–88.

25. Moroz P, Le MT, Norman PE. Homocysteine and abdominal aortic aneurysms. ANZ J Surg 2007; 77(5):329–32.

26. Caglayan AO, Dundar M. Inherited diseases and syndromes leading to aortic aneurysms and dissections. Eur J Cardiothorac Surg 2009;35(6):931–40.

27. Curci JA, Baxter BT, Thompson RW. Arterial aneurysms: etiologic considerations. In: Rutherford RB, editor. Vascular surgery. 6th edition. Philadelphia: Saunders; 2005.

28. Maiellaro K, Taylor WR. The role of the adventitia in vascular inflammation. Cardiovasc Res 2007;75(4): 640–8.

29. McCormick ML, Gavrila D, Weintraub NL. Role of oxidative stress in the pathogenesis of abdominal aortic aneurysms. Arterioscler Thromb Vasc Biol 2007;27(3):461–9.

30. Vollmar JF, Paes E, Pauschinger P, et al. Aortic aneurysms as late sequelae of above-knee amputation. Lancet 1989;2(8667):834–5.

31. Khanafer KM, Bull JL, Upchurch GR Jr, et al. Turbulence significantly increases pressure and fluid shear stress in an aortic aneurysm model under resting and exercise flow conditions. Ann Vasc Surg 2007;21(1):67–74.

32. Thompson RW, Geraghty PJ, Lee JK. Abdominal aortic aneurysms: basic mechanisms and clinical implications. Curr Probl Surg 2002;39(2):110–230.

33. Yeung JJ, Kim HJ, Abbruzzese TA, et al. Aortoiliac hemodynamic and morphologic adaptation to chronic spinal cord injury. J Vasc Surg 2006; 44(6):1254–65.

34. Cosford PA, Leng GC. Screening for abdominal aortic aneurysm. Cochrane Database Syst Rev 2007;(2):CD002945.

35. Takagi H, Tanabashi T, Kawai N, et al. Regarding "Screening for abdominal aortic aneurysm reduces both aneurysm-related and all-cause mortality." J Vasc Surg 2007;46(6):1311–2.

36. Vascular medicine: a companion to Braunwald's heart disease. Philadelphia: Elsevier; 2006.

37. Barnett SB, Ter Haar GR, Ziskin MC, et al. International recommendations and guidelines for the safe use of diagnostic ultrasound in medicine. Ultrasound Med Biol 2000;26(3):355–66.

38. Lederle FA, Wilson SE, Johnson GR, et al. Variability in measurement of abdominal aortic aneurysms. Abdominal Aortic Aneurysm Detection and Management Veterans Administration Cooperative Study Group. J Vasc Surg 1995;21(6):945–52.

39. Available at: http://www.cdc.gov/obesity/data/trends.html. Accessed October 22, 2009.

40. Lindholt JS, Juul S, Fasting H, et al. Screening for abdominal aortic aneurysms: single centre randomised controlled trial [comment]. BMJ 2005; 330(7494):750 [Erratum appears in BMJ 2005; 331(7521):876].

41. Norman PE, Jamrozik K, Lawrence-Brown MM, et al. Population based randomised controlled trial on impact of screening on mortality from abdominal aortic aneurysm [comment]. BMJ 2004;329(7477): 1259 [Erratum appears in BMJ 2005;330(7491): 596].

42. DRB. Aneurysms of the abdominal aorta. In: AB, editor. Abram's angiography: vascular and interventional radiology. 4th edition. Boston: Little, Brown and Company; 1997.

43. Greenhalgh RM, Forbes JF, Fowkes FG, et al. Early elective open surgical repair of small abdominal aortic aneurysms is not recommended: results of the UK Small Aneurysm Trial. Steering Committee. Eur J Vasc Endovasc Surg 1998;16(6):462–4.

44. Bown MJ, Sutton AJ, Bell PR, et al. A meta-analysis of 50 years of ruptured abdominal aortic aneurysm repair. Br J Surg 2002;89(6):714–30.

45. Macedo TA, Stanson AW, Oderich GS, et al. Infected aortic aneurysms: imaging findings. Radiology 2004;231(1):250–7 [Erratum appears in Radiology 2006;238(3):1078].

46. Arrive L, Correas JM, Leseche G, et al. Inflammatory aneurysms of the abdominal aorta: CT findings [comment]. AJR Am J Roentgenol 1995;165(6):1481–4.

47. Rakita D, Newatia A, Hines JJ, et al. Spectrum of CT findings in rupture and impending rupture of abdominal aortic aneurysms. Radiographics 2007;27(2):497–507.

48. Baxter BT, Terrin MC, Dalman RL. Medical management of small abdominal aortic aneurysms. Circulation 2008;117(14):1883–9.

49. Crawford ES, Beckett WC, Greer MS. Juxtarenal infrarenal abdominal aortic aneurysm. Special diagnostic and therapeutic considerations. Ann Surg 1986;203(6):661–70.

50. Qvarfordt PG, Stoney RJ, Reilly LM, et al. Management of pararenal aneurysms of the abdominal aorta. J Vasc Surg 1986;3(1):84–93.

51. Johnston KW, Rutherford RB, Tilson MD, et al. Suggested standards for reporting on arterial aneurysms. Subcommittee on Reporting Standards for Arterial Aneurysms, Ad Hoc Committee on Reporting Standards, Society for Vascular Surgery and North American Chapter, International Society for Cardiovascular Surgery [comment]. J Vasc Surg 1991;13(3):452–8.

52. Ayari R, Paraskevas N, Rosset E, et al. Juxtarenal aneurysm. Comparative study with infrarenal abdominal aortic aneurysm and proposition of a new classification. Eur J Vasc Endovasc Surg 2001;22(2):169–74.

53. Karkos CD, Bruce IA, Thomson GJ, et al. Retroaortic left renal vein and its implications in abdominal aortic surgery. Ann Vasc Surg 2001; 15(6):703–8.

54. Greenhalgh RM, Powell JT. Endovascular repair of abdominal aortic aneurysm. N Engl J Med 2008; 358(5):494–501.

55. Olsen PS, Schroeder T, Agerskov K, et al. Surgery for abdominal aortic aneurysms. A survey of 656 patients. J Cardiovasc Surg 1991;32(5):636–42.

56. Nachbur BH, Inderbitzi RG, Bar W. Isolated iliac aneurysms. Eur J Vasc Surg 1991;5(4):375–81.

57. Sukhija R, Aronow WS, Sandhu R, et al. Mortality and size of abdominal aortic aneurysm at long-term follow-up of patients not treated surgically and treated with and without statins. Am J Cardiol 2006;97(2):279–80.

58. Monge M, Eskandari MK. Strategies for ruptured abdominal aortic aneurysms. J Vasc Interv Radiol 2008;19(6 Suppl):S44–50.

59. Hinchliffe RJ, Hopkinson BR. Ruptured abdominal aortic aneurysm. Time for a new approach. J Cardiovasc Surg 2002;43(3):345–7.

60. Parodi JC, Palmaz JC, Barone HD. Transfemoral intraluminal graft implantation for abdominal aortic aneurysms. Ann Vasc Surg 1991;5(6):491–9.

61. Schwartz SA, Taljanovic MS, Smyth S, et al. CT findings of rupture, impending rupture, and contained rupture of abdominal aortic aneurysms. AJR Am J Roentgenol 2007;188(1):W57–62.

62. Adam DJ, Bradbury AW, Stuart WP, et al. The value of computed tomography in the assessment of suspected ruptured abdominal aortic aneurysm. J Vasc Surg 1998;27(3):431–7.

63. Gloviczki P, Pairolero PC, Mucha P Jr, et al. Ruptured abdominal aortic aneurysms: repair should not be denied [comment]. J Vasc Surg 1992;15(5):851–7 [discussion: 857–9].

64. Siegel CL, Cohan RH, Korobkin M, et al. Abdominal aortic aneurysm morphology: CT features in patients with ruptured and nonruptured aneurysms. AJR Am J Roentgenol 1994; 163(5):1123–9.

65. Arita T, Matsunaga N, Takano K, et al. Abdominal aortic aneurysm: rupture associated with the high-attenuating crescent sign [comment]. Radiology 1997;204(3):765–8.

66. Halliday KE, al-Kutoubi A. Draped aorta: CT sign of contained leak of aortic aneurysms [comment]. Radiology 1996;199(1):41–3.

67. Jones CS, Reilly MK, Dalsing MC, et al. Chronic contained rupture of abdominal aortic aneurysms. Arch Surg 1986;121(5):542–6.

68. De Bakey ME, Cooley DA. Treatment of aneurysms of the aorta by resection and restoration of continuity with aortic homograft. Angiology 1954;5(3): 251–4.

69. Eliason JL, Upchurch GR Jr. Endovascular abdominal aortic aneurysm repair. Circulation 2008; 117(13):1738–44.

70. Tan JW, Yeo KK, Laird JR. Food and Drug Administration-approved endovascular repair devices for abdominal aortic aneurysms: a review. J Vasc Interv Radiol 2008;19(6 Suppl):S9–S17.

71. Sakamoto I, Sueyoshi E, Hazama S, et al. Endovascular treatment of iliac artery aneurysms. Radiographics 2005;25(Suppl 1):S213–27.

72. Leon LR Jr, Mills JL, Psalms SB, et al. A novel hybrid approach to the treatment of common iliac aneurysms: antegrade endovascular hypogastric stent grafting and femorofemoral bypass grafting. J Vasc Surg 2007;45(6):1244–8.

73. Stanley BM, Semmens JB, Lawrence-Brown MM, et al. Fenestration in endovascular grafts for aortic aneurysm repair: new horizons for preserving blood flow in branch vessels [comment]. J Endovasc Ther 2001;8(1):16–24.

74. Chuter TA. Fenestrated and branched stent-grafts for thoracoabdominal, pararenal and juxtarenal aortic aneurysm repair. Semin Vasc Surg 2007; 20(2):90–6.

75. Greenhalgh RM, Brown LC, Kwong GP, et al. Comparison of endovascular aneurysm repair with open repair in patients with abdominal aortic aneurysm (EVAR trial 1), 30-day operative mortality results: randomised controlled trial. Lancet 2004; 364(9437):843–8.

76. Maldonado TS, Ranson ME, Rockman CB, et al. Decreased ischemic complications after endovascular aortic aneurysm repair with newer devices. Vasc Endovascular Surg 2007;41(3):192–9.

77. Greenberg RK, Chuter TA, Lawrence-Brown M, et al. Analysis of renal function after aneurysm repair with a device using suprarenal fixation (Zenith AAA Endovascular Graft) in contrast to open surgical repair. J Vasc Surg 2004;39(6):1219–28 [Erratum appears in J Vasc Surg 2004;40(1):23].

78. Walsh SR, Tang TY, Boyle JR. Renal consequences of endovascular abdominal aortic aneurysm repair. J Endovasc Ther 2008;15(1):73–82.

79. Lederle FA, Johnson GR, Wilson SE, et al. Relationship of age, gender, race, and body size to infrarenal aortic diameter. The Aneurysm Detection and Management (ADAM) Veterans Affairs Cooperative Study Investigators. J Vasc Surg 1997;26(4):595–601.

80. Lipski DA, Ernst CB. Natural history of the residual infrarenal aorta after infrarenal abdominal aortic aneurysm repair. J Vasc Surg 1998;27(5):805–11 [discussion: 811–2].

81. Illig KA, Green RM, Ouriel K, et al. Fate of the proximal aortic cuff: implications for endovascular aneurysm repair. J Vasc Surg 1997;26(3):492–9 [discussion: 499–501].

82. Dick F, Brown LC, Powell JT, et al. Appraisal era for endovascular repair of abdominal aortic aneurysms. Acta Chir Belg 2008;108(3):288–91.

83. Napoli V, Sardella SG, Bargellini I, et al. Evaluation of the proximal aortic neck enlargement following endovascular repair of abdominal aortic aneurysm: 3-years experience. Eur Radiol 2003; 13(8):1962–71.

84. Badger SA, O'Donnell ME, Makar RR, et al. Aortic necks of ruptured abdominal aneurysms dilate

more than asymptomatic aneurysms after endovascular repair. J Vasc Surg 2006;44(2):244–9.

85. Zarins CK, Bloch DA, Crabtree T, et al. Stent graft migration after endovascular aneurysm repair: importance of proximal fixation. J Vasc Surg 2003;38(6):1264–72 [discussion: 1272].

86. May J, White GH, Ly CN, et al. Endoluminal repair of abdominal aortic aneurysm prevents enlargement of the proximal neck: a 9-year life-table and 5-year longitudinal study. J Vasc Surg 2003;37(1):86–90.

87. Corbett TJ, Callanan A, Morris LG, et al. A review of the in vivo and in vitro biomechanical behavior and performance of postoperative abdominal aortic aneurysms and implanted stent-grafts. J Endovasc Ther 2008;15(4):468–84.

88. Sadat U, Boyle JR, Walsh SR, et al. Endovascular vs open repair of acute abdominal aortic aneurysms—a systematic review and meta-analysis [comment]. J Vasc Surg 2008;48(1):227–36.

89. Lovegrove RE, Javid M, Magee TR, et al. A meta-analysis of 21,178 patients undergoing open or endovascular repair of abdominal aortic aneurysm. Br J Surg 2008;95(6):677–84.

90. Lederle FA, Freischlag JA, Kyriakides TC, et al. Outcomes following endovascular vs open repair of abdominal aortic aneurysm: a randomized trial. JAMA 2009;302(14):1535–42.

91. Hobo R, Buth J, collaborators E. Secondary interventions following endovascular abdominal aortic aneurysm repair using current endografts. A EUROSTAR report. J Vasc Surg 2006;43(5): 896–902.

92. van Marrewijk C, Buth J, Harris PL, et al. Significance of endoleaks after endovascular repair of abdominal aortic aneurysms: the EUROSTAR experience. J Vasc Surg 2002;35(3):461–73.

93. Stavropoulos SW, Charagundla SR. Imaging techniques for detection and management of endoleaks after endovascular aortic aneurysm repair. Radiology 2007;243(3):641–55.

94. Bashir MR, Ferral H, Jacobs C, et al. Endoleaks after endovascular abdominal aortic aneurysm repair: management strategies according to CT findings. AJR Am J Roentgenol 2009;192(4): W178–186.

95. Tolia AJ, Landis R, Lamparello P, et al. Type II endoleaks after endovascular repair of abdominal aortic aneurysms: natural history. Radiology 2005; 235(2):683–6.

96. Napoli V, Bargellini I, Sardella SG, et al. Abdominal aortic aneurysm: contrast-enhanced US for missed endoleaks after endoluminal repair. Radiology 2004;233(1):217–25.

97. Gorich J, Rilinger N, Sokiranski R, et al. Leakages after endovascular repair of aortic aneurysms: classification based on findings at CT, angiography, and radiography. Radiology 1999;213(3):767–72.

98. Drury D, Michaels JA, Jones L, et al. Systematic review of recent evidence for the safety and efficacy of elective endovascular repair in the management of infrarenal abdominal aortic aneurysm. Br J Surg 2005;92(8):937–46.

99. ACC/AHA 2005 Practice guidelines for the management of patients with peripheral arterial disease (lower extremity, renal, mesenteric, and abdominal aortic). A collaborative report from the American Association for Vascular Surgery/Society for Vascular Surgery,* Society for Cardiovascular Angiography and Interventions, Society for Vascular Medicine and Biology, Society of Interventional Radiology, and the ACC/AHA Task Force on Practice Guidelines (Writing Committee to Develop Guidelines for the Management of Patients With Peripheral Arterial Disease).

100. Orton DF, LeVeen RF, Saigh JA, et al. Aortic prosthetic graft infections: radiologic manifestations and implications for management. Radiographics 2000;20(4):977–93.

101. Calligaro KD, Veith FJ. Diagnosis and management of infected prosthetic aortic grafts. Surgery 1991; 110(5):805–13.

102. Abdulla A, Yee L. The clinical spectrum of *Clostridium sordellii* bacteraemia: two case reports and a review of the literature. J Clin Pathol 2000; 53(9):709–12.

103. Silva ME, Malogolowkin MH, Hall TR, et al. Mycotic aneurysm of the thoracic aorta due to *Aspergillus terreus*: case report and review. Clin Infect Dis 2000;31(5):1144–8.

104. Belair M, Soulez G, Oliva VL, et al. Aortic graft infection: the value of percutaneous drainage. AJR Am J Roentgenol 1998;171(1):119–24.

105. Sharma P, Kyriakides C. Surveillance of patients post-endovascular aneurysm repair. Postgrad Med J 2007;83(986):750–3.

106. Armerding MD, Rubin GD, Beaulieu CF, et al. Aortic aneurysmal disease: assessment of stent-graft treatment-CT versus conventional angiography. Radiology 2000;215(1):138–46.

107. van der Laan MJ, Bakker CJ, Blankensteijn JD, et al. Dynamic CE-MRA for endoleak classification after endovascular aneurysm repair. Eur J Vasc Endovasc Surg 2006;31(2):130–5.

108. Rozenblit AM, Patlas M, Rosenbaum AT, et al. Detection of endoleaks after endovascular repair of abdominal aortic aneurysm: value of unenhanced and delayed helical CT acquisitions [comment]. Radiology 2003;227(2):426–33.

109. Iezzi R, Cotroneo AR, Filippone A, et al. Multidetector CT in abdominal aortic aneurysm treated with endovascular repair: are unenhanced and delayed phase enhanced images effective for endoleak detection? [comment]. Radiology 2006;241(3): 915–21.

110. Trimarchi S, Tsai T, Eagle KA, et al. Acute abdominal aortic dissection: insight from the International Registry of Acute Aortic Dissection (IRAD). J Vasc Surg 2007;46(5):913–9.

111. Jonker FH, Schlosser FJ, Moll FL, et al. Dissection of the abdominal aorta. Current evidence and implications for treatment strategies: a review and meta-analysis of 92 patients [comment]. J Endovasc Ther 2009;16(1):71–80.

112. Brewster DC. Clinical and anatomical considerations for surgery in aortoiliac disease and results of surgical treatment. Circulation 1991;83(2 Suppl):I42–52.

113. Norgren L, Hiatt WR, Dormandy JA, et al. Inter-Society Consensus for the Management of Peripheral Arterial Disease (TASC II). J Vasc Surg 2007; 45(Suppl S):S5–67.

114. Albrecht T, Foert E, Holtkamp R, et al. 16-MDCT angiography of aortoiliac and lower extremity arteries: comparison with digital subtraction angiography. AJR Am J Roentgenol 2007; 189(3):702–11.

115. Catalano C, Fraioli F, Laghi A, et al. Infrarenal aortic and lower-extremity arterial disease: diagnostic performance of multi-detector row CT angiography. Radiology 2004;231(2):555–63.

116. Heijenbrok-Kal MH, Kock MC, Hunink MG. Lower extremity arterial disease: multidetector CT angiography meta-analysis. Radiology 2007;245(2): 433–9.

117. Willmann JK, Mayer D, Banyai M, et al. Evaluation of peripheral arterial bypass grafts with multidetector row CT angiography: comparison with duplex US and digital subtraction angiography. Radiology 2003;229(2):465–74.

118. Hayashi H, Matsuoka Y, Sakamoto I, et al. Penetrating atherosclerotic ulcer of the aorta: imaging features and disease concept. Radiographics 2000;20(4):995–1005. A review publication of the Radiological Society of North America, Inc.

119. Nucifora G, Hysko F, Vasciaveo A. Blunt traumatic abdominal aortic rupture: CT imaging. Emerg Radiol 2008;15(3):211–3.

120. Mullinix AJ, Foley WD. Multidetector computed tomography and blunt thoracoabdominal trauma. J Comput Assist Tomogr 2004;28(Suppl 1):S20–27.

121. Gotway MB, Araoz PA, Macedo TA, et al. Imaging findings in Takayasu's arteritis. AJR Am J Roentgenol 2005;184(6):1945–50.

122. Sueyoshi E, Sakamoto I, Hayashi K. Aortic aneurysms in patients with Takayasu's arteritis: CT evaluation. AJR Am J Roentgenol 2000;175(6):1727–33.

CT Angiography of the Hepatic and Pancreatic Circulation

Rocio Perez-Johnston, MD, Dipti K. Lenhart, MD,
Dushyant V. Sahani, MD*

KEYWORDS

- Multidetector computed tomography angiography
- Hepatic imaging • Pancreatic imaging

The technological development of the multidetector computed tomography (MDCT) scanner allows not only a more rapid acquisition of axial images but also volumetric scanning in a desired anatomic area during selected phases of contrast enhancement. MDCT angiography (MDCTA) has become an established noninvasive imaging method to define vascular anatomy and pathology affecting vascular structures, as well as for presurgical treatment planning.[1,2]

The liver and pancreas are part of the mesenteric circulation and have inherently complex vascular anatomy. Therefore, to facilitate treatment decisions for tumors and minimize inadvertent surgical complications, adequate definition of the vascular structures of each organ is crucial.

The MDCT technology itself is constantly evolving and to exploit the full potential of these new developments in MDCT, scan protocol optimization has become paramount. This review focuses on various technical factors integral to MDCT protocols for CTA applications in the liver and pancreas (Table 1).

MDCT TECHNIQUES

Recent advances in MDCT scanners have provided multiphasic acquisition of abdominal organs in the optimal phase of enhancement and with improved 2-dimensional (2D) and 3D image display. In general, fast acquisition with appropriate thin slices and scanning delays are crucial components of an optimal MDCTA protocol.

Technical Factors

Distention of the stomach and duodenum is usually beneficial and in our practice patients drink from 500 to 1000 mL of water 20 to 30 minutes before the scan, and an additional 300 to 500 mL is administered immediately before the scan. Water or other oral contrast materials with neutral attenuation are preferred over radiopaque contrast, as the latter can interfere with high-attenuation structures such as hyperenhancing tumors and vessels in the vicinity of the stomach and duodenum on the 2D and 3D image display. Moreover, the natural density of water on CT also more confidently defines the periampullary anatomy and adjacent lesions.

Unenhanced CT

In our institution, unenhanced images are acquired first, using 5- to 10-mm slice thickness and a low mA (150–250) approach to cover the organ of interest. The role of unenhanced CT is controversial but usually helps with selecting the coverage for the CTA portion. It is agreed that it has a limited diagnostic role.

Contrast media protocol

Good intravenous access with an 18- to 20-gauge catheter is recommended to sustain faster

Disclosure: The authors have nothing to disclose.
Division of Abdominal Imaging and Intervention, Department of Imaging, Massachusetts General Hospital, 270 White, 55 Fruit Street, Boston, MA 02114, USA
* Corresponding author.
E-mail address: dsahani@partners.org

Radiol Clin N Am 48 (2010) 311–330
doi:10.1016/j.rcl.2010.02.021

Table 1
Major indications of MDCTA of the liver and pancreas

	Indication
Liver	Surgical planning: hepatic transplantation, primary and metastatic neoplasms Vascular pathology: arterial (aneurysms), portal (thrombosis, aneurysms), venous (Budd-Chiari syndrome) Pseudolesions: arterial and venous shunts Neoplasms: HCC
Pancreas	Pancreatic adenocarcinoma staging Hypervascular lesions (neuroendocrine tumor and metastases) Complications of pancreatitis

Abbreviations: HCC, hepatocellular carcinoma; MDCTA, multidetector computed tomography angiography.

injection for the CTA. Typically 100 to 120 mL of nonionic iodinated contrast material (CM) (300–370 mg of iodine/mL) is bolus injected at a rate of 4 to 5 mL per second. The initial arterial/pancreatic phase is acquired using slice thickness of 0.625 to 1.250 mm, covering the upper abdomen only. The venous phase is acquired subsequently at a delay of 65 to 70 seconds using 2.5- to 5.0-mm-thick slices. The technical parameters are listed in Table 2.

The newest MDCT technology offers flexibility with scan parameters and therefore a stringent scanning approach is not always needed. However, the overall quality of MDCTA is dependent on adequately selecting appropriate scanning and CM protocol variables. It is generally agreed that thinner collimation is desired for small lesion detection and local staging. In addition, the processed 2D and 3D image quality is also influenced by near isotropic data and a collimation of 1.25 to 2.50 mm is considered optimal to meet these objectives.[3]

With the advent of newer MDCT scanners from various vendors that offer 64 detector rows and more, the technical parameters vary and these have been listed in Table 3.

Image acquisition
Arterial phase Early or true arterial phase images are generally preferred for vascular/arterial imaging to map vascular anatomy, such as in preoperative evaluation for living liver donor evaluation (Box 1). This phase occurs within seconds of CM arrival in the abdominal aorta. A late arterial phase is advocated when hypervascular lesions of the liver or pancreas are suspected (Figs. 1 and 2). The different phases for both liver and pancreas acquisitions are summarized in Fig. 1.

Hepatic phases The dual blood supply of the liver must to be taken into consideration for protocol

Table 2
Technical parameter for MDCTA scanning with fixed delays as used in our institution

	Slice Thickness (mm)	Slice Interval (mm)	kV	mA	Pitch-Tube Rotation(s)	Fixed Delay Rate Injection (mL/s)	Delay (s)	Retro Recon
Unenhanced	5	5	120	150–450	1.375–0.5			
MDCTA-arterial phase	0.625	0.625	120–140	150–715	1.375–0.5	5 4 3	20 25 30	2.5 mm
MDCTA-pancreatic phase	0.625	0.625	120–140	150–715	1.375–0.5	5 4 3	40 45 50	2.5 mm
Portal venous phase	2.5	2.5	120	150–450	1.375–0.5	5 4 3	40 45 50	5.0 mm

Abbreviation: MDCTA, multidetector computed tomography angiography.

Table 3
Proposed MDCTA scanning parameters according to different vendors

	GE LightSpeed VCT	Philips Brilliance 64	Siemens Sensation 64	Toshiba Aquilion 64
Detector configuration (inner rows)	64 × 0.625 mm	64 × 0.625 mm	32 × 0.6 mm	64 × 0.5 mm
Detector configuration (outer rows)	NA	NA	8 × 1.2 mm	NA
Z-axis detector length (64-slice mode), mm	40	40	19.2	32
Fastest gantry rotation, s	0.4	0.40	0.33	0.40
Scan field of view, mm	25, 50	25–50	50 (option to 70)	18,24,32,40,50
Coverage in 1 second with a pitch of 1 in 64-slice mode, mm	80	80	38.4	80
X-ray generator power, kW	100	60	80	60
Anode heat capacity, MHU	8	8	Equivalent to 30	8
Maximum mA at 120 kV	800	500	665	500
Matrix	512	512,768,1028	512	512
Automatic dose reduction	3D dose modulation	Dose right	Care dose 4D	Sure exposure
Simultaneous ATCM in x-y and z-planes	Yes	Yes	Yes	Yes
Cone beam reconstruction algorithm	3 D	3 D	3 D	3 D
Automatic reformation in multiple planes	Source axial images	Source axial images	Raw data	Source axial images
Simultaneous functions	Yes	Yes	Yes	Yes
Speed of reconstruction, frame/s	22	14	2	2

Abbreviations: ATCM, automated tube current modulation; GE, General Electric Medical Systems, Milwaukee, WI; MDCTA, multidetector computed tomography angiography; NA, not applied; Philips, Philips Medical Systems, Best, the Netherlands; Siemens, Siemens Medical Solutions, Forchheim, Germany; Toshiba Medical Systems, Tochigi, Japan.

optimization. Typically the liver derives about 20% to 25% of its supply from arterial circulation and the remaining dominant 75% to 80% blood flow from the portal venous system. Liver tumors and other hypervascular lesions obtain their blood supply preferentially from the hepatic arteries, having an earlier enhancement than the rest of the parenchyma, best depicted in a late arterial phase at 15 seconds after the CM is in the aorta or 35 to 45 seconds after CM injection.[4]

Maximal enhancement of the liver parenchyma occurs in the portal phase, approximately 40 to 50 seconds after aortic enhancement or approximately 65 to 75 seconds after start of injection, depending of the rate of CM injection and the patient's cardiac status (Fig. 3).

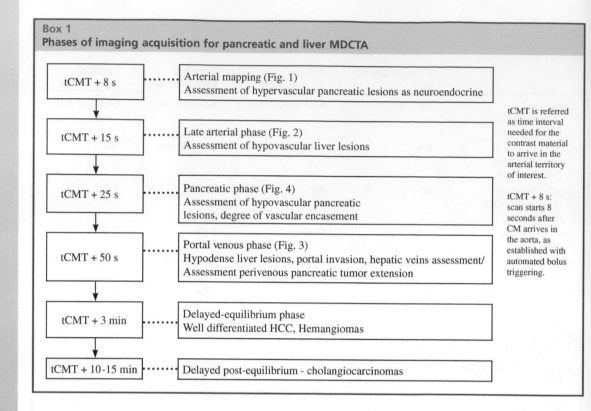

Box 1
Phases of imaging acquisition for pancreatic and liver MDCTA

tCMT + 8 s	Arterial mapping (Fig. 1) Assessment of hypervascular pancreatic lesions as neuroendocrine
tCMT + 15 s	Late arterial phase (Fig. 2) Assessment of hypovascular liver lesions
tCMT + 25 s	Pancreatic phase (Fig. 4) Assessment of hypovascular pancreatic lesions, degree of vascular encasement
tCMT + 50 s	Portal venous phase (Fig. 3) Hypodense liver lesions, portal invasion, hepatic veins assessment/ Assessment perivenous pancreatic tumor extension
tCMT + 3 min	Delayed-equilibrium phase Well differentiated HCC, Hemangiomas
tCMT + 10-15 min	Delayed post-equilibrium - cholangiocarcinomas

tCMT is referred as time interval needed for the contrast material to arrive in the arterial territory of interest.

tCMT + 8 s: scan starts 8 seconds after CM arrives in the aorta, as established with automated bolus triggering.

A delayed/equilibrium phase at 3 to 5 minutes after injection can complement the previous phases improving the characterization of certain liver lesions as hepatocellular carcinomas, especially in cirrhotic livers.

Pancreatic phases If a hypervascular pancreatic lesion is suspected or is being followed, the scanning protocol should be focused on an arterial phase of acquisition at 10 to 15 seconds after aortic opacification (similar to the protocol for hypervascular liver lesions).[5]

Because MDCTA for the pancreas is often undertaken for neoplasm staging, optimal parenchymal lesion conspicuity and vascular enhancement are 2 critical prerequisites. Hypovascular lesions such as adenocarcinoma are best appreciated when the pancreatic parenchyma enhancement is maximized (**Fig. 4**). Several approaches have been proposed to achieve optimal pancreatic

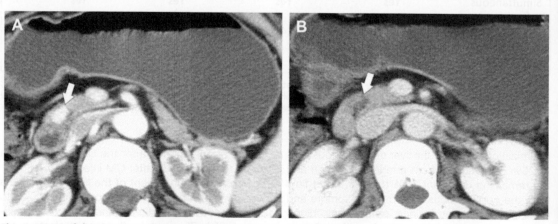

Fig. 1. MDCT of the pancreas of a 41-year-old female patient. (*A*) MDCTA image through the pancreas acquired in the arterial phase demonstrates a hypervascular mass (*arrow*) in the uncinate process, which becomes iso-hypodense (*arrow*) and less conspicuous in the portal venous phase (*B*).

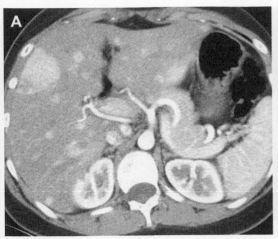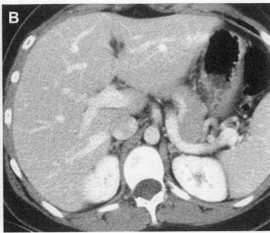

Fig. 2. MDCT axial images from the arterial (*A*) and portal (*B*) phase from a 69-year-old patient with terminal ileum carcinoid are shown. On the arterial phase image, multiple hyperdense lesions are noted that become isodense to liver parenchyma in the portal phase and therefore are difficult to visualize. This case highlights the value of optimal phase imaging for detecting hypervasular tumors.

phase acquisition. Using a CM test bolus or automated scan triggering approach, the best lesion-to-background contrast can be achieved between 20 and 25 seconds after CM arrival in the aorta.[6] However, most investigators advocate scanning in the late pancreatic phase using an empiric delay of 40 to 50 seconds from CM injection to achieve a late pancreatic phase of enhancement.[7] This delay also facilitates adequate vascular enhancement along with tumor detection for assessing local staging.

The portal venous phase is considered best for detecting metastases to liver and elsewhere in the abdomen and for portal vein enhancement.

Contrast Material

Volume

High-quality MDCTA requires sufficient contrast enhancement, which depends on iodine administration rate and injection duration, as well as the cardiac output and body weight of the patient.[5] It is preferable to adjust the CM volume based on its iodine concentration and body weight. For example, for CM of 300 mgI/mL, a total of 100- to 150-mL range can be used, whereas when a higher concentration of CM of 350 to 370 mgI/mL is being used, a CM dose of 80 to 120 mL is sufficient.[8]

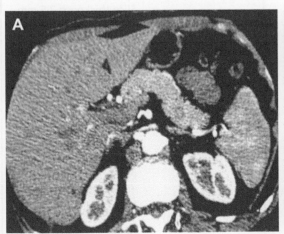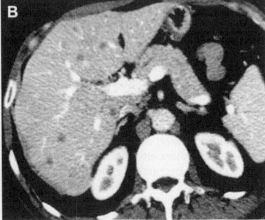

Fig. 3. Liver metastases detection on MDCT examination. (*A*) Arterial phase image shows subtle hypodense lesions in the liver without discernable tumors. (*B*) However, on the portal venous phase, multiple small hypodense tumors are now obvious.

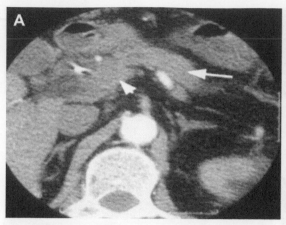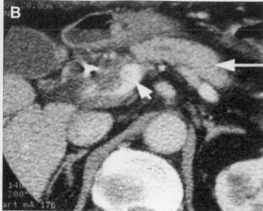

Fig. 4. CTA images from a patient with pancreatic adenocarcinoma. (*A*) Arterial image demonstrates suboptimal SMV enhancement (*short arrow*) and poor conspicuity of the tumor in the pancreatic head as the pancreatic parenchyma is not yet enhancing (*long arrow*). (*B*) In the corresponding pancreatic phase, the parenchymal enhancement is now improved (*long arrow*) with better conspicuity of the adenocarcinoma in the head of the pancreas, that is also partially involving the SMV (*short arrow*).

Iodine flux/rate of administration

Generally, CM injections at 3 to 5 mL/s have been shown to work effectively in obtaining a good-quality CTA examination. However, with the faster MDCT scanners, a rate of 5 mL/s is preferred because of its benefits for shortening the injection duration to match up with the scanning duration, thereby influencing CTA quality and optimal vascular enhancement.[9–11] Although injection rates as high as 8 mL/s have been used in clinical studies to improve tumor-to-parenchyma contrast, in general their use is not supported in the outpatient clinical practice owing to inherent increase in CM extravasation risks.[6]

Scan delay

The timing of CM delivery with respect to scan acquisition is crucial and there are several methods to determine an appropriate scan delay. An empiric delay that is fixed and based on the average organ circulation time for a given contrast medium injection rate is the most commonly used approach (as in our institution) (see Table 2). Alternatively, a small bolus of CM can be injected to determine the peak enhancement time in the desired vessel and adjust the scan delay accordingly (see Fig. 1).

Maintaining a fixed delay to match the expected phase of CM enhancement is the most commonly used technique because of ease of use and practical application in the outpatient setting. However, variable CM injection and cardiac output are not always accounted for by this approach, affecting the quality of vascular/organ enhancement in certain patients. With faster MDCT scanners, most centers with a high-volume MDCTA practice

use a test bolus or automated bolus-tracking technique.

Automated bolus tracking is more often used than the test-bolus technique because it is simpler to perform and it reduces the total CM dose. With bolus-tracking technique, scan acquisition can be performed sequentially during the respective phases of arterial, venous, and organ enhancement.[12]

Table 4 Adjustment of the protocol according to patient's weight, venous access, and renal function	
Large patients >300 pounds	kVP: 120–140 Maximize mA Speed rotation: 0.8–1.0 s Slice thickness: 2.5 mm Rate of injection: 5.5–6.0 mL/s
Patients <200 pounds	kVP: 80–100 in arterial phase
Compromised renal function (eGFR 30–45 mL/min/m²)	Pre-scan: IV saline hydration Volume contrast: 60–75 mL Saline flush: 40 mL Rate of injection: 3.5–4.5 mL/s Post-scan: IV saline hydration
Poor venous access (over 20 gauge)	Rate of injection: 2.5–3 mL/s Delay: use automated trigger

Abbreviation: IV, intravenous.

Irrespective of the use of scan delay technique, it is generally agreed that a saline chaser/flush of 30 to 40 mL not only decreases the artifacts in the subclavian vein, it also improves the iodine flux and provides more uniform vascular enhancement.[13]

Special Considerations

There are certain circumstances in which the defined protocols should be modified (Table 4).

Large body habitus

Patient body size and weight can affect the performance of CTA examination. Typically, image quality degradation from excessive noise as a result of inadequate beam penetration and field of view restrictions is the main concern in these patients. In our practice, for patients weighing more than 300 pounds, we increase the radiation delivery and beam penetration by using a kVP of 140 and increasing the effective mA to the maximum allowed on the scanner. Likewise, the rotation of the gantry is decreased to 0.8 to 1.0 second and the slice thickness is set at more than 2 mm to decrease image noise. The CM injection rate is increased by 0.5 to 1.0 mL/s faster than the standard rate of injection.

Compromised renal function

In patients with an estimated glomerular filtration rate (eGFR) less than 45 mL/min/m^2, risk of CM-induced nephropathy (CIN) can be minimized by adequate intravenous (IV) hydration before and after the IV CM injection. It is also recommended that the CM load be decreased by 20% to 30% of the calculated dose. It has been shown that the use of 60 to 75 mL of CM administered at 3.5 to 4.5 mL/s combined with the use of a 50-mL saline flush provides an adequate-quality examination. In our practice, eGFR of 30 mL/min/m^2 or less is considered a contraindication for IV CM administration.

Venous access issues

In patients with poor IV access, CM injection rate should be adjusted to 3 mL/s to minimize the risks of extravasation and arterial phase imaging initiated at 45 to 55 seconds or determined using automatic bolus triggering.

POSTPROCESSING TECHNIQUES

The liver and pancreas have complex diagnostic and management needs; therefore, imaging postprocessing is now integral to all CTA applications in these organs.[14] Although a variety of postprocessing protocols have been advocated, the most frequently used approaches include multiplanar reconstruction (MPR), maximum intensity projections (MIP), minimum intensity projections (MinIP), volume rendering (VR), 3D, and curved planar reformation (CPR). Each has a specific role for assessing regional anatomy and relationship of lesions in the vicinity (Fig. 5). The postprocessing protocols used in our institution are listed in Tables 5 and 6.

Modern hepatic and pancreatic surgery is based on knowledge of the distribution and variations of vasculature. Preoperative MDCTA provides essential information for planning the surgical procedures and routes of access.

The celiac trunk is the first major aortic branch below the diaphragm, giving rise to 3 vessels:

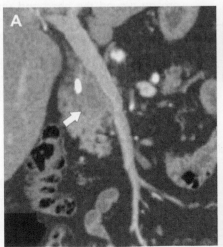
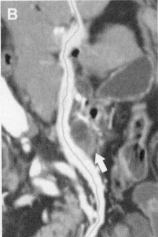

Fig. 5. MDCTA visualization tools for assessing tumor-vascular relationship. (A, B) Images from 2 different patients with adenocarcinoma of the pancreas that were created along the SMV–portal vein axis enable more obvious assessment of the tumor relationship with the critical venous structures in the vicinity (arrow).

Table 5
Postprocessed views for liver MDCTA

Anatomic structure assessed	Best postprocessing view
Hepatic artery	3D vascular maps
Portal pedicle	Coronal MPR and VR
Hepatic veins and IVC	Axial and coronal MPR and MIP
Biliary ductal anatomy	Coronal oblique MPR, VR, and MinIP

Abbreviations: IVC, inferior vena cava; MDCTA, multidetector computed tomography angiography; MinIP, minimum intensity projections; MIP, maximum intensity projections; MPR, multiplanar reconstruction; VR, volume rendering; 3D, 3-dimensional.

common hepatic artery, splenic artery, and left gastric artery. The superior mesenteric and inferior mesenteric arteries are the next anterior visceral branches.

The hepatic artery originates from the celiac trunk and divides into right and left branches; its branches classically follow the portal vein and bile duct distribution. The most frequent anatomic variation of the arterial hepatic system is a replaced right hepatic artery (arising from the superior mesenteric artery), present in up to 18% of patients (Fig. 6). The next most common variation is a replaced left hepatic artery arising from the left gastric artery.

The portal vein is formed by the confluence of the superior mesenteric vein (SMV) and splenic vein posterior to the neck of the pancreas. Most commonly, it divides into the right and left portal veins at the porta hepatis. The right portal vein

Table 6
Postprocessed views of pancreas MDCTA

Anatomic structure assessed	Best postprocessing view
Portal vein and superior mesenteric vein	CPR, MIP, VR
Celiac trunk and branches	Coronal and sagittal MPR, coronal VR
Superior mesenteric artery	CPR, MIP, VR
Pancreatic duct, common bile duct	CPR

Abbreviations: CPR, curved planar reformation; MDCTA, multidetector computed tomography angiography; MIP, maximum intensity projections; MPR, multiplanar reconstruction; VR, volume rendering.

divides into anterior and posterior branches that subdivide into superior and inferior branches to supply the segments of the right lobe. The left portal vein initially has a horizontal course to the left and then turns medially and anteriorly toward the ligamentum teres, supplying the lateral segments of the left lobe. It courses anteriorly in a concave curve to end in the superior and inferior branches supplying the medial segments of the left lobe (Fig. 7).

There are 3 hepatic veins. The right hepatic vein drains segments V, VI, and VII; the middle hepatic vein drains segments IV, V, and VIII; and the left vein drains segments II and III. In more than 60% of the population, the middle and left hepatic veins form a common vessel that drains directly into the inferior vena cava (IVC). An inferior accessory right hepatic vein is not uncommon and drains hepatic segment VI. Anatomic variations are important to appreciate before hepatic transplantation.

The arterial blood supply of the pancreas is derived from the celiac trunk and the superior mesenteric artery (SMA). The splenic artery courses along the superior margin of the pancreas, giving rise to the dorsal pancreatic artery, pancreatica magna artery, and distal arterial branches to the tail. The SMA arises from the aorta just below the celiac trunk and posterior to the pancreatic neck; it courses inferiorly to become anterior to the uncinate process of the pancreas, alongside the SMV (Fig. 8). In a minority of patients, the dorsal pancreatic artery arises from the SMA.

The gastroduodenal artery, which arises from the common hepatic artery, branches into the anterior and superior pancreatoduodenal arteries, which in turn anastomose with the inferior pancreaticoduodenal branch of the SMA, forming an arcade around the head and uncinate process. The transverse pancreatic artery connects the pancreaticoduodenal arcade, dorsal pancreatic, and pancreatica magna arteries.

The splenic vein is posterior to the body and tail of the pancreas and joins the SMV behind the neck to form the portal vein (see Fig. 8).

LIVER MDCTA
Surgical Planning

Hepatic transplantation
MDCTA is now the standard of care in the surgical planning for living liver donors, in which most of the right hepatic lobe with accompanying vessels and ducts is removed for transplantation to the recipient. This knowledge provides a better outcome for the recipient and minimizes risk to the donor. It is critical that the residual liver in the donor has sufficient volume and intact vascular supply and

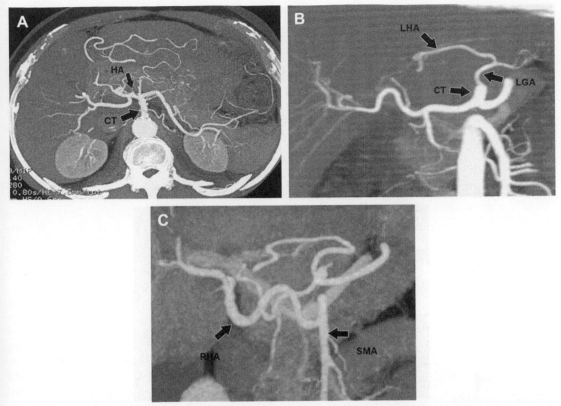

Fig. 6. MDCTA of the liver in arterial phase demonstrating arterial vascular anatomy from 3 different patients. (*A*) Axial MIP image showing the hepatic artery (HA) arising from the celiac trunk (CT). (*B, C*) Replaced left and right hepatic arteries (LHA and RHA) from the left gastric artery and SMA, respectively. Preoperative knowledge of this vascular variant is important before liver transplantation of the recipient and before placement of an intrarterial chemotherapy infusion pump.

biliary and venous drainage to sustain the donor's metabolic needs.[15] Relevant anatomic variants that can influence patient selection and surgical technique are summarized in **Table 7**, but their details are outside the scope of this review.

Other surgical procedures
In patients requiring major hepatectomies for primary neoplasms or metastatic disease, detailed assessment of the tumor and its relationship to critical vascular structures and the biliary tree are often needed to facilitate successful liver resection and obviate inadvertent injury to remaining liver parenchyma.[16]

In patients considered for intra-arterial (IA) chemotherapy pump placement for treatment of primary or metastatic disease, success depends on device placement, in turn dependent upon knowledge of hepatic arterial anatomy as well as tumor sensitivity to the chemotherapy agent.[17] Anomalous arteries may require ligation/

embolization or might render a patient unsuitable for IA pump placement.

Hepatocellular Carcinoma
Hepatocellular carcinoma (HCC) is the most frequent liver malignancy worldwide. Although not a prerequisite, most HCCs develop in the setting of chronic liver disease or cirrhotic livers. HCC may present as a solitary mass, multifocal nodules, or diffuse disease throughout the liver (**Fig. 9**). When infiltrative, HCCs usually have irregular borders and indistinct margins with invasion of the portal or hepatic veins.

Several recent studies have reported the overall sensitivity of dual-phase MDCT for HCC detection of about 86%. However, MDCT performance is dependent on tumor size, as it drops to about 60% for tumors with a diameter of 2 cm or smaller.[18,19]

On CT, an early arterial phase enhancement with a rapid washout in the portal venous phase with or

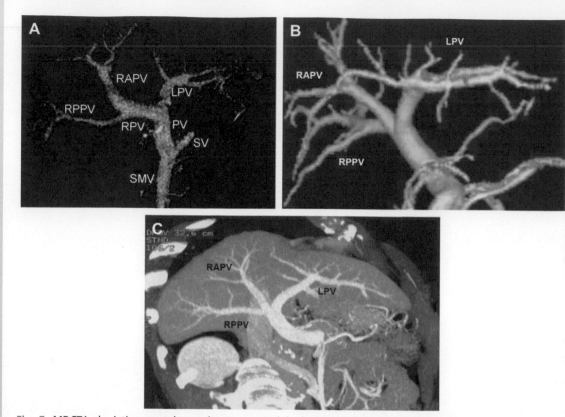

Fig. 7. MDCTA depicting portal vascular anatomy. (*A*) Three-dimensional vascular mapping showing normal portal anatomy. Main portal vein divides into right and left portal veins. The right portal vein (RPV) branches into anterior (RAPV) and posterior (RPPV) branches; the left portal vein (LPV) branches into medial and lateral branches. (*B, C*) Coronal MIP and 3D volume rendering images in the portal venous phase demonstrating portal trifurcation into the right anterior portal vein (RAPV), right posterior portal vein (RPPV), and left portal vein (LPV). This anatomic variant is important in presurgical planning of living donor liver transplantation.

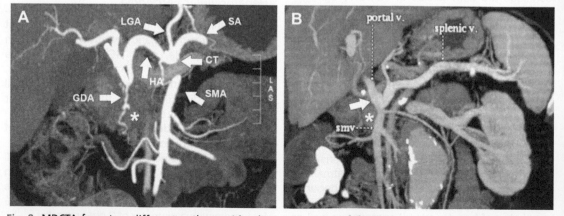

Fig. 8. MDCTA from two different patients with adenocarcionoma of the pancreas showing vascular structures with close relationship to the tumor. Coronal MIP images demonstrating pancreatic tumor (*) encasing the gastroduodenal artery (GDA) (*arrow* in image *A*) and portosplenic confluence vein (*arrow* in image *B*).

Table 7
Relevant anatomic variants of hepatic vasculature for pretransplant assessment and tumor resection planning

	Liver Transplant Donor	Liver Neoplasms
Hepatic arterial variants	MHA from RHA CHA trifurcation into RHA, LHA, and GDA	Replaced RHA and LHA Accessory RHA and LHA Origin of hepatic trunk from SMA or LGA
Hepatic venous variants	Accessory inferior RHV	Segment VIII drainage into MHV Accessory MHV draining directly into IVC Accessory inferior hepatic veins of segments V and VI draining directly into IVC
Portal variants	Trifurcation of portal vein	Trifurcation of portal vein Right and left portal veins supplying segment VIII

Abbreviations: CHA, common hepatic artery; GDA gastroduodenal artery; IVC, inferior vena cava; LGA, left gastric artery; RHA, MHA, and LHA, right, middle, and left hepatic arteries; RHV, MHV, and LHV, right, middle, and left hepatic veins; SMA, superior mesenteric artery.

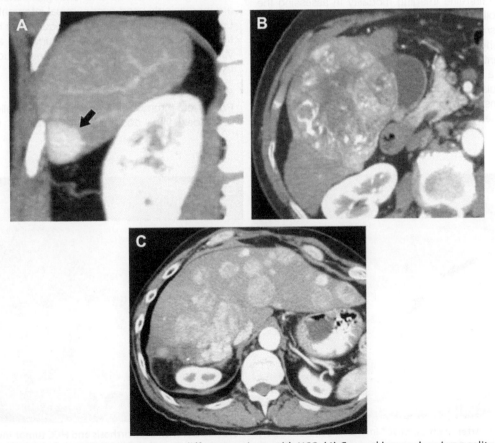

Fig. 9. Arterial phase MDCT images from 3 different patients with HCC. (*A*) Coronal image showing a solitary 2.5-cm homogeneously enhancing HCC (*arrow*). (*B*) In another patient, a large, heterogeneously enhancing mass with central hypoattenuating area, corresponding to central necrosis, is shown. (*C*) Multifocal tumors showing arterial phase enhancement are scattered throughout the liver parenchyma.

without a pseudocapsule is a typical presentation. However, tumor vascularity is dependent on the grade of malignancy and neoangiogenesis.[20]

Low-grade tumors smaller than 2 cm in diameter may have relatively limited arterial blood supply, demonstrate delayed enhancement in the early portal phase, and become more conspicuous as hypoenhancing lesions on delayed equilibrium phase images at 3 minutes. Some investigators advocate the routine use of delayed equilibrium phase images, as this increases diagnostic performance and may help differentiate HCC from arterioportal shunts in cirrhotic livers.[21]

A minority of patients develop HCC in the absence of cirrhosis or known risk factors. These tumors generally occur in younger patients, and are usually larger, solitary, and encapsulated masses or dominant lesions with satellite tumors.[22]

Hepatic resection is the mainstay of curative therapy for localized HCC. MDCTA by demonstrating the relationship of the tumor to major intrahepatic vessels, tumor invasion of the IVC or main portal vein, and the presence of satellite nodules, is the first-line imaging modality in assessing the feasibility of hepatic resection. For cirrhotic patients with small HCCs, liver transplantation has been established as an alternative curative treatment. It is currently agreed that patients with solitary HCC with a diameter smaller than 5 cm without gross vascular invasion, or the presence of fewer than 3 lesions measuring smaller than 3 cm in diameter, are the best candidates for this approach.[23,24]

Vascular Liver Pathology

Hepatic artery aneurysm

Hepatic artery aneurysms are the second most common visceral artery aneurysms. The most common causes reported are mediolysis, trauma, iatrogenic, and mycotic aneurysms.[25] Up to 80% of spontaneous hepatic artery aneurysms are solitary and have an extrahepatic location at the level of the common hepatic or right hepatic arteries. Often, these are incidentally detected on imaging studies but when symptomatic, they frequently present because of rupture or gastrointestinal bleeding. Intrahepatic aneurysms may rupture into the hepatobiliary system leading to the classic triad of biliary colic, hematobilia, and jaundice.[26] On MDCTA, aneurysms of the hepatic artery may be viewed as fusiform dilatation of the vessel or as a saccular arterial enhancing structure connecting with the hepatic artery.

Management is usually dependent on the size of the lesion and the regional vascular anatomy. Catheter-based endovascular approaches, including embolization and endograft exclusion, are increasingly used over surgical intervention.[27] Large proximal aneurysms may require liver resection. Extrahepatic aneurysm may undergo aneurysmorrhaphy, resection, and interposition or bypass grafting.

Portal vein thrombosis

Portal vein thrombosis is frequently a complication of preexisting abdominal malignancy (HCC,

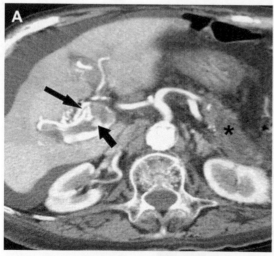 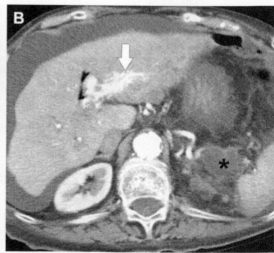

Fig. 10. Arterial phase MDCT images (*A, B*) from a 59-year-old patient with liver cirrhosis and HCC tumor invasion into the portal vein (primary tumor not shown). In the arterial phase, a large filling defect is seen in the right portal vein (*thin arrow*). Note focal areas of thrombus enhancement, indicating tumor thrombus. Early enhancement of the left portal vein (*white arrow*) due to arterioportal fistula in the tumor thrombus in the left lobe. A synchronous pancreatic neoplasms (*) was diagnosed.

pancreatic carcinoma) or abdominal inflammation such as pancreatitis, diverticulitis, or appendicitis.[28]

On MDCTA, an acute portal vein thrombus can be hyperdense and obscured on contrast-enhanced MDCTA. Chronic portal vein thrombus is relatively hypodense to adjacent soft tissues, presenting as a clearly defined filling defect within the enhanced portal vein lumen. The hepatic segment supplied by the occluded venous branch appears hyperdense on arterial phase imaging owing to compensatory arterial flow, and hypodense in comparison with the remaining hepatic parenchyma on the portal venous phase imaging (Fig. 10).[29]

Portal venous invasion is one of the most important prognostic factors affecting recurrence and survival after surgical resection of hepatic malignancies.[30] Diagnostic features are neovascularity and enhancement of an expansile intraluminal portal vein.[31] Intense enhancement is more associated with HCC over other malignancies (Fig. 11).[32]

When segmental occlusion of the portal venous system occurs, local collateral venous pathways form relatively quickly in response to occlusion of the main portal vein or one of its intrahepatic branches. Cavernous transformation of the portal vein is defined as a masslike network of intertwined veins in the hepatoduodenal ligament and porta hepatis that provide an alternative pathway around an occluded main portal vein or lobar branch. Compensatory arterial flow to the peripheral segments of the liver deprived of portal venous flow occurs and results in hyperattenuation in the arterial phase.

The central portion of the liver enhances in the portal phase as the cavernoma provides adequate flow to the central liver.

Other than in the setting of malignancy or inflammatory processes, portal cavernomas have also been reported as a congenital malformation in a nondeveloped portal vein and in patients with hemangioma of the portal vein.[33]

Budd-Chiari syndrome

Budd-Chiari syndrome represents a spectrum of disease resulting from hepatic venous outflow obstruction, which can occur at the level of the hepatic veins, IVC, or right atrium. The most common causes are myeloproliferative disorders such as polycythemia vera and use of oral contraceptives. Other less common known associated pathologies are hepatitis, hepatic abscesses, trauma, polycystic liver disease.[34]

The MDCTA imaging findings of Budd-Chiari syndrome depend on whether the disease is acute or chronic. In acute presentation, the parenchyma is enlarged and diffusely hypodense in unenhanced phase. The IVC and hepatic veins can be hyperdense because of the presence of thrombus. On arterial phase, there is early enhancement of the caudate lobe and central portion of the liver, as well as decreased peripheral enhancement (Fig. 12). On portal venous phase, no collateral veins are present and there is reverse pattern of enhancement, in which the central area of the liver is hypodense and the periphery displays increased attenuation with accumulation of contrast material in the subcapsular veins.

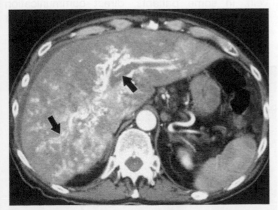

Fig. 11. A 63-year-old man with multifocal hepatocellular carcinoma and tumor invasion in the portal vein. CECT image obtained in the arterial phase demonstrates multiple enhancing tumor foci in both lobes of the liver along with enhancing thrombus in right and left branches of the portal vein causing portal vein expansion (*arrows*).

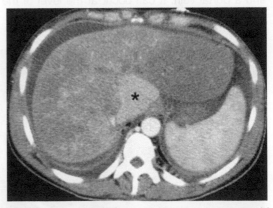

Fig. 12. Acute Budd-Chiari syndrome in a 53-year-old female patient. Axial contrast-enhanced image in arterial phase, with early enhancement of the caudate lobe (*) as well as central portion of the liver, and heterogeneous diminished perfusion of the peripheral hepatic segments.

In chronic Budd-Chiari syndrome, the liver appears irregular, with caudate lobe hypertrophy and atrophy of the peripheral segments, resulting in a caudate lobe to right lobe ratio of more than 0.55.[35] On arterial phase, there is heterogeneous enhancement of the parenchyma, with regenerative macronodules (ranging from 1 to 4 cm) that enhance homogeneously with or without a hypoattenuating rim.[36] Collateral circulatory portosystemic and intrahepatic pathways develop, with obliteration of the IVC, hepatic veins, or both. Other extrahepatic findings are ascites and splenomegaly.

In the setting of chronic disease, it is important to distinguish macronodules from small HCC, which usually enhance heterogeneously in the arterial phase and demonstrate washout in the portal venous phase. The morphologic characteristics of the liver and the clinical setting should help in differentiating them.[36]

It is critical to adequately diagnose Budd-Chiari syndrome, because if untreated, it has a mortality rate of 80%, with liver failure as the primary cause of death.[37] If patients with Budd-Chiari syndrome deteriorate despite medical treatment, decompressive portosystemic transjugular or surgical shunting must be considered. Before these procedures, patients need accurate vascular mapping and evaluation with MDCTA or magnetic resonance angiography to evaluate patency of hepatic, portal, and splanchnic veins.[38]

Pseudolesions/Shunts

Arterioportal shunts

An arterioportal (AP) shunt is defined as a direct communication between a hepatic arterial branch and a portal vein. It can occur at the level of the portal trunk, sinusoids, or peribiliary venules.[39]

AP shunts can occur following trauma, instrumentation, in association with a liver lesion, or can be congenital (as in Rendu-Osler-Weber disease). Spontaneous small arterioportal shunts may occur in a cirrhotic liver. In the setting of a liver lesion, they are associated with HCC and small hemangiomas. On MDCTA, the arterial phase shows a small, peripheral, enhancing focus, occasionally wedge-shaped, displaying early enhancement of the portal vein before the opacification to the main portal vein (Fig. 13). The arterioportal shunt becomes isoattenuating to the liver and vasculature in the portal venous phase.[40] The most important role of imaging when an early-enhancing focus is observed is to differentiate it from a small HCC, which is usually hypodense when compared with the parenchyma on portal venous phases (Fig. 14). When doubt persists, a follow-up in 6 months should be established, or complementary imaging should be performed with MR.[41]

Portosystemic shunts

An intrahepatic portosystemic venous shunt is a rare condition defined as communication between a systemic vein and a portal vein via an anomalous channel. It can be congenital or acquired. The most frequent portosystemic shunt occurs between the right portal vein and the IVC.[42] Clinical manifestation depends on shunt flow; a low-flow shunt can be asymptomatic, whereas a high-flow shunt can cause encephalopathy and hypoglycemia. On MDCTA, the most common finding on the portal venous phase is asymmetric enhancement of the draining hepatic vein. In some patients, direct communication between the portal vein branch and adjacent hepatic vein can be demonstrated.

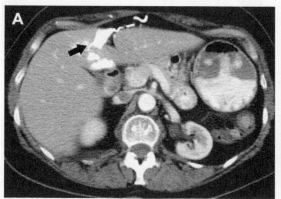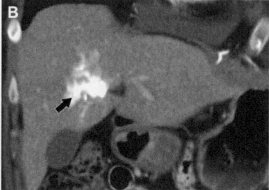

Fig. 13. Axial (*A*) and coronal (*B*) images showing an arterioportal shunt in the liver in a patient with SVC obstruction. Note early hepatic enhancement adjacent to the falciform ligament (*arrow*) and collaterals along the anterior chest wall.

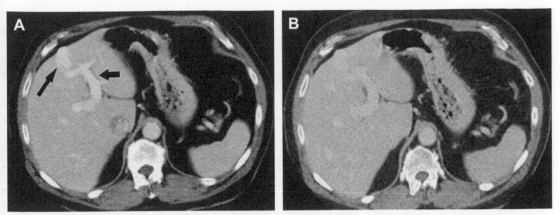

Fig. 14. Small arteriovenous shunts and pseudoaneursyms secondary to a previous biopsy in a 72-year-old male (A) Axial contrast-enhanced image in portal venous phase showing a markedly enhanced peripheral liver lesion (arrow) that is isointense to the aorta as well as early opacification of an enlarged portal venous branch (short arrow). (B) In the delayed image, the lesion is isointense to the rest of the parenchyma, differentiating it from an HCC.

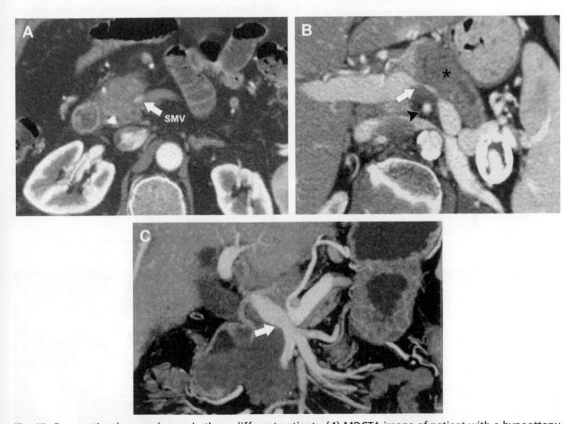

Fig. 15. Pancreatic adenocarcinoma in three different patients. (A) MDCTA image of patient with a hypoattenuating adenocarcinoma in the neck of the pancreas, encasing the superior mesenteric vein. (B) Reformatted image along the portal vein. Encasement and narrowing of the lumen of the portal vein (arrow) secondary to invasion from pancreatic adenocarcinoma located in the body and neck (*). Encasement of the superior mesenteric artery is also noted (arrowhead). (C) Coronal MIP image in a patient with invasive adenocarcinoma of the head and neck of the pancreas with encasement of the portal confluence (arrow).

Table 8
Criteria established for unresectable and borderline pancreatic carcinoma

Unresectable	Distant metastasis
	Invasion of adjacent organs other than duodenum
	Vascular invasion:
	more than 50% of tumor contiguity with celiac artery, hepatic artery, superior mesenteric artery
	Occlusion of superior mesenteric vein at portal confluence extending inferiorly to involve middle colic, gastroploploic, and jejunal veins
Borderline resectable	Tumor abuts the superior mesenteric artery or common hepatic artery over a short segment.
	Focal occlusion of the superior mesenteric vein (SMV)-portal vein (PV) confluence with suitable vein above and below such that venous reconstruction is possible.

PANCREATIC MDCTA
Pancreatic Neoplasm

Ductal adenocarcinoma is the most common neoplasm of the pancreas and it is the fourth leading cause of death from cancer. The 5-year survival rate decreases from 6% in a IIB stage in which surgical treatment is advocated, compared with 1% in a stage IV presenting with distant metastasis.[43] Imaging plays an important role in early detection, accurate staging, and correct selection of surgical candidates.

Most patients with pancreatic carcinoma have a focal mass at presentation with a small minority approximating 5% presenting with diffuse gland involvement. The characteristic finding on MDCTA of pancreatic adenocarcinoma is a mass that is hypoattenuating compared with the normal-enhancing parenchyma, in both arterial and venous phases (Fig. 15). In a small number of cases the lesions can be isodense to the rest of the parenchyma. In these cases, it is important to rely on secondary signs as loss of the lobulated contour of the parenchyma and abrupt cutoff of a dilated pancreatic duct.[44]

MDCTA is the imaging modality of choice for staging pancreatic adenocarcinoma, with an excellent negative predictive value (NPV) for vascular invasion (100%) and good NPV (87%) for tumor resectability.[45] Criteria for unresectable tumors are described in Table 8 (Fig. 16).

Over the past several years, a distinct subset of patients defined as "borderline resectable" has been reported. These patients were previously considered unresectable and now may be appropriate candidates for surgical resection after neoadjuvant therapy (see Table 8).[46]

When performing MDCTA of the pancreas for cancer staging, adenopathy, peritoneal implants, and liver metastases should be assessed. The latter will usually appear as low-attenuation lesions compared with the normal-enhancing parenchyma, being best depicted in the portal venous phase.

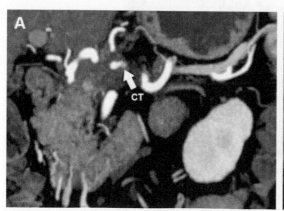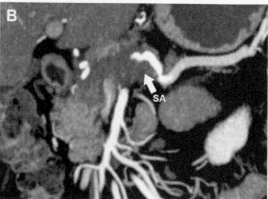

Fig. 16. Unresectable pancreatic adenocarcinoma. MIP coronal images demonstrating a hypodense tumor extending from the pancreatic neck and body, involving the celiac trunk (CT) (*A*) and the splenic artery (SA) (*B*).

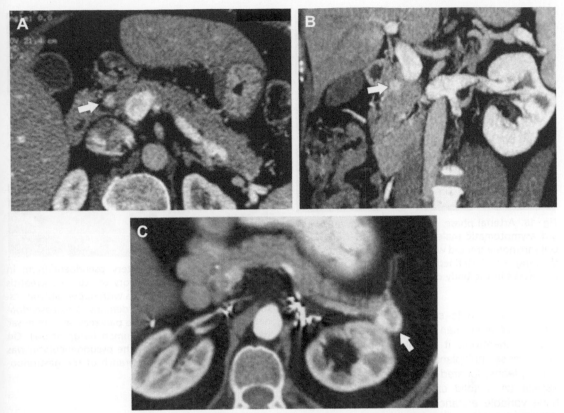

Fig. 17. Arterial phase MDCT images of pancreas from 2 different patients with suspected neuroendocrine tumors. (*A, B*) Images from a patient with a suspected gastrinoma show a hyperattenuating round lesion in the expected location of gastroduodenal artery (*arrow*). (*B*) However, the coronal reformatted image demonstrates its location in the head of the pancreas and the absence of tubular morphology of a vessel (*arrow*). (*C*) In another patient with insulinoma, a well-defined and avidly enhancing mass is noted in the tail (*arrow*).

Hypervascular Tumors

Neuroendocrine tumors

Neuroendocrine tumors account for most hypervascular tumors in the pancreas. Hypervascular lesions are supplied by systemic arterial supply, demonstrating earlier enhancement than the normal pancreatic parenchyma. Accordingly, neuroendocrine tumors appear as hyperattenuating lesions during arterial and portal venous phases and can become isodense to the surrounding parenchyma in the later phases (Fig. 17).

Like the primary neoplasms, lymph nodes and metastases are hypervascular as well. As with the primary neoplasm, nodal metastases are hypervascular. As neuroendocrine neoplasms grow, they may undergo central necrosis and less frequently cystic degeneration.[47]

Neuroendocrine tumors are classified into functioning and nonfunctioning. Functional neoplasms, which are categorized based on the main hormone they produce, are diagnosed at an earlier stage

because of their clinical manifestations. Nonfunctional tumors are detected when they are large and produce mass effect. Insulinomas are the most common neuroendocrine tumor, only 6% to 10% being malignant, followed by gastrinomas (60% malignant), glucagonomas, VIPomas, somatostatinomas, and corticotropinomas. No difference in the pattern of enhancement has been described according to functional status. The overall sensitivity of MDCTA for detecting islet tumors ranges from 64% to 82%, although it is lower for very small lesions.[48]

Hypervascular metastases

Isolated metastatic cancer to the pancreas accounts for approximately 2% to 3% of all pancreatic neoplasms. The most common primary cancer to metastasize to the pancreas is renal cell carcinoma, which can occur up to 10 years after the diagnosis (Fig. 18).[49] Less common hypervascular metastases include thyroid cancer, carcinoid tumors, melanoma, and breast cancer.[50]

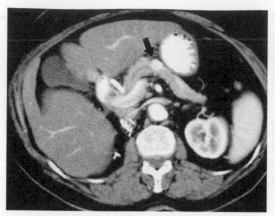

Fig. 18. Arterial phase, MDCT image from a 67-year-old asymptomatic male with history of right renal cell carcinoma treated with nephrectomy 3 years prior showing a well-defined, homogeneously enhancing metastasis in the body of the pancreas (*arrow*).

Vascular variants such as focal tortuosity of the splenic artery can mimic small hypervascular lesions; therefore, it is important to construct and assess multiplanar reconstructions. Accessory spleens, located in the pancreatic tail, can appear as a solid enhancing mass. They can have variable enhancement patterns, making it difficult to accurately distinguish them from pancreatic hypervascular lesions.[51]

Vascular Complications of Pancreatitis

Extravasation of pancreatic enzymes causes vascular and hemorrhagic complications in patients with pancreatitis. Venous thrombosis is the most common complication affecting the splenic, portal, or SMV. An incidence of 19% of splenic vein thrombosis in patients with pancreatitis has been reported, often associated with dilated short gastric and gastroepiploic veins.[52]

Pseudoaneurysm formation is a rare complication and results from autodigestions of the arterial wall by extravasated pancreatic enzymes. The splenic, gastroduodenal, and pancreaticoduodenal arteries are most commonly affected. Hemorrhage from a ruptured pseudoaneurysm is the most dreaded complication and has an incidence of 10%.[53] Although most cases present as a pseudoaneurysm bleeding into a pseudocyst, some patients may present with upper gastrointestinal bleeding. Hemosuccus pancreaticus is referred when communication between the pancreatic duct and the pseudocyst exists. Less commonly ruptured pseudoaneurysms may cause hemoperitoneum or retroperitoneal bleed.

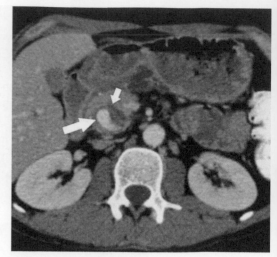

Fig. 19. Gastroduodenal artery pseudoaneurysm in a 34-year-old male with history of acute pancreatitis 6 months prior; now presents with upper gastrointestinal tract hemorrhage. CECT demonstrates a pseudoaneurysm in the region of the pancreas, aneurysm sac (*small arrows*) and patent lumen (*large arrow*). On conventional angiography, the pseudoaneurysm was confirmed to arise from a branch of the gastroduodenal artery.

MDCTA has a sensitivity of 80% to 100% for detecting pseudoaneurysm.[54] Pseudoaneurysms appear as well-defined, densely enhancing lesions related to a peripancreatic artery, isolated or in conjunction with a pseudocyst (Fig. 19). Angiography is indicated for diagnosing small pseudoaneurysms as well as for endovascular treatment with embolization, with a success rate of 75% to 100%.[55]

SUMMARY

In summary, MDCTA is an effective, high-resolution, noninvasive imaging technique that readily demonstrates the presence of vascular and neoplastic pathology, with a direct impact on treatment decisions including patient selection for surgical management.

REFERENCES

1. Frenchel S, Boll DT, Fleiter TR, et al. Multislice helical CT of the pancreas and spleen. Eur J Radiol 2003; 45(Suppl 1):S59–72.
2. Kamel IR, Liapi E, Fishman EK. Liver and biliary system. Evaluation by multidetector CT. Radiol Clin North Am 2005;43:977–97.
3. Miyoshi T, Kanematsu M, Kondo H, et al. Abdomen: angiography with 16-detector CT-comparison of

image quality and radiation dose between studies with 0.625mm and those with 1.25mm collimation. Radiology 2008;249:142–50.

4. Foley WD, Mallisee TA, Hohenwalter MD, et al. Multiphase hepatic CT with a multirow detector CT scanner. Am J Roentgenol 2000;175:679–85.

5. Fleishmann D, Kamaya A. Optimal vascular and parenchymal contrast enhancement: the current state of the art. Radiol Clin North Am 2009;47:13–26.

6. Shueller G, Schima W, Schueller-Weidekamm C, et al. Multidetector CT of the pancreas: effects of contrast material flow rate and individualized scan delay on enhancement of pancreas and tumor contrast. Radiology 2006;241:441–8.

7. Fletcher JG, Wiersema MJ, Farrell MS, et al. Pancreatic malignancy value of arterial, pancreatic, and hepatic phase imaging with multidetector row CT. Radiology 2003;229:81–90.

8. Furuta A, Ito K, Fujita T, et al. Hepatic enhancement in multiphasic contrast-enhancement MDCT: comparison of high and low-iodine-concentration contrast medium in same patients with chronic liver disease. Am J Roentgenol 2004;183:157–62.

9. Pannu HK, Maley WR, Fishman EK. Liver transplantation: preoperative CT. Radiographics 2001;21: S133–46.

10. Horton KM, Fishman EK. 3D CT angiography of the celiac and superior mesenteric arteries with multidetector CT data sets: preliminary observations. Abdom Imaging 2000;25:523–5.

11. Tanikake M, Shimizu T, Narabayashi I, et al. Three-dimensional angiography of the hepatic artery: use of multi-detector row helical CT and contrast agent. Radiology 2003;227:883–9.

12. Kondo H, Kanematsu M, Goshima S, et al. MDCT of the pancreas: optimizing scanning delay with a bolus-tracking technique for pancreatic, peripancreatic vascular, and hepatic contrast enhancement. Am J Roentgenol 2007;188:751–6.

13. Tatsugami F, Matsuki M, Kani H, et al. Effect of saline pushing after contrast material injection in abdominal multidetector computed tomography with the use of different iodine concentrations. Acta Radiol 2006;47(2):192–7.

14. Singh AK, Sahani DV, Blake MA, et al. Assessment of pancreatic tumor resectability with multidetector computed tomography semiautomated console-generated images versus dedicated workstation generated images. Acad Radiol 2008;15: 1058–68.

15. Catalano O, Singh A, Uppot R, et al. Vascular and biliary variants in the liver: implications for liver surgery. Radiographics 2008;28:359–78.

16. Sahani D, Mehta A, Blake M, et al. Preoperative hepatic vascular evaluation with CT and MR angiography: implications for surgery. Radiographics 2004; 24:1367–80.

17. Allen PJ, Nissan A, Picon AI, et al. Technical complications and durability of hepatic artery infusion pumps for unresectable colorectal liver metastases: an institutional experience of 544 consecutive cases. J Am Coll Surg 2005;201(1):57–65.

18. Murakami T, Kim T, Takamura M, et al. Hypervascular hepatocellular carcinomas: detection with double arterial phase multi-row helical CT. Radiology 2001; 218:763–7.

19. Lim JH, Kim CK, Lee WJ, et al. Detection of hepatocellular carcinomas and dysplastic nodules in cirrhotic livers: accuracy of helical CT in transplant patients. Am J Roentgenol 2000;175:693–8.

20. Tajima T, Honda H, Taguchi K, et al. Sequential hemodynamic change in hepatocellular carcinoma and dysplastic nodules: CT angiography and pathologic correlation. Am J Roentgenol 2002;178:885–97.

21. Iannaccone R, Laghi A, Catalano C, et al. Hepatocellular carcinoma: role of unenhanced and delayed phase multi-detector row helical CT in patients with cirrhosis. Radiology 2005;234:460–7.

22. Brancatelli G, Federle MP, Grazioli L, et al. Hepatocellular carcinoma in noncirrhotic liver: CT, clinical, and pathologic findings in 39 US residents. Radiology 2002;222:89–94.

23. Poon RT-P, Fan ST. Hepatectomy for hepatocellular carcinoma: patient selection and postoperative outcome. Liver Transpl 2004;10(Suppl 1):S39–45.

24. Figueras J, Jaurrieta E, Valls C, et al. Resection or transplantation for hepatocellular carcinoma in cirrhotic patients: outcomes based on indicated treatment strategy. J Am Coll Surg 2000;190:580–7.

25. Shanley CJ, Shah NL, Messina LM. Common splanchnic artery aneurysms: splenic, hepatic and celiac. Ann Vasc Surg 1996;10(3):315–22.

26. Pasha SF, Gloviczki P, Stanson AW, et al. Splanchnic artery aneurysms. Mayo Clin Proc 2007;82(4):472–9.

27. Rossi M, Rebonato A, Greco L, et al. Endovascular exclusion of visceral artery aneurysms with stent-grafts: technique and long-term follow-up. Cardiovasc Intervent Radiol 2008;31(1):36–42.

28. Cohen J, Edelman RR, Chopra S. Portal vein thrombosis: a review. Am J Med 1992;92:173–82.

29. Parvey R, Raval B, Sandler C. Portal vein thrombosis: imaging findings. Am J Roentgenol 1994;162:77–81.

30. Ikai I, Arii S, Kojiro M, et al. Reevaluation of prognostic factors for survival after liver resection in patients with hepatocellular carcinoma in a Japanese nationwide survey. Cancer 2004;101:769–802.

31. Tublin M, Dodd GD, Baron R. Benign and malignant portal vein thrombosis: differentiation by CT characteristics. Am J Roentgenol 1997;168:719–23.

32. Shah Z, McKernan MG, Hahn P, et al. Enhancing and expansile portal vein thrombosis value in the diagnosis of hepatocellular carcinoma in patients with multiple hepatic lesions. Am J Roentgenol 2007;188:1320–3.

33. De Gaetano AM, Lafotune M, Patriquin H, et al. Cavernous transformation of the portal vein: patterns of intrahepatic and splachnic collateral circulation detected with Doppler sonography. Am J Roentgenol 1995;165:1151–5.

34. Denninger MH, Chait Y, Casadevall N, et al. Causes of portal or hepatic venous thrombosis in adults: the role of multiple concurrent factors. Hepatology 2000; 31:587–91.

35. Kim TK, Chung JW, Han JK, et al. Hepatic changes in benign obstruction of the hepatic inferior vena cava: CT findings. Am J Roentgenol 1999;173: 1235–42.

36. Brancatelli G, Federle MP, Grazioli L, et al. Large regenerative nodules in Budd-Chiari syndrome and other vascular disorders of the liver: CT and MR imaging findings with clinico-pathologic correlation. Am J Roentgenol 2002;178:877–83.

37. Valla DC. The diagnosis and management of the Budd-Chiari syndrome: consensus and controversies. Hepatology 2003;38:793–803.

38. Mancuso A, Fung K, Mela M, et al. TIPS for acute and chronic Budd-Chiari syndrome: a single center experience. J Hepatol 2003;38:751–4.

39. Quiroga S, Sebastia C, Pallisa E, et al. Improved diagnosis of hepatic perfusion disorders value of hepatic arterial phase imaging during helical CT. Radiographics 2001;21:65–81.

40. Kamel IR, Liapi E, Fishman EK. Incidental nonneoplastic hypervascular lesions in the noncirrhotic liver: diagnosis with 16 MDCT and 3D angiography. AJR Am J Roentgenol 2006;187:682–7.

41. Torabi M, Hosseinzadeh K, Federle M. CT of nonneoplastic hepatic vascular and perfusion disorders. Radiographics 2008;28:1967–82.

42. Lane MJ, Jeffrey RB Jr, Katz DS. Spontaneous intrahepatic vascular shunts. Am J Roentgenol 2000; 174:125–31.

43. American Cancer Society. Cancer facts and figures 2008. Atlanta (GA): American Cancer Society; 2008.

44. Prokesh RW, Chow LC, Beaulieu CT, et al. Isoattenuating pancreatic adenocarcinoma at multidetector row CT: secondary signs. Radiology 2002;224:764–8.

45. Vargas R, Nino-Murcia M, Trueblood W, et al. MDCT in pancreatic adenocarcinoma: prediction of vascular invasion and respectability using a multiphasic technique with curved planar reformations. Am J Roentgenol 2004;182(2):419–25.

46. Katz M, Pisters P, Evans D, et al. Borderline resectable pancreatic cancer: the importance of this emerging stage of disease. J Am Coll Surg 2008; 206:833–46.

47. Brugge WR, Lauwers GY, Sahani D, et al. Cystic neoplasms of the pancreas. N Engl J Med 2004; 351:1218–26.

48. Ichikawa T, Peterson MS, Federle MP, et al. Islet tumor of the pancreas: biphasic CT versus MR imaging in tumor detection. Radiology 2000;216:163–71.

49. Ng CS, Loyer EM, Iyer RB, et al. Metastases to the pancreas from renal cell carcinoma: finding on three-phase contrast-enhanced helical CT. Am J Roentgenol 1999;172:1555–9.

50. Ferrozzi F, Bova D, Campodonico F, et al. Pancreatic metastases: CT assessment. Eur Radiol 1997;7: 241–5.

51. Mortele KJ, Mortele B, Silverman SG. CT features of the accessory spleen. Am J Roentgenol 2004;183: 1653–7.

52. Mortele KJ, Mergo PJ, Taylor HM, et al. Peripancreatic vascular abnormalities complicating acute pancreatitis: contrast enhanced helical CT findings. Eur Radiol 2004;52:67–72.

53. Balthazar EJ, Fisher LA. Hemorrhagic complications of pancreatitis: radiologic evaluation with emphasis on CT imaging. Pancreatology 2001;1:306–13.

54. Savastano S, Feltrin GP, Antonio T, et al. Arterial complications of pancreatitis: diagnostic and therapeutic role of radiology. Pancreas 1993;8:687–92.

55. De Perrot M, Berney T, Buhler L, et al. Management of bleeding pseudoaneurysms in patients with pancreatitis. Br J Surg 1999;86:29–32.

CT Angiography of the Mesenteric Circulation

Karen M. Horton, MD[a],*, Elliot K. Fishman, MD[b]

KEYWORDS

• Mesentery • Three-dimensional imaging • CT angiography

Significant advancements in computed tomography (CT) scanner technology along with the development of powerful and affordable 3-dimensional (3D) software have resulted in new applications for CT imaging. The mesenteric vasculature was traditionally imaged with conventional angiography, but can now easily be imaged rapidly and safely using multidetector-row CT (MDCT) scanners and 3D imaging software. CT can now be used to visualize the normal mesenteric vasculature, both arteries and veins, identify important anatomic variants, and evaluate a wide range of pathology.

TECHNIQUE

For optimal visualization of the mesenteric vessels, MDCT is necessary to provide high-resolution, thin, submillimeter collimation, and fast scanning speeds. Using their 64-slice MDCT scanner (Siemens Sensation 64, Siemens Medical Solutions Malvern, PA, USA) the authors typically use a 64 × 0.6-mm collimator setting; this allows creation of 0.75-mm slices, which can be reconstructed every 0.5 mm to obtain high-quality 3D data sets. A second set of reconstructions is also performed, usually 3- to 5-mm slices, for review of the entire data set. Similar protocols are used on dual-source scanners such as the Flash (Siemens Medical Systems), although this ultrafast scanner does require some changes in data acquisition protocols and bolus timing.

Because both the mesenteric arterial and venous systems must be adequately evaluated, dual-phase imaging is usually necessary. One hundred to 120 mL of nonionic contrast is administered through a peripheral catheter placed in the antecubital fossa at a rate of 4 to 5 mL per second. Images are obtained from the diaphragm through the synthesis pubis. Arterial phase acquisition is usually obtained 25 to 30 seconds after the start of the injection. The venous phase is obtained 50 to 60 seconds after the start of the injection.

When imaging patients with suspected pathology of the mesenteric vasculature, water is used for oral contrast. One liter of water given over an interval of 20 minutes is usually adequate; this allows excellent visualization of the enhancing bowel wall. In addition, the use of water will allow easy editing of the 3D volume set, without the need to edit out the high-density bowel.[1,2] Using high-density oral contrast such as barium suspensions or iodinated solutions is cumbersome when editing and postprocessing, and also limits evaluation of bowel wall enhancement. Other low-density oral agents are available, including methylcellulose agents or diluted barium agents.

Given the complexity of the mesenteric vasculature, 3D imaging is extremely valuable. For 3D imaging, the thin slices (0.75 mm) are transferred to the 3D workstation. The use of the submillimeter collimator creates isotropic data sets and therefore the 3D images of mesenteric arteries and veins are of excellent quality. At the authors' institution, all images are reviewed using InSpace software (Siemens Medical Solutions, Malvern, PA, USA), which allows

[a] Department of Radiology, Johns Hopkins Medical Institutions, 601 North Caroline Street, Room 3253, Baltimore, MD 21287, USA
[b] Department of Radiology, Johns Hopkins Medical Institutions, 601 North Caroline Street, Room 3254, Baltimore, MD 21287, USA
* Corresponding author.
E-mail address: kmhorton@jhmi.edu

Radiol Clin N Am 48 (2010) 331–345
doi:10.1016/j.rcl.2010.02.004

multiplanar reconstruction (MPR) as well as interactive 3D volume rendering. The brightness, opacity, window width, and level can be adjusted in real time to accentuate the wall of the gastrointestinal (GI) tract or optimize visualization of the vessels. Manipulating trapezoidal transfer functions interactively modifies the image contrast and relative pixel attenuations in the final image. This function assigns color and opacity to each voxel and can be adjusted to alter the display instantaneously.[3] The transfer function is applied to a histogram of the data set, with the x-axis representing Hounsfield units and the y-axis color or opacity. All voxels are incorporated into the display. Sliding the trapezoid higher along the x-axis excludes lower attenuation voxels from the display, therefore yielding images of the high-attenuation collecting system.[3] The process can be simplified by creating "presets" that can be applied quickly, and then only minor adjustments are needed. In the authors' experience, review of the 3D scan can usually be completed in approximately 5 minutes.

When evaluating a patient for suspected pathology of the mesenteric vessels, it is usually helpful to use a combination of both volume rendering and maximum-intensity projection (MIP). In addition, simple MPR can sometimes be helpful for a global view of the anatomy and pathology. The origin of the celiac axis and superior mesenteric artery (SMA) are best visualized using a sagittal or sagittal oblique projection (Fig. 1).[4] This projection offers excellent visualization of the first few centimeters of both vessels, which is critical when evaluating patients with ischemia or atherosclerotic disease. The inferior mesenteric artery (IMA) is also seen at its origin using a sagittal projection. Although the sagittal view is typically adequate to look at the origin of these mesenteric arteries, their branches are best visualized using coronal, coronal oblique, or axial oblique projections (Fig. 2), which can be easily done in real time using clip planes. The opacity and densities can be adjusted to maximize visualization of the branches. In many cases, the very distal branches can be visualized to the level of the bowel wall. MIP using thin slabs is often helpful to visualize the vasa recta (Fig. 3).

For 3D imaging of the mesenteric veins the anatomy is slightly simpler, and usually a combination of coronal or coronal oblique projections is adequate (Fig. 4).[4] The most proximal portion of the superior mesenteric vein (SMV) with its confluence to the splenic vein and portal vein is usually an important area of pathology.

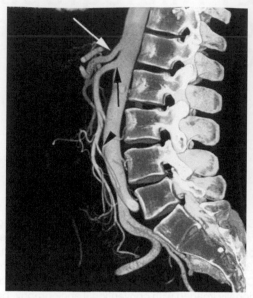

Fig. 1. Volume-rendered 3D image in sagittal projection shows the normal appearance of the origin of the celiac axis (*white arrow*), superior mesenteric artery (*black arrow*), and inferior mesenteric artery (*black arrowhead*).

Although volume rendering is often excellent, the authors have found that maximum intensity projection, especially when using thin slabs, can sometimes better display all the complex collaterals that can occur when splenic vein or SMV thrombosis or occlusion is present.

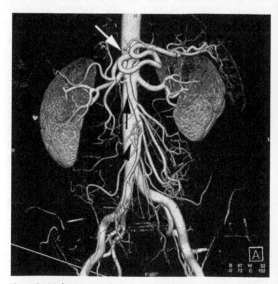

Fig. 2. Volume-rendered 3D image in a coronal projection, after bone editing, shows the normal anatomy and branching pattern of the celiac axis (*white arrow*), superior mesenteric artery (*black arrow*), and inferior mesenteric artery (*black arrowhead*).

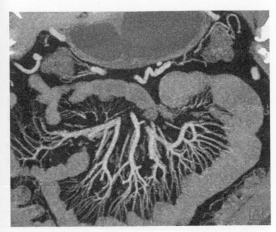

Fig. 3. Thin-slab MIP images of the vasa recta, supplying the small bowel.

NORMAL ANATOMY AND VARIANTS
Arteries

The celiac axis is the first major branch of the abdominal aorta, usually arising at the T12-L1 vertebral body level (see **Figs. 1** and **2**). The left gastric is classically the first branch off the celiac trunk, supplying the stomach. The celiac then bifurcates into the common hepatic artery and splenic artery. This branching pattern is present in approximately 70% of patients.[5] In approximately one-third of patients, a trifurcation of the celiac axis will be seen into the common hepatic artery, splenic artery, and left gastric artery.[6] Other variants include a common celiomesenteric trunk (**Fig. 5**), the hepatic artery arising from the SMA or aorta, the left gastric artery arising directly

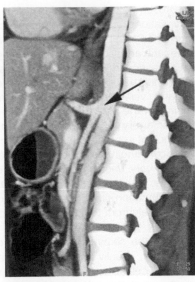

Fig. 5. Volume-rendered 3D image in sagittal projection shows variant anatomy, a common celiomesenteric trunk (*arrow*).

from the aorta, or the splenic artery arising directly off the aorta or off the SMA. In very rare cases, the splenic artery and hepatic artery can arise directly from the aorta (**Fig. 6**).[6]

As noted earlier, the common hepatic artery classically originates from the celiac trunk. The gastroduodenal artery is the first branch in a posterior position. The proper hepatic artery continues on into the porta. The right gastric artery branch arises from the proper hepatic artery, before the proper hepatic artery trifurcates into the left, middle, and right hepatic arteries. Variations are common. Variations in the hepatic artery anatomy

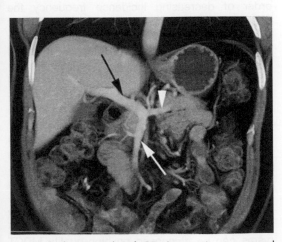

Fig. 4. Volume-rendered 3D image in a coronal projection shows the normal anatomy of the portal vein (*black arrow*), splenic vein (*white arrowhead*), and the superior mesenteric vein (*white arrow*).

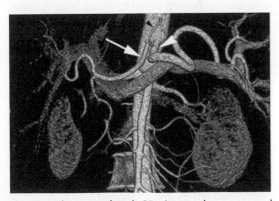

Fig. 6. Volume-rendered 3D image in a coronal projection shows variant anatomy with the common hepatic artery arising directly from the aorta (*white arrow*). The splenic artery (*white arrowhead*) arises directly fro the aorta and the left gastric artery (*black arrowhead*) arises from the proximal splenic artery.

occur in 40% of the population.[6] The most common variations include the right hepatic artery arising from the SMA, the left hepatic or an accessory left hepatic artery arising from the left gastric artery, an accessory right hepatic artery arising off the SMA, the left hepatic artery arising directly off the aorta and, very rarely, the common hepatic artery arising off the SMA.[6]

The splenic artery is the most tortuous and the longest branch of in celiac axis. The splenic artery can have its own origin off the aorta or off the SMA, but these are very uncommon. As noted earlier, the left gastric can originate off the celiac axis before the bifurcation or can originate directly off the aorta, or rarely from the gastrohepatic or gastrosplenic trunk.[6,7]

The SMA is the second major branch off the abdominal aorta, usually arising approximately 1 cm below the celiac trunk.[8] The SMA supplies the midgut, consisting of the third and fourth portions of the duodenum; the jejunum, ileum, and right colon; and the transverse colon to approximately the splenic flexure (see Fig. 2). The vascular supply to the transverse colon to the level of the splenic flexure can be variable, sometimes arising from the SMA or IMA.[8]

There are usually 4 to 6 jejunal arteries arising from the left side of the SMA, which are often difficult to visualize adequately on axial images because they run in an oblique course. The ileocolic artery arises from the right side of the SMA, marking the transition from jejunal to ileal arteries, of which there are typically 8 to 12.[9] The branching pattern of the last jejunal artery, ileocolic artery, and ileal arteries varies. The ileocolic artery has branches to the terminal ileum, cecum, and lower ascending The right colic artery can arise from the SMA to aid the ileocolic and middle colic arteries in supplying blood to the ascending colon. However, it is absent in up to 80% of individuals.[9] The middle colic artery usually arises from the right side of the SMA just before it enters the mesentery; it descends into the right lower quadrant, where it anastomoses with the ileocolic artery. Other branches that may arise from the SMA include an artery for the right angle of the colon and one for the transverse colon. Aberrant branches from the SMA are relatively common, and include the common hepatic artery, right hepatic artery, splenic artery, celiac trunk, cystic artery, gastroduodenal artery, right gastroepiploic artery, and left gastric artery.[6,8,9]

The third major artery, the IMA, usually arises 4 to 7 cm below the level of the SMA (see Figs. 1 and 2).[8,9] The IMA supplies the colon from approximately the splenic flexure to the rectum, and has several branches: the left colic, marginal, sigmoid, and superior hemorrhoidal arteries. The rectum itself has a variable supply from the hemorrhoidal arteries, which originate from the IMA as well as a supply from the internal iliac arteries.[6]

There are also several common collateral pathways between the mesenteric arteries. The gastroduodenal artery, for example, is an important collateral pathway between the celiac axis and the SMA (Fig. 7). The most significant collateral pathways between the SMA and IMA are the marginal artery of Drummond and the arc of Riolan (or paracolic arcade).[6]

Veins

The main trunk of the SMV is of variable length, usually between 5 and 50 mm, before its division into 2 main intestinal branches. The main trunk can be absent, with 2 large intestinal branches draining directly into the splenic vein.[8,9] The gastrocolic trunk is a tributary of the SMV that can drain directly into the main SMV trunk or into the right intestinal branch. Jejunal branches typically drain into the main trunk or left intestinal branches.

The inferior mesenteric vein (IMV) can drain directly into the splenic vein, into the SMV, or at the angle of the splenoportal confluences. The left colic vein, which usually drains the left colon and flexure, is often visible draining into the IMV.

SMV tributaries include ileocolic, gastrocolic, right colic, and middle colic veins. IMV tributaries include the superior hemorrhoidal vein and sigmoid vein, which join to form the left colic vein.[9]

ARTERIAL PATHOLOGY
Aneurysms

Splanchnic artery aneurysms are relatively rare. In order of decreasing incidence frequency the arteries involved are splenic (60%) (Fig. 8), hepatic (20%) (Fig. 9), superior mesenteric (5.5%), celiac (4%), pancreatic (2%), and gastroduodenal (1.5%).[10,11] Splanchnic artery aneurysms are clinically important due to the risk of rupture and bleeding. Depending on the location of the aneurysm, mortality rates can be as high as 20% to 75%.[10,11]

These aneurysms were traditionally diagnosed with catheter angiography. However, with the increasing use and increased speed and resolution of cross-sectional imaging modalities such as MDCT and magnetic resonance, these aneurysms are being detected with greater frequency and even in asymptomatic patients. Visceral aneurysms can be diagnosed on high-quality MDCT data sets using fast intravenous contrast infusion and thin collimation. Large aneurysms are usually easy to detect on axial images, but small

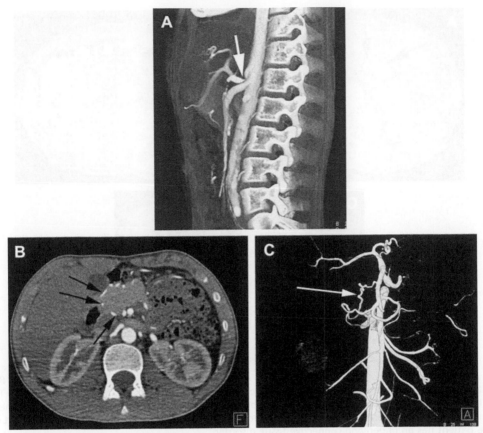

Fig. 7. A patient with median arcuate ligament syndrome. (A) Volume-rendered 3D image in sagittal projection shows stenosis of the proximal celiac artery (*arrow*). This stenosis has a characteristic hooklike appearance with poststenotic dilatation. (B) Axial contrast-enhanced image shows prominent vessels around the pancreatic head (*arrows*). (C) Coronal volume-rendered image shows that the prominent vessels are actually a dilated gastroduodenal artery (*arrow*), which is now supplying the celiac axis through the SMA.

aneurysms are often much better visualized on MPR and 3D imaging.[12] Also, 3D computed tomographic angiography (CTA) is essential to map out the anatomy and to detect anatomy variants, which may be important especially if endovascular repair is anticipated.[12]

Treatment depends on the location, size, and type of the aneurysm as well as on the medical

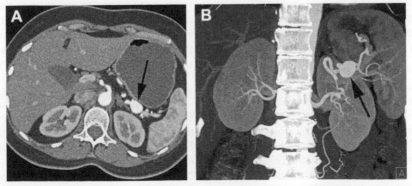

Fig. 8. A 63-year-old woman with an incidental splenic artery aneurysm. (A) Axial contrast-enhanced image shows a splenic 1.8-cm aneurysm (*arrow*). (B) Coronal MIP image better displays the aneurysm (*arrow*) and its relationship to the splenic artery. This CTA can be used for treatment planning.

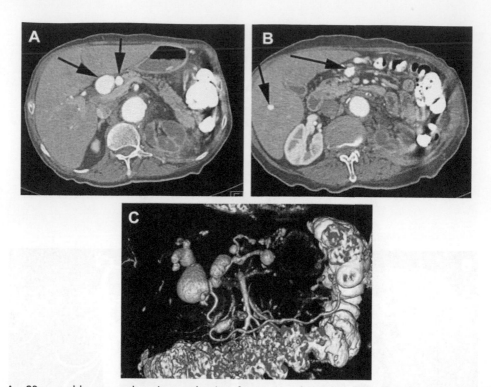

Fig. 9. An 80-year-old man undergoing evaluation for repair of thoracoabdominal aneurysm. (*A, B*) Axial contrast-enhanced images show dilated vascular structures (*arrows*) in the porta, mesentery, and liver. The left kidney is infarcted. Residual barium is present in the colon. (*C*) Volume-rendered CTA shows numerous aneurysms involving the celiac axis, splenic artery, left gastric artery and hepatic artery, and gastroduodenal artery. It is likely that the patient has an underlying connective tissue disorder.

condition of the patient.[13] In the literature there is general agreement that these aneurysms should often be treated, even in asymptomatic patients, especially if the aneurysm is twice the diameter of the normal vessels, is rapidly growing, or if the patient is a woman of childbearing age. Treatment is also recommended in patients with symptoms attributable to the aneurysm.[14] Either surgical repair or endovascular procedures are acceptable treatment options. The type of treatment often depends on the location of the aneurysm, underlying patient condition, as well as individual patient anatomy and vascular variations.[15,16]

Dissection

The celiac artery and SMA can be involved in patients with aortic dissection. The dissection flap can extend into the proximal portion of the vessels and therefore can decrease blood flow or, rarely, result in complete obstruction of blood flow through these arteries. This situation is typically best appreciated using 3D imaging. Volume rendering is especially useful for visualizing the flap and its course. In addition to aortic dissections

with involvement of the mesenteric arteries, there have been case reports of spontaneous dissection of the SMA (**Fig. 10**).[17] This condition rare, with a relatively high mortality rate.[18] Patients can present with acute abdominal pain. The dissection flap is confined to the proximal segment of the SMA, but does not extend into the aorta. The flap is easily detected on high-quality CTA.[19] The exact origin of this condition is not known, but may be related to underlying connective tissue disease. Treatment is typically surgical repair, and in some cases endovascular stenting may be possible. In addition, isolated dissection of the celiac axis has been reported (**Fig. 11**).

Superior Mesenteric Artery Syndrome

SMA syndrome is a rare condition in which there is narrowing of the space between the aorta and SMA, resulting in compression and/or obstruction of the third portion of the duodenum. Patients typically present with intermittent abdominal pain (worse after meals), nausea, vomiting, and weight loss.[20–22] This condition has been reported to occur with increased frequency in patients after

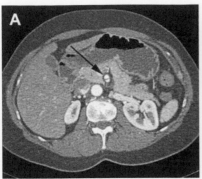
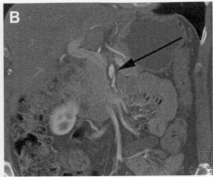

Fig. 10. A 54-year-old woman undergoing evaluation for acute abdominal pain. (*A*) Axial contrast-enhanced image and (*B*) Coronal volume-rendered 3D image show a focal dissection in the SMA (*arrow*). There is no associated aortic dissection.

rapid weight loss (also known as cast syndrome)[23] and in patients with anorexia.

Upper gatrointestinal series can be helpful in suggesting the diagnosis by demonstrating gastric distension and dilatation of the first and second portion of the duodenum with a linear area of extrinsic pressure along the third portion of the duodenum.[23] However, these findings on fluoroscopy are not specific for SMA syndrome. Therefore, CTA is usually also performed to directly visualize the arterial anatomy to measure the aorta-SMA angle and the distance between the aorta and SMA, and its effect on the third portion of the duodenum (Fig. 12).[24] In normal patients, the aorta-SMA angle has been reported to be 25° to 60° and the aorta-SMA distance 10 to 28 mm. In studies of patients with SMA syndrome using angiography, the aorta-SMA angle ranged between 6° and 22° and the aorta-SMA distance was 2 to 8 mm.[21,24,25] Similar differences in the

aorta-SMA distance have been reported using thin collimation CTA and by those who used CTA combined with 3D reconstruction.[24,26]

Segmental Arterial Mediolysis

Segmental arterial mediolysis is a rare noninflammatory vascular condition of the visceral arteries of unknown origin. Segmental arterial mediolysis primarily involves the outer layer of the media resulting in disruption, intramural hemorrhage, and periadventitial fibrin disposition.[27] Patients may present with abdominal pain, intra-abdominal hemorrhage, or lower GI bleeding. The typical features of the condition were first described by Heritz and colleagues[28] on conventional angiography in 1990 and include focal aneurysms, vascular beading, and focal areas of narrowing involving the splanchnic and renal arteries. These findings can be very similar to those seen with

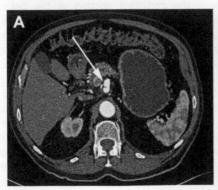
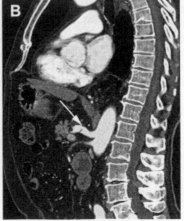

Fig. 11. An 83-year-old man with upper gatrointestinal bleeding of unknown cause. (*A*) Axial contrast enhanced scan and (*B*) sagittal MPR show a small focal dissection (*arrow*) in the proximal celiac artery.

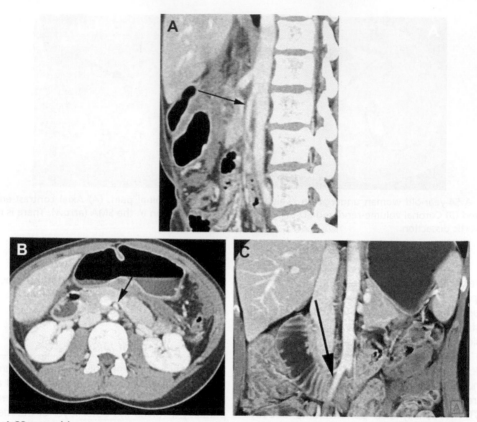

Fig. 12. A 22-year-old woman presenting with weight loss and abdominal pain. The patient is status post resection of a retroperitoneal sarcoma 12 months previously. (*A*) Sagittal volume-rendered and (*B*) axial image show narrowing of the space between the SMA and aorta (*arrow*). (*C*) Coronal volume-rendered image shows distention of the stomach and duodenum, with an abrupt transition and obstruction of the duodenum (*arrow*) at the level where it crosses under the SMA.

fibromuscular dysplasia and are considered by some investigators to be a variant of that condition.[27] According to a retrospective study by Michael and colleagues,[27] the investigators evaluated the potential role of CTA. In that study the SMA or its branches were affected in all patients. Three of 5 patients also had involvement of the celiac axis or branches and 2 of 5 patients demonstrated renal involvement.[27]

The natural history of the condition is unknown, and treatment usually consists of either surgical or endovascular interventions to manage complications such as vascular occlusion, thrombosis, or hemorrhage. Long-term follow-up of patients is lacking in the literature.

Median Arcuate Ligament Syndrome

The median arcuate ligament is a fibrous band that unites the crura on both sides of the aortic hiatus. The ligament typically crosses superior to the origin of the celiac axis. However, in some people there is variant anatomy in which the ligament crosses more inferiorly and thus can cross over the proximal portion of the celiac axis.[29] This variant can be minor and cause no symptoms. In a small number of people with this variant, the median arcuate ligament can cause compression of the celiac axis, resulting in a celiac stenosis and pain, especially if there is not good collateral flow through the gastroduodenal artery from the SMA. The diagnosis, traditionally made with catheter angiography, can now be made with 3D CTA.[30] The median arcuate ligament causes characteristic findings in the CT angiogram, which can allow accurate diagnosis. The sagittal plane typically is optimal to visualize the proximal portion of the celiac axis, and in many cases 3D imaging also allows identification of the actual median arcuate ligament. On CTA, patients with median arcuate ligament syndrome demonstrate a characteristic focal narrowing in the proximal celiac axis with a hook appearance (see **Fig. 7**). Also, the presence of associated poststenotic dilatation or collaterals may signify actual pathology and warrant clinical correlation.

Once the disorder has been diagnosed, surgery can be performed to relieve the compression; in some patients the ligamentous constriction of the celiac axis causes vascular damage that may require vascular reconstruction. Surgical treatment is more likely to relieve symptoms in those patients with postprandial pain, greater than 20 lb weight loss, are between 40 and 60 years of age, or with poststenotic dilatation and vascular collaterals.[31] Detection of a low-lying median arcuate ligament even in asymptomatic patients can be important, especially if patients are due undergo certain abdominal surgeries, such as a Whipple. In this scenario, if not corrected, decreased perfusion to the liver or bowel can result.

Acute Mesenteric Ischemia

Acute mesenteric ischemia is caused by an abrupt reduction of either arterial or venous blood flow to the gut, and is associated with a high morbidity and mortality rate. The condition requires urgent diagnosis and treatment.[32] Almost all patients present with severe abdominal pain. In patients with emboli as the cause the onset of pain is usually sudden, whereas patients with thombotic etiology may have a more insidious onset of symptoms. Nausea, vomiting, and diarrhea are also common complaints.[32]

CTA is an excellent modality to evaluate patients with suspected acute mesenteric ischemia. CT in combination with 3D CTA can evaluate the mesenteric vasculature as well as bowel enhancement,

and is therefore a comprehensive study. There are 4 major causes of acute mesenteric ischemia: SMA embolus, SMA thrombus, mesenteric venous thrombus, and nonocclusive mesenteric[33] ischemia.[34]

Acute emboli to the SMA are the most common origin of acute mesenteric ischemia, occurring in 40% to 50% of cases.[35] Most emboli originate in the heart and will lodge in the SMA a few centimeters distal to the origin, typically near the origin of the middle colic artery. Smaller emboli lodge more distally and may affect only small segments of bowel.[35,36] The arterial thrombus is visible as a low-density filling defect on CT. Proximal thrombi are best visualized on the sagittal reconstructions, while distal thrombi may only be visible using volume rendering with comprehensive interrogation of all the distal mesenteric branches (**Fig. 13**).[37,38] Regardless of the cause of the ischemia, the affected small bowel loops may be dilated and fluid filled, as a result of an interruption in normal peristalsis and increased secretions (**Fig. 14**). The wall may be thickened, but in some cases will actually be normal or thinned (see **Fig. 14**). Ischemia usually causes circumferential thickening of the bowel wall. The ischemic bowel wall is typically to 8 to 9 mm thick, but in some cases becomes as thick as 1.5 cm. Bowel wall thickening is more pronounced in cases of venous thrombosis than in cases of arterial thrombosis.[39] Therefore, a bowel wall measuring 1.5 cm, in the setting of suspected ischemia, most likely signals obstruction of venous blood flow. Complete lack of mural enhancement has been reported but is an unusual finding, given the redundant blood supply to the gut. The bowel wall may appear of low density, reflecting decreased perfusion (see

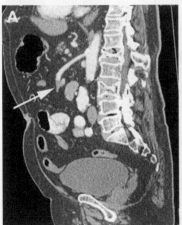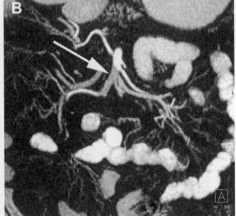

Fig. 13. An 80-year-old man presenting with acute abdominal pain. (*A*) Sagittal MPR and (*B*) Coronal MIP show a large thrombus in the mid SMA (*arrow*); this was embolic, presumably from a cardiogenic source. Surgical embolectomy was performed.

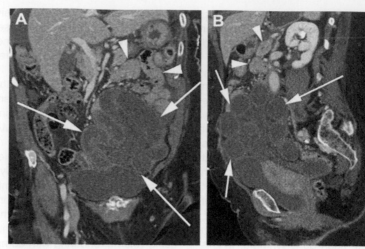

Fig. 14. An 80-year-old woman with an acute closed loop small bowel obstruction. (*A*) Coronal MPR and (*B*) sagittal MPR show dilated fluid-filled small bowel loops. The wall appears thinned and has decreased enhancement (*arrows*) compared with the more proximal and unaffected small bowel loops (*arrowheads*).

Fig. 14) and edema, or may appear increased in density relative to normal bowel loops, related to hemorrhage or hyperemia. The halo sign may be present. Intramural hemorrhage may be present, and is often only appreciated if noncontrast scans are obtained.[40] After intravenous contrast is administered, intramural hemorrhage may be misinterpreted as enhancement.[41] Pneumatosis is a late finding, indicating transmural infarction, and may be accompanied by air in the mesenteric veins and/or portal vein (Fig. 15). In patients with acute arterial ischemia, there may be stranding in the mesentery and ascites, also indicating severe ischemia and usually transmural infarction.[41]

Thrombosis of the SMA usually occurs in the setting of atherosclerotic disease, likely as the result of rupture of an unstable atherosclerotic plaque. Thrombosis of the SMA is estimated to be responsible for up to 30% of all cases of acute

ischemia.[42] Unlike emboli, thrombi typically develop at the origin of the SMA and within the first 2 cm, best visualized using sagittal reconstructions (Fig. 16). There is usually a combination of calcified plaque with superimposed thrombus. Because SMA thrombosis often occurs in the setting of patients with chromic ischemia, there may be associated arterial collaterals, which can be visualized well using CTA. Mesenteric venous thrombosis is another recognized cause of acute mesenteric ischemia (see later discussion).

Nonocclusive mesenteric ischemia is thought to represent up to 25% of cases and is associated with a high mortality rate, up to 70%.[43] Nonocclusive mesenteric ischemia occurs in patients with hypotension or cardiogenic shock. Severe hypoperfusion of the gut will cause severe vasoconstriction of the mesenteric arteries. The findings on CT may be subtle. For example, the SMA and

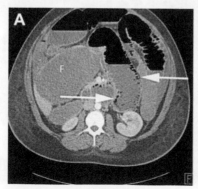
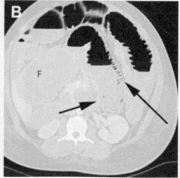

Fig. 15. A 37-year-old postpartum woman with severe abdominal pain. Axial contrast-enhanced CT with soft tissues windows (*A*) and lung windows (*B*) shows a small bowel obstruction and pneumatosis (*arrows*). F, large necrotic uterine fibroid.

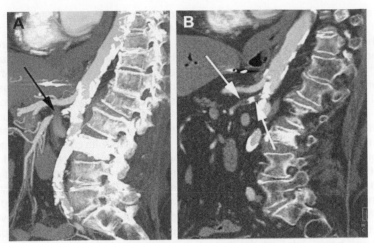

Fig. 16. An 83-year-old woman with acute abdominal pain. (*A*) Sagittal MIP shows extensive calcified atherosclerotic disease involving aorta and proximal SMA (*arrow*). (*B*) There is also a filling defect in the proximal SMA (*arrows*), which is acute thrombus that has form in a region of calcified plaque.

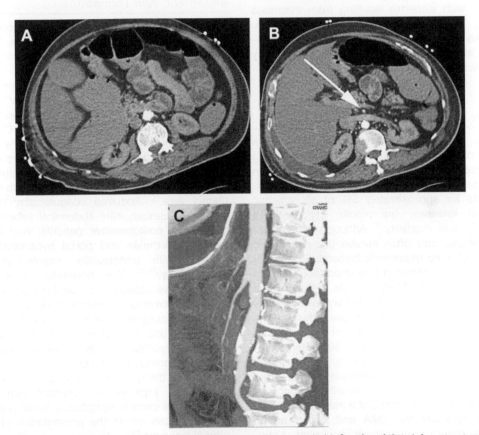

Fig. 17. A 65-year-old man in cardiogenic shock after an acute myocardial infarction. (*A*) Axial contrast-enhanced image through the mid abdomen shows dilated small bowel and colon as well as poor perfusion of the kidneys. (*B*) Axial contrast-enhanced image shows a small-caliber SMA (*arrow*). A right pleural effusion is also present. (*C*) Sagittal MIP image shows the small-caliber celiac axis and SMA, a typical finding in patients with hypotension.

its branches will appear small in caliber and there may be delayed opacification of the mesenteric veins (Fig. 17). The bowel is often dilated and fluid filled. The bowel wall may also be thickened.[35–37,44] In severe cases pneumatosis or portomesenteric venous gas is present, indicating transmural infarction, which carries a dismal prognosis.

In patients with suspected infarcted bowel resulting from emboli, therapy for acute mesenteric ischemia consists of exploratory laparotomy with resection of the nonviable bowel and reestablishment of blood flow to the intestines. However, advancements in interventional radiology techniques offer an effective, less invasive therapeutic alternative for patients with ischemia but no clear evidence of infarcted bowel. Intra-arterial thrombolysis, angioplasty, and stent placement are all available and effective.[45] Venous thrombosis can be treated with systemic, anticoagulation, or percutaneous transhepatic delivery of thrombolytics. Nonocclusive mesenteric ischemia can often by treated with selective arterial administration of vasodilating agents (ie, papaverine).[45] Patients with ischemia resulting from thrombus forming in the setting of chronic mesenteric ischemia may require a combination of percutaneous and systemic therapies, and ultimately may need stenting or surgical revascularization.

Chronic Mesenteric Ischemia

Chronic mesenteric ischemia is almost always a result of severe atherosclerotic disease involving the mesenteric arteries, and therefore occurs in older patients. Chronic mesenteric ischemia accounts for approximately 5% of all ischemic intestinal illnesses, but results in significant morbidity and mortality.[46] Although atherosclerotic disease can often involve the mesenteric arteries, chronic mesenteric ischemia is actually a relatively uncommon but an important cause of abdominal pain in elderly patients.[35] Even in the absence of symptoms, patients may have clinically significant atherosclerotic disease affecting the mesenteric arteries. Up to 18% of patients older than 65 years have greater than 50% stenosis of a mesenteric artery, usually without symptoms.[47]

Patients with significant atherosclerotic stenosis of the mesenteric arteries will usually only become asymptomatic when least 2 of 3 major mesenteric vessels, typically the SMA and celiac artery, become severely stenotic or occluded. Long-term studies have shown that as many as 86% of asymptomatic patients with greater than 50% stenosis of the mesenteric arteries eventually develop symptoms.[48] Mortality is approximately 40%.

Standard treatment for chronic mesenteric ischemia involves revascularization, which can be surgical or catheter based. After surgical treatment, the recurrence rate of mesenteric ischemia symptoms at 3 years is approximately 11%.[49] Percutaneous interventions include embolectomy, thrombolysis, angioplasty, and stenting.[50]

In patients with chronic mesenteric ischemia, CT will show significant stenosis of at least 2 of the major mesenteric arteries, usually the celiac trunk and SMA. The stenosis is usually at the origin and may be a combination of calcified and noncalcified plaque. Because the process develops over a long period of time, collaterals are present. CTA and volume rendering in particular are especially valuable in detecting and quantifying the degree of stenosis and displaying the collaterals.[37] This technique can be used as a road map for the surgeon or interventional radiologist.

VENOUS PATHOLOGY
Mesenteric Vein Thrombosis

Mesenteric vein thrombosis (MVT) accounts for 5% to 15% of all mesenteric ischemias. Thrombosis usually involves the SMV, only rarely involving the IMV.[35,51]

MVT can be classified as either primary or secondary.[35,52] Primary or idiopathic MVT results when no underlying etiology can be identified. Secondary MVT is more common. Common causes include underlying coagulopathy, either hereditary or acquired. Hereditary factors include Factor III deficiency, deficiencies in protein C, protein S, or antithrombin, or patients with polycythemia vera.[52] Acquired coagulopathy is often related to cancer, intra-abdominal inflammatory conditions, postoperative patients, oral contraceptives, cirrhosis and portal hypertension, or patients with pancreatitis, sepsis, or after splenectomy.[35,52] The increased incidence in postoperative patients may be the result of transient hypovolemia or release of tissue thromboplastins at surgery. In a retrospective study by Warshauer and colleagues[53], 11 of 43 patients with SMV thrombosis were status post partial or total colectomies. Clinical presentation varies depending on the location, extent, and cause of the thrombosis. Patients can present with acute, subacute, or chronic symptoms. Acute presentation can often mimic the presentation of acute arterial ischemia.[52]

In acute presentations, patients present with severe pain and there is a high risk of both ischemia and infarction. Outcomes vary, based on the extent of thrombosis. Complete thrombosis carries a poor prognosis, as does extension of thrombus into other veins. Acute thrombosis can result in venous hypertension depending on the residual drainage from the intestines. Severe venous hypertension will compromise the viability and perfusion of the bowel.[35] On CT, thrombus will be visible in the mesenteric veins, typically associated with engorgement of the veins (Fig. 18).[35] The walls of the veins may be thickened with increased enhancement. Stranding in the mesentery and ascites are also often present. The bowel wall is usually thickening, often related to the venous obstruction. There may be decreased enhancement of the wall, or in some patients there may be increased enhancement due to hyperemia. A halo pattern has also been described.[35,52] Complete lack of bowel enhancement is uncommon, but does signify transmural infarction, especially when there is accompanying pneumatosis or portomesenteric gas.[35,52] In subacute situations, patients may have abdominal pain, but typically do not show associated signs of ischemia, likely related to the development of collaterals.

Treatment in acute and subacute cases usually includes anticoagulation, alone or in combination with surgery.[35] Conservative treatment usually consists of anticoagulation, supportive measures, and bowel rest. Surgery may be required in patients with peritonitis and signs of ischemia/infarcted bowel. Surgery may include resection of the small bowel, although the goal is to conserve as much bowel as possible. In select cases, thrombectomy or mechanical and percutaneous clot lysis can be performed. Overall, MVT carries a high mortality rate (20%–50%). The principal cause of the high mortality is delay in diagnosis. The condition is often misdiagnosed as gastroenteritis, small bowel obstruction, or inflammatory bowel disease. Even after treatment there is a high rate of occurrence, most commonly in the first 30 days after treatment.

Chronic MVT, often in cirrhotic patients, typically causes little symptoms because of the development of an extensive collateral network. However, these patients are at increased risk for GI bleeding related to the presence of the collaterals. In patients with chromic MVT, treatment may include propranolol to help decrease the risk of variceal bleeding.

On CT, chronic MVT will appear as a low-density intraluminal clot. Enlargement of the vein and bowel wall thickening, as well as mesenteric

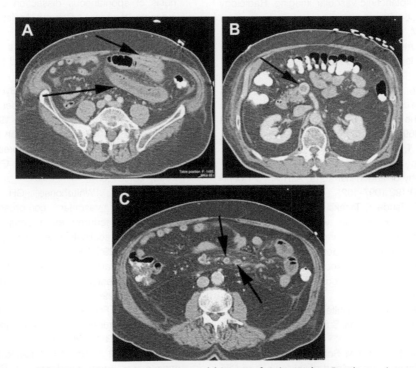

Fig. 18. An 80-year-old man with abdominal pain and history of Osler-Weber-Rendu syndrome. (A) Contrast-enhanced axial CT shows small bowel thickening (arrows). (B) Axial image through the superior mesenteric vein shows a large clot (arrow). (C) Axial contrast-enhanced image through the mid abdomen shows extensive thrombus (arrows) in the branches of the SMV.

stranding and edema are typical associated findings. Multiple veins may be involved. Venous collaterals may also be present.[52]

SUMMARY

MDCT and 3D imaging are now accepted as an excellent first-line imaging modality in patients with a wide array of suspected pathology. The examination is rapid, high-resolution, and comprehensive, allowing visualization of the arteries, veins, and bowel simultaneously. MDCT examinations provide crucial information that guides medical and surgical management.

REFERENCES

1. Horton KM, Fishman EK. Volume-rendered 3D CT of the mesenteric vasculature: normal anatomy, anatomic variants, and pathologic conditions. Radiographics 2002;22:161–72.

2. Horton KM, Fishman EK. 3D CT angiography of the celiac and superior mesenteric arteries with multidetector CT data sets: preliminary observations. Abdom Imaging 2000;25:523–5.

3. Johnson PT, Heath DG, Kuszyk BS, et al. CT angiography with volume rendering: advantages and applications in splanchnic vascular imaging. Radiology 1996;200:564–8.

4. Horton KM, Fishman EK. Mutidetector row and 3D CT of the mesenteric vasculature: normal anatomy and pathology. Semin Ultrasound CT MR 2003;24: 353–63.

5. Vandamme JP, Bonte J, Van der Schueren G. A revaluation of hepatic and cystic arteries. The importance of the aberrant hepatic branches. Acta Anat (Basel) 1969;73:192–209.

6. Hazirolan T, Metin Y, Karaosmanoglu AD, et al. Mesenteric arterial variations detected at MDCT angiography of abdominal aorta. AJR Am J Roentgenol 2009;192:1097–102.

7. Kumano S, Tsuda T, Tanaka H, et al. Preoperative evaluation of perigastric vascular anatomy by 3-dimensional computed tomographic angiography using 16-channel multidetector-row computed tomography for laparoscopic gastrectomy in patients with early gastric cancer. J Comput Assist Tomogr 2007;31:93–7.

8. Kornblith PL, Boley SJ, Whitehouse BS. Anatomy of the splanchnic circulation. Surg Clin North Am 1992; 72:1–30.

9. Rosenblum JD, Boyle CM, Schwartz LB. The mesenteric circulation. Anatomy and physiology. Surg Clin North Am 1997;77:289–306.

10. Chiesa R, Astore D, Guzzo G, et al. Visceral artery aneurysms. Ann Vasc Surg 2005;19:42–8.

11. Rokke O, Sondenaa K, Amundsen S, et al. The diagnosis and management of splanchnic artery aneurysms. Scand J Gastroenterol 1996;31:737–43.

12. Horton KM, Smith C, Fishman EK. MDCT and 3D CT angiography of splanchnic artery aneurysms. AJR Am J Roentgenol 2007;189:641–7.

13. Pilleul F, Beuf O. Diagnosis of splanchnic artery aneurysms and pseudoaneurysms, with special reference to contrast enhanced 3D magnetic resonance angiography: a review. Acta Radiol 2004;45: 702–8.

14. Gabelmann A, Gorich J, Merkle EM. Endovascular treatment of visceral artery aneurysms. J Endovasc Ther 2002;9:38–47.

15. O'Driscoll D, Olliff SP, Olliff JF. Hepatic artery aneurysm. Br J Radiol 1999;72:1018–25.

16. Liu Q, Lu JP, Wang F, et al. Visceral artery aneurysms: evaluation using 3D contrast-enhanced MR angiography. AJR Am J Roentgenol 2008; 191:826–33.

17. Barmeir E, Halachmi S, Croitoru S, et al. CT angiography diagnosis of spontaneous dissection of the superior mesenteric artery. AJR Am J Roentgenol 1998;171:1429–30.

18. Krupski WC, Effeney DJ, Ehrenfeld WK. Spontaneous dissection of the superior mesenteric artery. J Vasc Surg 1985;2:731–4.

19. Corbetti F, Vigo M, Bulzacchi A, et al. CT diagnosis of spontaneous dissection of the superior mesenteric artery. J Comput Assist Tomogr 1989; 13:965–7.

20. Jones SA, Carter R, Smith LL, et al. Arteriomesenteric duodenal compression. Am J Surg 1960;100: 262–77.

21. Mansberger AR Jr, Hearn JB, Byers RM, et al. Vascular compression of the duodenum. Emphasis on accurate diagnosis. Am J Surg 1968;115:89–96.

22. Marchant EA, Alvear DT, Fagelman KM. True clinical entity of vascular compression of the duodenum in adolescence. Surg Gynecol Obstet 1989;168:381–6.

23. Griffiths GJ, Whitehouse GH. Radiological features of vascular compression of the duodenum occurring as a complication of the treatment of scoliosis (the cast syndrome). Clin Radiol 1978;29:77–83.

24. Konen E, Amitai M, Apter S, et al. CT angiography of superior mesenteric artery syndrome. AJR Am J Roentgenol 1998;171:1279–81.

25. Gustafsson L, Falk A, Lukes PJ, et al. Diagnosis and treatment of superior mesenteric artery syndrome. Br J Surg 1984;71:499–501.

26. Applegate GR, Cohen AJ. Dynamic CT in superior mesenteric artery syndrome. J Comput Assist Tomogr 1988;12:976–80.

27. Michael M, Widmer U, Wildermuth S, et al. Segmental arterial mediolysis: CTA findings at

presentation and follow-up. AJR Am J Roentgenol 2006;187:1463–9.

28. Heritz DM, Butany J, Johnston KW, et al. Intraabdominal hemorrhage as a result of segmental mediolytic arteritis of an omental artery: case report. J Vasc Surg 1990;12:561–5.

29. Lindner HH, Kemprud E. A clinicoanatomical study of the arcuate ligament of the diaphragm. Arch Surg 1971;103:600–5.

30. Horton KM, Talamini MA, Fishman EK. Median arcuate ligament syndrome: evaluation with CT angiography. Radiographics 2005;25:1177–82.

31. Reilly LM, Ammar AD, Stoney RJ, et al. Late results following operative repair for celiac artery compression syndrome. J Vasc Surg 1985;2:79–91.

32. Park WM, Gloviczki P, Cherry KJ Jr, et al. Contemporary management of acute mesenteric ischemia: Factors associated with survival. J Vasc Surg 2002;35:445–52.

33. Lee R, Tung HK, Tung PH, et al. CT in acute mesenteric ischaemia. Clin Radiol 2003;58:279–87.

34. Oldenburg WA, Lau LL, Rodenberg TJ, et al. Acute mesenteric ischemia: a clinical review. Arch Intern Med 2004;164:1054–62.

35. Shih MC, Hagspiel KD. CTA and MRA in mesenteric ischemia: part 1, role in diagnosis and differential diagnosis. AJR Am J Roentgenol 2007;188: 452–61.

36. Shih MC, Angle JF, Leung DA, et al. CTA and MRA in mesenteric ischemia: part 2, normal findings and complications after surgical and endovascular treatment. AJR Am J Roentgenol 2007;188:462–71.

37. Horton KM, Fishman EK. Multidetector CT angiography in the diagnosis of mesenteric ischemia. Radiol Clin North Am 2007;45:275–88.

38. Horton KM, Fishman EK. Multi-detector row CT of mesenteric ischemia: can it be done? Radiographics 2001;21:1463–73.

39. Kim JY, Ha HK, Byun JY, et al. Intestinal infarction secondary to mesenteric venous thrombosis: CT-pathologic correlation. J Comput Assist Tomogr 1993;17:382–5.

40. De Filippo M, Sagone C, Zompatori M. Unenhanced MDCT findings of acute bowel ischemia. AJR Am J Roentgenol 2008;190:W271.

41. Furukawa A, Kanasaki S, Kono N, et al. CT diagnosis of acute mesenteric ischemia from various causes. AJR Am J Roentgenol 2009;192:408–16.

42. Lock G. Acute mesenteric ischemia: classification, evaluation and therapy. Acta Gastroenterol Belg 2002;65:220–5.

43. Bassiouny HS. Nonocclusive mesenteric ischemia. Surg Clin North Am 1997;77:319–26.

44. Wildermuth S, Leschka S, Alkadhi H, et al. Multislice CT in the pre- and postinterventional evaluation of mesenteric perfusion. Eur Radiol 2005; 15:1203–10.

45. Berland T, Oldenburg WA. Acute mesenteric ischemia. Curr Gastroenterol Rep 2008;10:341–6.

46. Cognet F, Ben Salem D, Dranssart M, et al. Chronic mesenteric ischemia: imaging and percutaneous treatment. Radiographics 2002;22:863–79. [discussion: 879–80].

47. Roobottom CA, Dubbins PA. Significant disease of the celiac and superior mesenteric arteries in asymptomatic patients: predictive value of Doppler sonography. AJR Am J Roentgenol 1993;161:985–8.

48. Thomas JH, Blake K, Pierce GE, et al. The clinical course of asymptomatic mesenteric arterial stenosis. J Vasc Surg 1998;27:840–4.

49. Park WM, Cherry KJ Jr, Chua HK, et al. Current results of open revascularization for chronic mesenteric ischemia: a standard for comparison. J Vasc Surg 2002;35:853–9.

50. Matsumoto AH, Angle JF, Spinosa DJ, et al. Percutaneous transluminal angioplasty and stenting in the treatment of chronic mesenteric ischemia: results and longterm followup. J Am Coll Surg 2002;194: S22–31.

51. Stoney RJ, Cunningham CG. Acute mesenteric ischemia. Surgery 1993;114:489–90.

52. Bradbury MS, Kavanagh PV, Bechtold RE, et al. Mesenteric venous thrombosis: diagnosis and noninvasive imaging. Radiographics 2002;22: 527–41.

53. Warshauer DM, Lee JK, Mauro MA, et al. Superior mesenteric vein thrombosis with radiologically occult cause: a retrospective study of 43 cases. AJR Am J Roentgenol 2001;177(4):837–41.

CT Angiography of the Renal Circulation

Peter S. Liu, MD*, Joel F. Platt, MD

KEYWORDS

- CT angiography • Kidney • Renal circulation
- Preoperative evaluation • Renal artery stenosis

Computed tomographic angiography (CTA) has evolved over the past 2 decades from a technical curiosity into a robust, noninvasive method for angiographic investigation of suspected renal disease. Although catheter angiography remains the accepted gold standard for imaging of the renal vascular system, rapid progress in cross-sectional imaging techniques has caused a paradigm shift in many diagnostic algorithms toward noninvasive techniques such as CTA.[1,2] Whereas catheter angiography is limited to luminal vascular imaging, cross-sectional imaging techniques provide an opportunity for comprehensive renal investigation, including renal parenchymal and excretory imaging that would be impossible with angiography alone. While other competing noninvasive technologies such as ultrasound and magnetic resonance angiography can be used successfully in renal imaging, the benefits of CTA are substantial, including high spatial and temporal resolution, widespread availability, implantable device compatibility, and easy technical reproducibility.[3,4] This article describes the technical considerations relevant to CTA of the renal vascular system, postprocessing algorithms for volumetric data, and numerous specific applications, including renal artery stenosis, acute occlusive disease, aneurysms, preoperative evaluation, and postprocedural follow-up.

TECHNIQUE
Computed Tomography Acquisition

Because the kidneys are of relatively small volume but receive up to a quarter of cardiac output, renal transit time is rapid, with approximately 6 seconds between initial renal arterial and renal venous opacification.[5] Four phases of renal enhancement have been reported, including an arterial vascular phase, combined venous/angionephrogram phase, nephrographic phase, and an excretory phase; these all occur across a relatively narrow temporal window from 15 to 25 seconds after contrast administration through 180 to 300 seconds. This requirement for high temporal scan resolution makes accurate imaging of renal enhancement technically challenging. The advent of helical scan technique and evolution of multidetector computed tomography (CT) technology has dramatically transformed CTA by facilitating volumetric data acquisition with isotropic submillimeter resolution and rapid scan speeds that permit highly accurate timing, including for angiographic evaluation.[3,4]

The use of iodinated contrast material is mandatory for intravascular opacification on CT. Because iodinated contrast material can be nephrotoxic in patients with marginal renal function, using the lowest possible volume of contrast is desirable to minimize any potential renal insult. The greater scan coverage provided by multidetector-row CT (MDCT) versus conventional single-detector CT systems results in much shorter acquisition times. As a result, shorter acquisition times permit a finer acquisition window, which means that less contrast is required for complete vascular opacification during a short acquisition window versus a long acquisition window.[2] As an example, when comparing a 4-slice and 16-slice MDCT system with equivalent gantry rotation times, a typical renal MDCT volume can be acquired on the 16-slice unit in approximately one-third of the acquisition time.[2] This temporal gain allows the

Department of Radiology, University of Michigan Medical Center, 1500 East Medical Center Drive, Ann Arbor, MI 48109-0030, USA
* Corresponding author.
E-mail address: peterliu@med.umich.edu

Radiol Clin N Am 48 (2010) 347–365
doi:10.1016/j.rcl.2010.02.005

administered contrast volume to decrease by approximately 20% to 35% of the original volume, depending on iodine concentration in the contrast medium. Power injectors allow rapid delivery of contrast medium at pressures unachievable by hand injection, creating a uniform contrast bolus. Dual-head injector models allow both contrast and saline injection in the same continuous bolus, allowing immediate saline flush after contrast injection, thereby maximizing contrast efficiency and decreasing dense venous contrast artifacts. However, as scanner speed increases and administered contrast volumes decrease, achieving accurate contrast bolus timing becomes even more essential. Fixed scan delays are satisfactory for routine CT imaging. The narrow temporal window for pure arterial imaging coupled with the variability in circulation time between individuals (particularly acutely ill patients or those with cardiovascular compromise) results in variable time to peak arterial enhancement.[4,6] As such, a small "test-bolus"/"mini bolus" preliminary injection or an automated bolus-tracking software is commonly used to accurately time scan acquisition in relation to contrast arrival time in the aortorenal circulation.

Current renal CTA protocols often rely on several scan acquisitions to provide comprehensive renal imaging. Precontrast imaging can be performed as part of a renal CTA protocol to aid to identify acute hemorrhage, vascular calcifications, collecting system calculi, and renal masses.[7] Noncontrast imaging can be accomplished with a low-dose technique and thick section acquisition, as this dataset is used as a complement to the contrast-enhanced dataset.[2] At the authors' institution, precontrast imaging is accomplished using the following technical parameters: acquisition volume starting 2 cm above the kidneys and extending through the aortic bifurcation; acquired image slice thickness is 5 mm; pitch of 1.375. Subsequently, thin-section arterial phase renal CTA is acquired using a similar acquisition volume, 0.625 mm slice thickness, with 0 mm gap, and pitch of 1.375; additional 2.5-mm thick slices are reconstructed from the helical dataset for routine axial interpretation (LightSpeed VCT, General Electric Healthcare, Milwaukee, WI, USA). Contrast injection is accomplished using a power injector capable of delivering 100 mL of iodinated contrast (Isovue-370, Bracco Diagnostics, Princeton, NJ, USA) material at a rate of 4 mL/s, followed by a 50-mL saline flush at the same rate. Automatic bolus-tracking software (SmartPrep, GE Healthcare, Milwaukee, WI, USA) is used for accurate contrast timing by monitoring enhancement in the suprarenal abdominal aorta.

Following completion of the arterial CTA data acquisition, a nephrographic phase dataset is obtained using similar scan parameters to the noncontrast dataset, with scan acquisition beginning approximately 100 seconds after contrast injection. A delayed scout image can be obtained at 4 to 7 minutes if an overview of collecting system morphology is desired, such as in the preoperative evaluation for potential renal donors.

Scan Postprocessing

Postprocessing techniques play a very important role in renal CTA. Because state of the art helical MDCT can result in several hundred images for a single imaging sequence, the use of postprocessing algorithms are used to easily display the 3-dimensional (3D) relationships of the acquired volumetric dataset.[8] Often an interactive approach is preferred for optimal evaluation of CTA datasets, with the interpreting physician doing the primary postprocessing manipulation. While a full review of the different reconstruction techniques is beyond the scope of this article, some general points are considered. The source axial images are an integral part of the study, providing important information about nonvascular findings related to the scan volume, and exposing artifacts that may confound or exaggerate apparent findings seen only on reconstructed images.[2] Early studies demonstrated that the axial source images and multiplanar reformatted images can be used to accurately identify high-grade arterial narrowing and accessory renal arteries.[9] As MDCT technology has matured and has become standard in most practices, other more complex postprocessing algorithms have been introduced for displaying volumetric data, including maximum-intensity projection (MIP), surface-shaded display (SSD), and volume rendering (VR). A study by Rubin and colleagues[10] demonstrated improved accuracy for stenosis grading using MIP postprocessing techniques versus SSD. Subsequently, it has been shown that VR and MIP postprocessing techniques demonstrate similar sensitivity for vessel stenosis, but increased specificity is afforded by the VR technique.[11] The primary advantage of a VR algorithm is the maintenance of the original 3D relationships between objects inherent in the volumetric data set; these relationships can be confused by a projectional technique such as MIP.[8] Additional projectional techniques that account for curvilinear object geometry, such as curved planar reformatted images (CPR), can be of value to "correct for" the degree of tortuosity shown on projectional images; there have been some limited published data to suggest that such newer curved projectional techniques are highly accurate.[12] At the authors' institution, renal CTA studies are postprocessed automatically by a 3D laboratory, as well as reviewed interactively by the primary interpreting physician on a 3D work-station. The authors' 3D laboratory protocol for renal CTA studies includes MIP, VR, and curved multiplanar reconstruction (MPR) images of the renal arteries. The additional diagnostic informa-tion gathered from the postprocessed data sets can help the interpreting physician understand complex anatomic relationships and subtle obli-que vascular narrowings. Furthermore, postpro-cessed images, especially VR images, often aid the referring physician by generating a recogniz-able anatomic image of the pathology in question.

APPLICATIONS
Renal Artery Stenosis

Evaluation of the renal circulation for suspected arterial stenosis is one of the major indications for noninvasive renal vascular imaging, such as CTA. Because of the critical role that renal perfu-sion plays in regulating systemic blood pressure, renal artery stenosis is seen as a potentially treat-able cause of systemic hypertension, which itself is a risk factor for morbid conditions such as stroke, arterial dissection, and myocardial infarc-tion. Unfortunately, renal artery stenosis accounts for only a small fraction (1%–5%) of all hyperten-sion cases in the general population.[13] Nonethe-less, when clinical selection criteria are applied to identify at-risk patients, the estimated preva-lence of renovascular-induced hypertension increases to 20% to 40%.[2,14] Furthermore, reno-vascular disease is a leading cause of end-stage renal disease (ESRD) among the elderly, accounting for approximately 15% to 24% of ESRD cases seen in patients older than 50 years.[15,16] Atherosclerosis accounts for 70% to 90% of all cases.[2,16,17] The next most common cause is fibromuscular dysplasia, accounting for the majority of remaining cases (10%–25%).[16,17] Other causes of renal artery stenosis such as neurofibromatosis, Takayasu arteritis, or radiation arteriopathy are considered rare. Progression of renal artery stenosis has been reported in 51% of patients with any degree of renal artery stenosis after 5 years, and faster 3-year progression rates seen have been shown in patients with higher degrees of stenosis.[18] Ultimately, 3% to 16% of all patients with renal artery stenosis will develop frank arterial occlusion.[16]

From an imaging standpoint, atherosclerotic disease and fibromuscular dysplasia have different characteristic appearances. Atherosclerotic renal artery disease generally manifests on CTA as a stenosis occurring at the vessel origin or in the proximal segment, usually within 2 cm of the vessel ostium (Figs. 1 and 2).[7,13] An atherosclerotic stenosis may be eccentric or concentric, and can demonstrate varying degrees of calcification. Concomitant poststenotic dilation may be seen in the vascular segment immediately downstream from the stenosis (Fig. 3). Fibromuscular dysplasia (FMD) is a collection of several fibrotic disorders that involve the different layers of medium-sized arteries.[13] The most common type (medial fibropla-sia) accounts for approximately 65% to 70% of FMD cases, and demonstrates similar character-istic imaging features on CTA as are seen on conventional angiography, namely, multiple sequential stenoses ("string of pearls" appear-ance) and aneurysm formation (Fig. 4).[17] A stenosis in the mid or distal portion of the renal artery in a young adult female patient would also be typical for FMD. Some subtypes of FMD lack patho-gnmonic radiographic features, whether by conventional angiography or CTA.

Early reports demonstrated a high accuracy of CTA for the detection of hemodynamically signif-icant renal artery stenosis outside of the renal hilum, including on axial images alone.[9] As previ-ously discussed, high sensitivity and specificity for significant narrowing have been reported using 3D postprocessing techniques, primarily including MIP and interactive VR. Similarly, several retrospective comparative studies have shown strong diagnostic performance of CTA in evaluating FMD that was later proven on catheter angiography, with reported sensitivity varying between 87% and 100%.[17,19] When consecutive patients were investigated by both CTA and digital subtraction angiography, 100% of patients with FMD identified on CTA were shown to have FMD on subsequent catheter angiography.[20] In fact, a meta-analysis of available data in 2001 showed exceptionally high diagnostic perfor-mance for renal CTA, with an area under the receiver-operating characteristic curve of 0.99.[21] In the light of such convincing data, consensus statements recommended CTA as a primary diag-nostic modality for the evaluation of suspected renal artery stenosis.[22] However, recent pub-lished data from the multicenter RADISH (Renal Artery Diagnostic Imaging Study in Hypertension) trial calls into question both the reproducibility and diagnostic efficacy of noninvasive renal vascular imaging, including CTA, with the investi-gators concluding that CTA is insufficient for eval-uation/exclusion of suspected renal artery stenosis.[23] Of note, the diagnostic performance of CTA did improve when only atherosclerotic

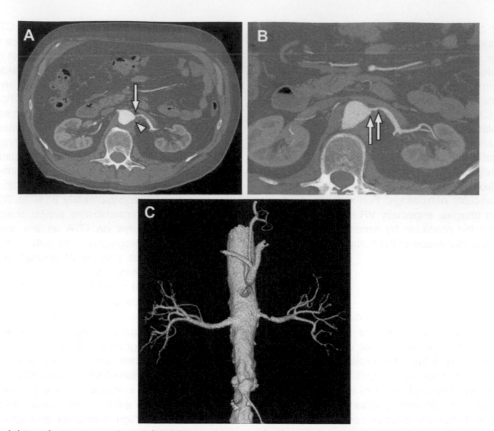

Fig. 1. (A) Renal artery stenosis. Axial CTA image shows moderate ostial narrowing of the left renal artery (arrow) with contiguous atherosclerotic soft plaque extending from the abdominal aorta into the left renal artery origin (arrowhead). (B) Renal artery stenosis. Oblique maximum intensity projection (MIP) image better shows the ostial narrowing, with at least 2 apparent stenoses contributing to the narrowed segment (arrows). (C) Renal artery stenosis. Volume-rendered (VR) image confirms narrowing seen on axial CTA and MIP images.

stenoses were considered, thereby excluding diagnosis of FMD by CTA. Although some have questioned certain technical aspects and population characteristics of the RADISH study, the results did renew interest in prospective trials of noninvasive renal vascular imaging. In fact, new randomized trials comparing CTA to digital subtraction angiography have validated it as a diagnostic technique, showing 94% sensitivity, 93% specificity, and a 99% negative predictive value.[14] These newer data also supported the high efficacy of CTA in the diagnosis of FMD, with all affected renal artery segments shown on CTA. Therefore, these new data would suggest that a negative renal CTA is unlikely to miss occult renovascular disease, though additional prospective studies should be considered.

Acute Renal Artery Occlusion

Acute occlusion of the main renal artery can rapidly lead to renal infarction, as the kidneys have a narrow reported revascularization window

of approximately 60 to 90 minutes and little collateral arterial supply of any clinical significance.[13] Unfortunately, the clinical manifestations of renal infarction are vague and protean, including back or flank pain, nausea, vomiting, and hematuria.[7,13] These ambiguous symptoms can delay accurate diagnosis. Although many different origins exist for acute renal infarction, the most common cause in elderly patients is thromboembolic disease, generally from a cardiac source.[13,24] Some autopsy studies have shown pathologic evidence of renal embolic disease in up to 15% of elderly patients.[25] Renal arterial dissection leading to acute renal artery occlusion should be considered in patients with a known history of connective tissue disease (such as Ehlers-Danlos syndrome), recent renal artery catheterization, established history of abdominal aortic dissection, or in patients with a history of cocaine abuse. It has been estimated that 8% of patients with an abdominal aortic dissection will have an ischemic renal complication.[26] Other causes of acute renal infarction include trauma, dehydration, and

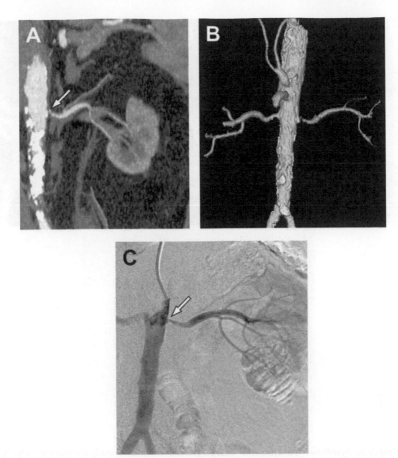

Fig. 2. (*A*) Renal artery stenosis. Oblique MIP image shows severe ostial narrowing of the left renal artery (*arrow*). (*B*) Renal artery stenosis. VR image reveals severe ostial narrowing of the left renal artery. (*C*) Renal artery stenosis. Digital subtraction angiography image confirms suspected ostial narrowing on renal CTA (*arrow*). Patient was treated with percutaneous angioplasty and renal artery stent placement.

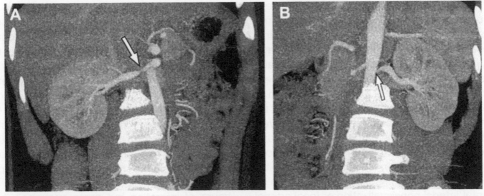

Fig. 3. (*A*) Medically refractory hypertension due to bilateral renal artery stenosis. Oblique MIP image shows severe segmental ostial and proximal narrowing of the right renal artery (*arrow*) with concomitant poststenotic dilation. (*B*) Medically refractory hypertension due to bilateral renal artery stenosis. Oblique MIP image shows severe focal ostial narrowing of the left renal artery (*arrow*) with concomitant poststenotic dilation. The patient underwent surgical revascularization to both kidneys, with marked improvement in blood pressure control.

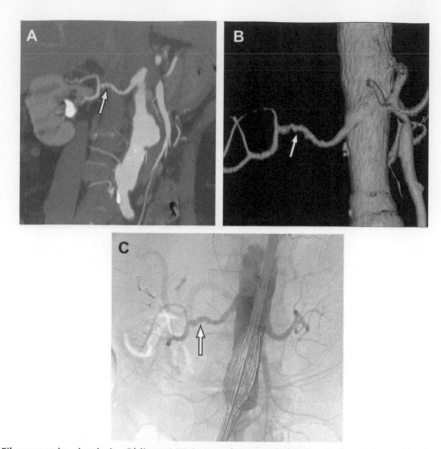

Fig. 4. (A) Fibromuscular dysplasia. Oblique MIP image shows multifocal web formation with tiny intervening aneurysms in the distal right main renal artery (arrow), compatible with fibromuscular dysplasia. (B) Fibromuscular dysplasia. VR image reveals concordant findings to MIP image, with multifocal narrowing of the mid-distal right main renal artery (arrow). (C) Fibromuscular dysplasia. Digital subtraction angiography shows "string of pearls" appearance of the right renal artery (arrow), confirming angiographic diagnosis of fibromuscular dysplasia.

hypercoagulable states such as nephrotic syndrome and Factor V Leiden disease. Acute thrombosis of a preexisting stenosis is less frequently associated with rapid loss of renal function, as chronic ischemia can promote some renal collateral formation.[13] If the diagnosis is made quickly, revascularization attempts can be made using either percutaneous or surgical techniques.

Although acute onset of back or flank pain is considered a "classic" clinical manifestation for renal infarction, there is considerable clinical overlap with retroperitoneal hematoma and renal stone disease, both of which are imaged using noncontrast techniques. As such, the vascular manifestations of acute thromboembolic occlusion, such as segmental arterial nonvisualization or focal arterial narrowing, are rarely imaged and sparsely reported in the literature (Fig. 5).[7,27] The CTA appearance of acute arterial dissection has been reported, including direct visualization of the

intimal flap, which is specific for the diagnosis of dissection.[26] Unfortunately, a severe narrowing with downstream vascular distention may be the only identifiable feature of renal arterial dissection, which overlaps considerably with thromboembolic disease. Often, the resulting parenchymal effects are the only demonstrable feature of ischemic insult, including wedge-shaped or global perfusion abnormalities, segmental mass effect, and perinephric inflammatory changes (Fig. 6).[25,28] Preserved blood flow via capsular collateral vessels to a rim of residual functioning subcapsular nephrons has been termed the "capsular rim" sign. This sign has been reported in approximately 19% of cases, and can develop within hours of infarction but more commonly is seen several days after the insult.[7,24] A more recent "flip-flop" enhancement pattern has also been observed in renal ischemia/infarction, postulated to result from increased cellular permeability

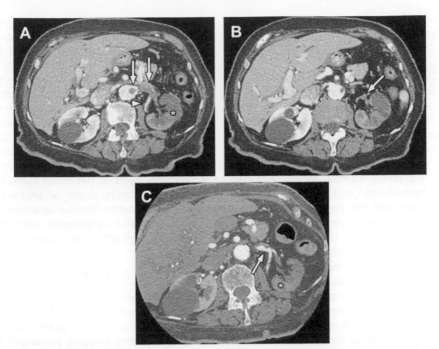

Fig. 5. (A) Acute embolism in patient with atrial fibrillation and new left flank pain. Axial CTA image shows expansile clot within the left main renal artery (*arrow*), which bulges into the aortic lumen itself. Acute embolism with rapid progressive thrombosis of the main renal circulation was diagnosed given the clinical and imaging findings. Asterisk indicates near-absent left nephrogram. There remains some residual flow in a posterior renal branch (*arrowhead*). (B) Acute embolism in patient with atrial fibrillation and new left flank pain. Axial CTA image shows expansile clot near the renal sinus with some preserved peripheral enhancement around the clot itself (*arrow*). (C) Acute embolism in patient with atrial fibrillation and new left flank pain. Axial CTA image obtained after 3 months of anticoagulation shows some clot lysis and restitution of flow within the left main renal artery (*arrow*). However, there remains almost complete absence of the left nephrogram, compatible with global infarction (*asterisk*).

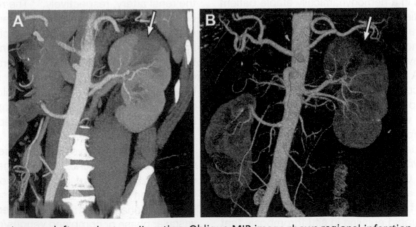

Fig. 6. (A) Spontaneous left renal artery dissection. Oblique MIP image shows regional infarction (*arrow*) in the left upper pole with decreased apparent arterial supply to the affected segment versus other normally perfused segments. Findings and diagnosis were confirmed on catheter angiography. (B) Spontaneous left renal artery dissection. VR image confirms oblique MIP image findings with regional infarction (*arrow*) and decreased arterial supply. Dissection flap was not discretely visualized on renal CTA due to complete downstream thrombosis.

during ischemia that results in leakage of contrast into the extracellular space.[25]

Renal Trauma

Traumatic renal injury is estimated to occur in approximately 8% to 10% of all abdominal traumatic injuries, with blunt traumatic injury accounting for 80% to 90% of cases and penetrating traumatic injury accounting for the remainder.[29] The majority of traumatic renal injuries will be minor injuries, which includes contusions, hematomas, and small lacerations that do not extend into the medulla or violate the collecting system.[7,29] However, major and catastrophic renal injuries can be physiologically devastating because of the substantial circulatory fraction that contributes to renal perfusion. Injuries that result in vascular disruption of the renovascular pedicle or active bleeding in the perinephric space are now considered Grade 4 injuries in the American Association of Surgeons in Trauma grading system, previously classified as a catastrophic category III injury using a radiologic classification system.[30,31] Although such renovascular injuries account for approximately 5% of all renal traumatic injuries, these injuries frequently necessitate emergent surgical management. Therefore, accurate imaging plays a critical role in the triage of suspected renal trauma. Renal CTA using MDCT technology is highly accurate in the depiction of a renovascular traumatic injury, including both blunt and penetrating trauma.[32] In fact, catheter angiography is now rarely indicated for the primary diagnostic evaluation of suspected traumatic renovascular injury. Catheter angiography is currently used only for clarification of ambiguous CTA findings in a hemodynamically stable patient or for potential therapeutic renovascular salvage via an endovascular approach.[7,29]

A comprehensive renal CTA protocol is a rapid method for evaluation of suspected renovascular trauma. CTA allows direct visualization of the primary vascular injury, and also delineates any associated parenchymal or collecting system injury, which would otherwise be occult on catheter angiography. Most renovascular injuries result from rapid deceleration that causes an arterial dissection with subsequent rapid distal thrombosis.[29] On CTA, renal arterial injury generally manifests as a focal cutoff or abrupt vessel termination. It can be difficult to actually identify the flap itself, as the rapid ensuing in situ thrombosis that occurs beyond the flap takeoff decreases the contrast resolution between the true lumen, flap, and false lumen. There are concomitant downstream ischemic changes in the renal parenchyma, including a decreased nephrogram that may be global or segmental in distribution, depending on the dissection location (Fig. 7). A capsular rim sign may be present.[7,29] Frank vascular transection or avulsion can be seen in substantial blunt trauma or penetrating trauma, leading to active extravasation of contrast material in the perinephric space or pseudoaneurysm formation.[13] Venous injury and in situ venous thrombosis are reported complications of renal trauma, both of which are rare.[29] Although CTA is relatively good at detecting acute intraluminal venous thrombosis, it can be problematic in the detection of subtle venous lacerations or shear injuries—catheter venography may be indicated if there is a high clinical suspicion.

Renal Artery Aneurysms

Renal artery aneurysms are rare lesions, with an estimated prevalence of 0.01% to 0.1%.[7] Renal aneurysms may be detected incidentally at autopsy or during imaging investigation for other indications. Renal aneurysms can be divided into several groups based on anatomic characteristics, such as location (extrarenal vs intrarenal) or morphology (saccular vs fusiform). The most common cause of renal artery aneurysms is atherosclerosis, particularly for aneurysms in an extrarenal location.[7] Other origins of aneurysm formation include FMD, connective tissue disease, mycotic disease, and vasculitis (such as Behcet disease and polyarteritis nodosa).[13] Renal aneurysms are frequently asymptomatic lesions; however, back pain and hypertension have been reported as a result of downstream embolic phenomenon and aneurysm sac compression of the renal artery, respectively.[13] The risk of rupture is increased when the diameter exceeds 2 cm and in pregnant patients.[33] Mural calcification may impart some mild protection against rupture.[13] Lesions smaller than 2 cm are generally managed conservatively. Larger lesions, symptomatic lesions, or lesions in women of childbearing age often require an individualized approach, with both surgical and endovascular repair methods described.[33]

Renal artery aneurysms can generally be well assessed on CTA. Noncontrast images can clearly show the presence of continuous or interrupted calcification about the aneurysm margin.[7] Contrast-enhanced images obtained during the vascular phase or combined venous/angionephrogram phase can show the amount of mural thrombus and internal enhancement evident within the aneurysm sac (Figs. 8 and 9). Thin-section MDCT and postprocessing techniques allow

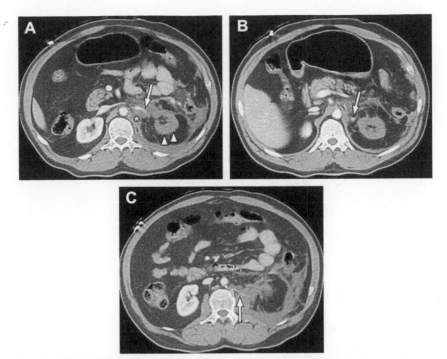

Fig. 7. (A) Motorcycle-versus-automobile trauma patient. Axial CTA image shows abrupt disruption of the left renal artery (arrow) with resulting retroperitoneal hematoma (asterisk). Note absent left nephrogram, indicative of acute renal ischemia (arrowheads). (B) Motorcycle-versus-automobile trauma patient. Axial CTA image shows active extravasation of arterial contrast into the left perinephric space (arrow). (C) Motorcycle-versus-automobile trauma patient. Axial CTA image shows dependent layering of extravasated contrast in retroperitoneal hematoma (arrow).

visualization of smaller aneurysms that may be easily missed on axial images due to the inherent tortuosity of the renal arterial circulation.[33] Comprehensive renal CTA protocols may show the downstream infarcted parenchymal changes if distal embolic phenomena are suspected. Unfortunately, the diagnostic utility of CTA in assessing microaneurysms of the intrarenal circulation is limited, as the spatial resolution and rapid background parenchymal enhancement in the renal cortex can render peripheral/distal aneurysms occult on CTA.[13] Therefore, while a comprehensive renal CTA protocol may show parenchymal infarcts or extrarenal hematomas in patients with

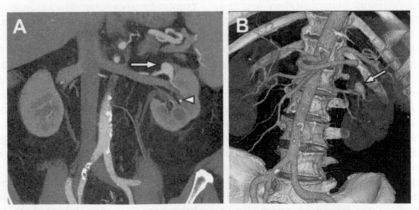

Fig. 8. (A) Renal artery aneurysm. Oblique MIP image shows a focal saccular aneurysm of the left renal artery near the left renal hilum (arrow). Nonobstructing renal calculus is also present (arrowhead). (B) Renal artery aneurysm. VR image also depicts left renal artery aneurysm (arrow). Interactive VR postprocessing technique allows the interpreting physician to delineate the relationship of the aneurysm sac to intrarenal branch arteries.

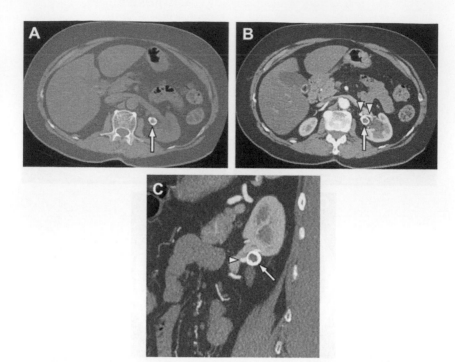

Fig. 9. (*A*) Thrombosed left renal artery aneurysm. Axial precontrast CT image shows a heavily calcified eccentric saccular aneurysm (*arrow*) of the left main renal artery near the renal hilum. (*B*) Thrombosed left renal artery aneurysm. Axial arterial phase CTA image shows patency of the left renal artery (*arrowheads*) coursing adjacent to the calcified aneurysm sac (*arrow*). (*C*) Thrombosed left renal artery aneurysm. Oblique MIP image confirms the adjacent vessel (*arrowhead*) passes anterior to the calcified aneurysm sac (*arrow*). No opacification is seen within the aneurysm sac itself, confirming thrombosis.

suspected tiny intrarenal aneurysms such as those with polyarteritis nodosa, catheter angiography may be required to directly visualize the aneurysms themselves.[13]

Preoperative Evaluation: Renal Donors

As a result of the marked discrepancy between patients awaiting renal transplantation and the availability of cadaveric grafts, the use of living renal donors has become an increasingly common surgical procedure.[34] Laparoscopic renal nephrectomy was introduced in 1995, and has become the standard method for renal harvesting in many transplant centers.[35] The advantages of a laparoscopic operative approach are many, including decreased blood loss, reduced postoperative pain and narcotic requirement, shorter hospital stay with faster return to regular activities, as well as an improved cosmetic result.[35,36] Outcomes data show similar graft survivals for transplants obtained via open surgery versus laparoscopic harvesting.[36] However, the limited operative field of view that results from laparoscopic exposure leads to technical challenges for the operating surgeon, particularly regarding the renal vascular supply.

Therefore, preoperative imaging has become critical to assist surgeons in selecting optimal donor candidates. Before the advent of modern CT technology, preoperative evaluation for potential living renal donors was accomplished via a combination of excretory urography, catheter angiography, and sometimes ultrasound examination.[34] At present, the modern MDCT technique allows comprehensive noninvasive evaluation of potential renal donors in a single study, with reported accuracy similar or superior to prior combination techniques.[37,38] A comprehensive renal CTA protocol can address numerous preoperative considerations, including potential vascular, parenchymal, and collecting system variance/abnormalities.

Arterial anatomic assessment has traditionally been the most critical aspect of preoperative imaging in patients undergoing transplant nephrectomy, including delineation of accessory renal arteries (**Figs. 10** and **11**) or parenchymal branches originating less than 1.5 to 2.0 cm from the renal artery origin, also called "prehilar" branches (**Fig. 12**).[13,35] Multiple renal arteries have a reported incidence of approximately 18% to 32%, but generally are not considered a contraindication to transplantation, especially when well

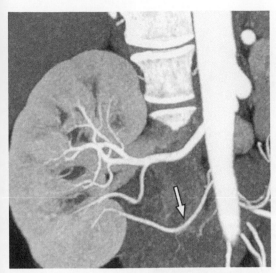

Fig. 10. Preoperative evaluation for potential renal donation. Oblique MIP image shows an accessory right renal artery (*arrow*).

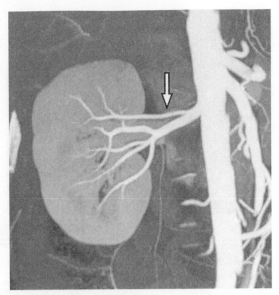

Fig. 12. Preoperative evaluation for potential renal donation. Oblique MIP image shows a prehilar branch originating from the right renal artery (*arrow*) that supplies the right upper pole.

depicted on preoperative imaging.[35,39] However, the presence of prehilar branches can jeopardize a technically adequate anastomosis, and has a reported prevalence of 10%, though recent imaging literature suggests an even higher incidence of 15% to 21%.[36,40] Therefore, it is critical to accurately define the presence of prehilar branches on preoperative imaging, particularly in patients undergoing laparoscopic nephrectomy. Renal CTA has been reported as highly accurate for identifying prehilar branches.[36,38]

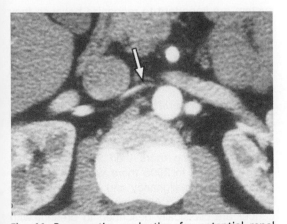

Fig. 11. Preoperative evaluation for potential renal donation. Axial CTA image shows a tiny accessory renal artery originating from the anterior aspect of the aorta (*arrow*). Tiny accessory arteries can be overlooked on coronal reformatted MIP images or VR images, particularly if originating from the anterior aspect of the aorta. Review of the native acquired axial CTA images is critical to avoid this error.

The left kidney is generally preferred for donor nephrectomy, because of its longer renal vein segment that makes recipient transplantation easier without necessitating complex venous reconstruction. The variance in renal venous anatomy is substantially less than that of arterial anatomy, with the majority of the population demonstrating single renal veins bilaterally.[35] The most common left renal vein anomaly is a circumaortic left renal vein, reported in up to 11% of patients in the clinical literature and in up to 17% of cadaveric studies (**Fig. 13**).[35] A retroaortic vein is uncommon, reported in 2% to 3% of the population.[41] Anomalies of the left renal vein are not a contraindication to transplantation, with similar reported patient/graft outcomes after transplantation as grafts with standard anatomy.[42] Duplicated or multiple renal veins are reportedly more frequent on the right side.[35,39] The presence of multiple right renal veins has been associated with higher incidence of graft renal vein thrombosis, and therefore can be considered a contraindication for renal harvesting.[43] Large systemic venous tributaries entering the left renal vein, including lumbar, gonadal, adrenal, or retroperitoneal veins, can also be well delineated on renal CTA. Identification of substantial venous channels can be important for laparoscopic planning, as lumbar tributaries can be easily overlooked due to the limited operative exposure.[36,44] Recent imaging literature suggests that retroperitoneal or gonadal varices (vessel diameter ≥ 5 mm) actually

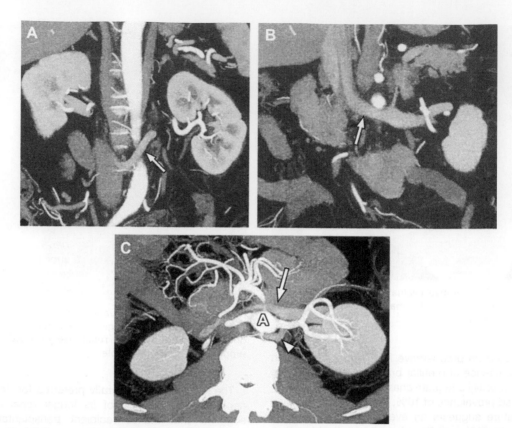

Fig. 13. (*A*) Preoperative evaluation for potential renal donation. Oblique MIP image shows the retroaortic component of a circumaortic left renal vein (*arrow*). (*B*) Preoperative evaluation for potential renal donation. Oblique MIP image shows the preaortic component of a circumaortic left renal vein (*arrow*). (*C*) Preoperative evaluation for potential renal donation. Thick-volume oblique MIP image shows both components of the circumaortic left renal vein, including the retroaortic component (*arrowhead*) and the preaortic component (*arrow*), which together encircle the aorta (A).

occur with a relatively high frequency.[40] This finding may be important, as some transplant centers use substantial retroperitoneal varices as an exclusion criteria for transplantation.[35]

In addition to potential vascular anomalies, a comprehensive renal CTA protocol can demonstrate possible renal parenchymal and collecting system pathology that may preclude transplantation. Developmental renal anomalies such as horseshoe kidney, agenesis, and ectopia are obvious contraindications for transplantation. Similarly, the presence of renal pathology, including renal neoplasm, medullary sponge kidney, polycystic kidney disease, or hydronephrosis—all demonstrable on CTA—can be considered a contraindication to transplantation.[35] The presence of nephrolithiasis is considered a relative contraindication for transplantation, but is well evaluated on a comprehensive renal CTA protocol.[38] Although relatively uncommon when compared with the incidence of vascular abnormalities, congenital anomalies of the collecting

system are important to recognize because they may substantially affect surgical planning.[35,38] At the authors' institution, collecting system abnormalities are easily evaluated on delayed scout imaging to minimize radiation exposure.

Preoperative Evaluation: Renal Tumors

Malignancies of the kidney account for only 1% to 2% of all malignancies, with renal cell carcinoma (RCC) constituting more than 90% of all renal malignancies.[45] In 2005 there were 36,160 new cases of renal malignancy and 12,660 deaths in the United States.[46] Although patients with renal cancer are classically described to present with a clinical triad of pain, hematuria, and flank mass, it is estimated that 30% to 50% of new renal cancer cases are now diagnosed incidentally during cross-sectional imaging for unrelated complaints. This high incidental detection rate has resulted in more early-stage lesions, which may be amenable to newer surgical techniques to maximize residual renal function, such as nephron-sparing surgery (NSS).[47] NSS has been shown to have similar success rates to radical nephrectomy for tumors smaller than 4 cm in patients with normal contralateral renal function, and very low local recurrence rates have been demonstrated.[48] The staging accuracy of CT for RCC has been reported to be 91%, making it an optimal test for both detection and staging purposes.[46] RCC is particularly prone to vascular invasion, with renal vein invasion demonstrated in 25% to 30% of cases and inferior vena cava (IVC) invasion present in 7% of cases. Therefore, accurate evaluation of the renal vasculature is critical for proper RCC staging. Moreover, the increased technical challenge of NSS mandates understanding the complex 3D relationship between the tumor and renal vasculature, particularly the renal arterial circulation.

Comprehensive renal CTA accurately depicts renal tumor for staging purposes, and clearly delineates the relevant preoperative vascular considerations, including renal vein thrombus and parasitized capsular arteries.[45] CT is useful in the direct depiction of renal vein thrombus, including both bland and tumor thrombus, with a positive predictive value of 92% and negative predictive value of 97%.[47] Bland thrombus is generally seen as a low-attenuation filling defect within the enhancing renal vein during the venous/angionephrogram or nephrograhic phase of enhancement. A caliber change of the main renal vein and clot extension into collateral veins are considered corroborative signs of tumor thrombus, but can be confounded by the increased venous return from large tumors.[47] Enhancing foci within the thrombus during arterial phase imaging are highly suggestive of tumor thrombus rather than bland thrombus (Fig. 14).[45] The presence of IVC involvement, including the location of the cephalad extent, is important for surgical planning, as extension into the intrahepatic IVC or supradiaphragmatic IVC will alter the surgical plan, potentially requiring cardiothoracic surgical consultation. Although some investigators believe magnetic resonance imaging (MRI) is somewhat superior to MDCT for depiction of IVC thrombus, MDCT with 3D reformatted images has been shown to accurately show the extent of IVC thrombus.[47,49] The use of renal CTA in depicting the renal arterial anatomy and tumor location and extent is very important for newer surgical approaches, including NSS. Preoperative identification of the renal tumor arterial supply is important because recruited capsular or aberrant vessels can be seen in 9% of cases, and may be an important source of hemorrhage if overlooked in a laparoscopic approach (Fig. 15). One study has reported 100% accuracy in the depiction of such recruited arterial supply.[45] Unfortunately, the accuracy of renal CTA for depicting arterial tumor infiltration about the renal hilum has been reported as much lower, with a specificity of approximately 40%.[46] This low value may be confounded on imaging by a sterile inflammatory response near the renal hilum that surrounds the artery, rather than actual perivascular tumor extension.

Preoperative Evaluation: Ureteropelvic Junction Obstruction

Ureteropelvic junction (UPJ) obstruction is a condition that encompasses both primary and secondary causes of potentially treatable narrowing at the base of the renal pelvis as it transitions

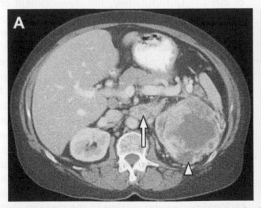
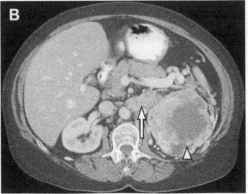

Fig. 14. (A) Left renal cell carcinoma. In addition to the large left renal mass (*arrowhead*), there is expansion of the left renal vein with heterogeneous enhancing tissue (*arrow*) in the renal vein itself, compatible with tumor thrombus. (B) Left renal cell carcinoma. In addition to the large left renal mass (*arrowhead*), there is expansion of the left renal vein with heterogeneous enhancing tissue (*arrow*) in the renal vein itself, compatible with tumor thrombus.

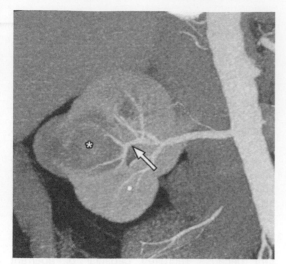

Fig. 15. Right renal cell carcinoma. Oblique MIP image shows a hypovascular mass in the interpolar region of the right kidney (*asterisk*). The vascular supply feeding the tumor is well delineated (*arrow*) on renal CTA.

to the proximal ureter. UPJ obstruction in children is often primary due to developmental problems of collagen and smooth muscle at the UPJ, whereas UPJ obstruction in adults is frequently secondary to acquired stenoses from infection, ischemia, or nephrolithiasis.[50] The emergence of endourologic techniques for the treatment of UPJ obstruction has led to decreased perioperative morbidity, including shorter hospitalization stays, decreased postoperative pain, and faster return to normal daily activity.[50] However, because the endourologic procedure requires a deep longitudinal cut through the UPJ, there is an increased risk of complications. Specifically, vascular complications are seen in up to 10% of cases, including hematoma, pseudoaneurysm, or arterial-venous fistula formation.[51] Both anatomic and imaging studies have shown crossing vessels near the UPJ in a variable proportion of the population, reported as between 29% and 75% of the population, depending on location from the UPJ itself.[51–53] Published data demonstrate a higher rate of endourologic treatment failure when crossing vessels are present.[54] However, the causative role of crossing vessels in UPJ obstruction and the relative risk posed by such vessels for proposed endovascular UPJ surgery are areas of substantial debate in the literature. As such, the need for preoperative assessment of crossing vessels near the UPJ may be debated. Nonetheless, identification of crossing vessels near the UPJ can affect surgical planning, with some surgeons preferring to use an open or

laparoscopic approach if crossing vessels are regarded as a contraindication to endourologic surgery.[53]

Renal CTA is highly effective at demonstrating the presence of crossing vessels in the setting of UPJ obstruction (**Fig. 16**). Evaluation of early CTA technology with 10-mm sections demonstrated 100% sensitivity and 97% specificity for detection of crossing vessels when compared with catheter angiography.[55] Subsequent studies have shown similar excellent diagnostic performance, with near perfect accuracy seen when modern thin-section protocols are implemented.[50,53] Renal CTA was able to correctly identify the crossing vessel as artery or vein in several published series.[50,53] Renal CTA is noninvasive, fast, and cheaper to perform when compared with catheter angiography. Furthermore, renal CTA creates volumetric datasets that can be postprocessed using MIP or VR techniques to easily demonstrate the 3D relationships of crossing vessels in relation to the UPJ obstruction, benefiting both interpreting radiologists and referring urologists.[53]

Postprocedural Evaluation: Renal Artery Stents

The use of renal artery stents to augment balloon angioplasty in percutaneous revascularization of renal artery stenosis is becoming increasingly common, particularly for treatment of ostial lesions. Although the procedure itself may treat the initial arterial stenosis, a meta-analysis demonstrated that approximately 17% of patients will develop in-stent restenosis, noting one series showing rates up to 39% using a particular type of stent.[56] Unfortunately, the development of in-stent restenosis can be clinically occult, often with ambiguous changes in clinical parameters (such as worsening blood pressure or declining renal function) that do not specifically indicate in-stent restenosis.[57] Therefore, direct anatomic surveillance is often frequently desired. Both MRI and ultrasound have been used as noninvasive methods for evaluating renal artery stents. However, sonographic evaluation of renal artery stents remains operator dependent and can be substantially limited by bowel gas, body habitus, or acoustic impedance from the stent itself.[58] Similarly, MRI evaluation can be heavily degraded by local dephasing related to the metallic stent itself, resulting in segmental vascular nonvisualization. Catheter angiography may be required for optimal evaluation, but is both invasive and time consuming.

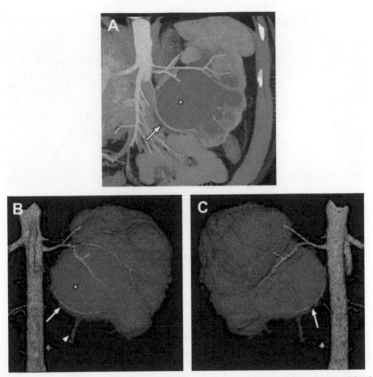

Fig. 16. (A) UPJ obstruction. Oblique subvolume MIP image shows UPJ obstruction with dilated renal pelvis (*asterisk*) and caliectasis. A crossing accessory renal artery is shown near the UPJ obstruction (*arrow*). (B) UPJ obstruction. Anterior projection of volume rendered image with variable transparency of background renal parenchyma/collecting system shows crossing artery (*arrow*) near the UPJ obstruction. Dilated renal pelvis (*asterisk*) and caliectasis is noted, while the proximal ureter (*arrowhead*) is nondilated. (C) UPJ obstruction. Posterior projection of VR image with variable transparency of background renal parenchyma/collecting system shows crossing artery (*arrow*) near the UPJ obstruction. Interactive evaluation of the VR 3D dataset allows proper localization of the crossing vessel to the anterior aspect of the UPJ obstruction. This relationship is suggested on posterior projectional VR image with the use of variable transparency.

Renal CTA has been proposed as a noninvasive method for anatomic evaluation of in situ stents. Mature MDCT technology permits isotropic imaging of the renal arteries in a narrow temporal window with high-resolution volumetric data. The beam-hardening artifacts associated with metal stents and dense atherosclerotic calcifications can be mitigated by thin-section MDCT, allowing visualization of the in-stent vascular lumen (Fig. 17).[58,59] Several studies have demonstrated

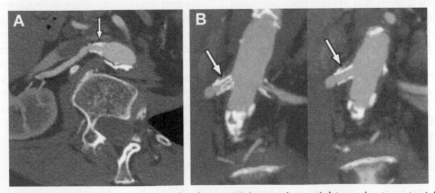

Fig. 17. (A) Right renal artery stent. Oblique subvolume MIP image shows right renal artery stent (*arrow*) with preserved in-stent patency. (B) Right renal artery stent. Oblique MPR images show right renal artery stent (*arrow*) with preserved in-stent patency.

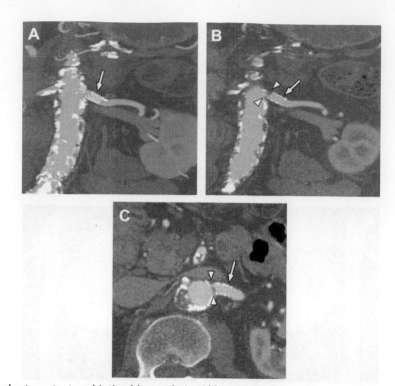

Fig. 18. (*A*) Renal artery stent and intimal hyperplasia. Oblique subvolume MIP image shows right renal artery stent (*arrow*). Note that intimal hyperplasia is not well depicted by MIP technique because of thick selected slab volume. (*B*) Renal artery stent and intimal hyperplasia. Oblique MPR image shows right renal artery stent (*arrow*) with focal low attenuation projecting near the proximal margin of the stent (*arrowhead*), compatible with intimal hyperplasia. (*C*) Renal artery stent and intimal hyperplasia. Oblique MPR image shows right renal artery stent (*arrow*) with focal low attenuation projecting near the proximal margin of the stent (*arrowhead*), compatible with intimal hyperplasia.

the efficacy of renal CTA as a noninvasive imaging technique for evaluation of renal stents. Initial studies using early-generation MDCT scanners underestimated the in-stent residual lumen on CTA versus conventional catheter angiography.[58] Some investigators have suggested using specific window-level combinations to optimally evaluate both the vascular lumen and the stent profile itself.[59] In addition, the use of postprocessing techniques including MPR and VR has been validated as reproducible and useful in evaluating stent patency.[60] A recent study has demonstrated very promising results using a modern 64-slice MDCT setup, with all cases of hemodynamically significant in-stent restenosis correctly identified on renal CTA, yielding a negative predictive value of 100% (**Fig. 18**).[57] This outstanding sensitivity is good validation for renal CTA as a viable screening test for in-stent restenosis.

SUMMARY

Renal CTA has become a widely used, robust, noninvasive method for evaluation of the renovascular system. Several technological advances,

including MDCT systems, power injectors, and accurate bolus-tracking mechanisms, have made acquisition of high-resolution volumetric renal CTA data sets a reality. Manipulation of these 3D data sets generally mandates the use of postprocessing techniques, providing valuable information about complex vascular spatial relationships. Renal CTA can be used effectively for investigation of primary renovascular disease, including occlusive and aneurysmal disease. In contrast to catheter angiography, renal CTA is a single study that can provide comprehensive evaluation of disease processes that involve both the renal parenchyma and the renovascular system, such as renal trauma, and preoperative evaluation of renal tumors. Renal CTA has many advantages over other imaging modalities in the postprocedural evaluation of renal artery stents, and can be used with high diagnostic accuracy.

REFERENCES

1. Kim TS, Chung JW, Park JH, et al. Renal artery evaluation: comparison of spiral CT angiography to intra-arterial DSA. J Vasc Interv Radiol 1998;9(4):553–9.

2. Fleischmann D. Multiple detector-row CT angiography of the renal and mesenteric vessels. Eur J Radiol 2003;45(Suppl 1):S79–87.

3. Glockner JF, Vrtiska TJ. Renal MR and CT angiography: current concepts. Abdom Imaging 2007; 32(3):407–20.

4. Liu PS, Williams DM. Understanding acute dissection. In: Matsumura JS, Morasch MD, Pearce WH, et al, editors. Techniques and outcomes in endovascular surgery. 1st edition. Evanston (IL): Greenwood Academic; 2009. p. 180–8.

5. Foley WD. Special focus session: multidetector CT: abdominal visceral imaging. Radiographics 2002; 22(3):701–19.

6. Fleischmann D. Use of high concentration contrast media: principles and rationale-vascular district. Eur J Radiol 2003;45(Suppl 1):S88–93.

7. Kawashima A, Sandler CM, Ernst RD, et al. CT evaluation of renovascular disease. Radiographics 2000;20(5):1321–40.

8. Fishman EK, Ney DR, Heath DG, et al. Volume rendering versus maximum intensity projection in CT angiography: what works best, when, and why. Radiographics 2006;26(3):905–22.

9. Galanski M, Prokop M, Chavan A, et al. Renal arterial stenoses: spiral CT angiography. Radiology 1993;189(1):185–92.

10. Rubin GD, Dake MD, Napel S, et al. Spiral CT of renal artery stenosis: comparison of three-dimensional rendering techniques. Radiology 1994; 190(1):181–9.

11. Johnson PT, Halpern EJ, Kuszyk BS, et al. Renal artery stenosis: CT angiography—comparison of real-time volume-rendering and maximum intensity projection algorithms. Radiology 1999;211(2):337–43.

12. Puchner S, Stadler A, Minar E, et al. Multidetector CT angiography in the follow-up of patients treated with renal artery stents: value of different reformation techniques compared with axial source images. J Endovasc Ther 2007;14(3):387–94.

13. Kaufman JA. Renal arteries. In: Kaufman JA, Lee MJ, editors. Vascular and interventional radiology: the requisites. 1st edition. Philadelphia: Mosby; 2004. p. 219–45.

14. Rountas C, Vlychou M, Vassiou K, et al. Imaging modalities for renal artery stenosis in suspected renovascular hypertension: prospective intraindividual comparison of color Doppler US, CT angiography, GD-enhanced MR angiography, and digital subtraction angiography. Ren Fail 2007; 29(3):295–302.

15. Scoble JE, Maher ER, Hamilton G, et al. Atherosclerotic renovascular disease causing renal impairment—a case for treatment. Clin Nephrol 1989; 31(3):119–22.

16. Safian RD, Textor SC. Renal-artery stenosis. N Engl J Med 2001;344(7):431–42.

17. Beregi JP, Louvegny S, Gautier C, et al. Fibromuscular dysplasia of the renal arteries: comparison of helical CT angiography and arteriography. AJR Am J Roentgenol 1999;172(1):27–34.

18. Caps MT, Perissinotto C, Zierler RE, et al. Prospective study of atherosclerotic disease progression in the renal artery. Circulation 1998;98(25):2866–72.

19. Sabharwal R, Vladica P, Coleman P. Multidetector spiral CT renal angiography in the diagnosis of renal artery fibromuscular dysplasia. Eur J Radiol 2007; 61(3):520–7.

20. Fraioli F, Catalano C, Bertoletti L, et al. Multidetector-row CT angiography of renal artery stenosis in 50 consecutive patients: prospective interobserver comparison with DSA. Radiol Med 2006;111(3): 459–68.

21. Vasbinder GB, Nelemans PJ, Kessels AG, et al. Diagnostic tests for renal artery stenosis in patients suspected of having renovascular hypertension: a meta-analysis. Ann Intern Med 2001; 135(6):401–11.

22. Olin JW, Kaufman JA, Bluemke DA, et al. Atherosclerotic vascular disease conference: writing group IV: imaging. Circulation 2004;109(21):2626–33.

23. Vasbinder GB, Nelemans PJ, Kessels AG, et al. Renal Artery Diagnostic Imaging Study in Hypertension (RADISH) Study Group. Accuracy of computed tomographic angiography and magnetic resonance angiography for diagnosing renal artery stenosis. Ann Intern Med 2004; 141(9):674–82.

24. Hazanov N, Somin M, Attali M, et al. Acute renal embolism. Forty-four cases of renal infarction in patients with atrial fibrillation. Medicine (Baltimore) 2004;83(5):292–9.

25. Suzer O, Shirkhoda A, Jafri SZ, et al. CT features of renal infarction. Eur J Radiol 2002;44(1):59–64.

26. Williams DM, Lee DY, Hamilton BH, et al. The dissected aorta: percutaneous treatment of ischemic complications—principles and results. J Vasc Interv Radiol 1997;8(4):605–25.

27. Raptis L, Androulaki M, Passas G, et al. CT evaluation of renal artery embolism with ectopic artery. Eur J Intern Med 2006;17(1):61–2.

28. Yoshida T, Ikehara N, Miyabe H, et al. Two cases with renal infarction diagnosed in the early course using contrast-enhanced CT. Hypertens Res 2004; 27(7):523–6.

29. Kawashima A, Sandler CM, Corl FM, et al. Imaging of renal trauma: a comprehensive review. Radiographics 2001;21(3):557–74.

30. Federle MP. Evaluation of renal trauma. In: Pollack HM, editor. Clinical urography. Philadelphia: Saunders; 1989. p. 1422–94.

31. Moore EE, Shackford SR, Pachter HL, et al. Organ injury scaling: spleen, liver, and kidney. J Trauma 1989;29:1664–6.

32. Federle MP, Brown TR, McAninch JW. Penetrating renal trauma: CT evaluation. J Comput Assist Tomogr 1987;11(6):1026–30.

33. Sabharwal R, Vladica P, Law WP, et al. Multidetector spiral CT renal angiography in the diagnosis of giant renal artery aneurysms. Abdom Imaging 2006;31(3): 374–8.

34. Rankin SC, Jan W, Koffman CG. Noninvasive imaging of living related kidney donors: evaluation with CT angiography and gadolinium-enhanced MR angiography. AJR Am J Roentgenol 2001; 177(2):349–55.

35. Kawamoto S, Fishman EK. MDCT angiography of living laparoscopic renal donors. Abdom Imaging 2006;31(3):361–73.

36. Holden A, Smith A, Dukes P, et al. Assessment of 100 live potential renal donors for laparoscopic nephrectomy with multi-detector row helical CT. Radiology 2005;237(3):973–80.

37. Platt JF, Ellis JH, Korobkin M, et al. Potential renal donors: comparison of conventional imaging with helical CT. Radiology 1996;198(2): 419–23.

38. Platt JF, Ellis JH, Korobkin M, et al. Helical CT evaluation of potential kidney donors: findings in 154 subjects. AJR Am J Roentgenol 1997;169(5): 1325–30.

39. Pollak R, Prusak BF, Mozes MF. Anatomic abnormalities of cadaver kidneys procured for purposes of transplantation. Am Surg 1986;52(5):233–5.

40. Raman SS, Pojchamarnwiputh S, Muangsomboon K, et al. Surgically relevant normal and variant renal parenchymal and vascular anatomy in preoperative 16-MDCT evaluation of potential laparoscopic renal donors. AJR Am J Roentgenol 2007;188(1):105–14.

41. Kawamoto S, Montgomery RA, Lawler LP, et al. Multidetector row CT evaluation of living renal donors prior to laparoscopic nephrectomy. Radiographics 2004; 24(2):453–66.

42. Lin CH, Steinberg AP, Ramani AP, et al. Laparoscopic live donor nephrectomy in the presence of circumaortic or retroaortic left renal vein. J Urol 2004;171(1):44–6.

43. Mandal AK, Cohen C, Montgomery RA, et al. Should the indications for laparoscopic live donor nephrectomy of the right kidney be the same as for the open procedure? Anomalous left renal vasculature is not a contraindication to laparoscopic left donor nephrectomy. Transplantation 2001;71(5):660–4.

44. Scatarige JC, Horton KM, Ratner LE, et al. Left adrenal vein localization by 3D real-time volume-rendering CTA before laparoscopic nephrectomy in living renal donors. Abdom Imaging 2001;26(5): 553–6.

45. Ferda J, Hora M, Hes O, et al. Assessment of the kidney tumor vascular supply by two-phase MDCT-angiography. Eur J Radiol 2007; 62(2):295–301.

46. Hallscheidt P, Wagener N, Gholipour F, et al. Multislice computed tomography in planning nephron-sparing surgery in a prospective study with 76 patients: comparison of radiological and histopathological findings in the infiltration of renal structures. J Comput Assist Tomogr 2006;30(6):869–74.

47. Sheth S, Scatarige JC, Horton KM, et al. Current concepts in the diagnosis and management of renal cell carcinoma: role of multidetector CT and three-dimensional CT. Radiographics 2001;21(Spec No): S237–54.

48. Coll DM, Herts BR, Davros WJ, et al. Preoperative use of 3D volume rendering to demonstrate renal tumors and renal anatomy. Radiographics 2000; 20(2):431–8.

49. Hallscheidt PJ, Bock M, Riedasch G, et al. Diagnostic accuracy of staging renal cell carcinomas using multidetector-row computed tomography and magnetic resonance imaging: a prospective study with histopathologic correlation. J Comput Assist Tomogr 2004;28(3):333–9.

50. Braun P, Guilabert JP, Kazmi F. Multidetector computed tomography arteriography in the preoperative assessment of patients with ureteropelvic junction obstruction. Eur J Radiol 2007; 61(1):170–5.

51. Quillin SP, Brink JA, Heiken JP, et al. Helical (spiral) CT angiography for identification of crossing vessels at the ureteropelvic junction. AJR Am J Roentgenol 1996;166(5):1125–30.

52. Sampaio FJ, Favorito LA. Ureteropelvic junction stenosis: vascular anatomical background for endopyelotomy. J Urol 1993;150(6):1787–91.

53. Khaira HS, Platt JF, Cohan RH, et al. Helical computed tomography for identification of crossing vessels in ureteropelvic junction obstruction-comparison with operative findings. Urology 2003; 62(1):35–9.

54. Van Cangh PJ, Wilmart JF, Opsomer RJ, et al. Long-term results and late recurrence after endoureteropyelotomy: a critical analysis of prognostic factors. J Urol 1994;151(4):934–7.

55. Rouvière O, Lyonnet D, Berger P, et al. Ureteropelvic junction obstruction: use of helical CT for preoperative assessment—comparison with intraarterial angiography. Radiology 1999;213(3):668–73.

56. Leertouwer TC, Gussenhoven EJ, Bosch JL, et al. Stent placement for renal arterial stenosis: where do we stand? A meta-analysis. Radiology 2000; 216(1):78–85.

57. Steinwender C, Schützenberger W, Fellner F, et al. 64-Detector CT angiography in renal artery stent evaluation: prospective comparison with selective catheter angiography. Radiology 2009; 252(1):299–305.

58. Behar JV, Nelson RC, Zidar JP, et al. Thin-section multidetector CT angiography of renal artery stents. AJR Am J Roentgenol 2002;178(5): 1155–9.

59. Willoteaux S, Negawi Z, Lions C, et al. Observations from multidetector CT imaging of different types of renal artery stents. J Endovasc Ther 2004;11(5): 560–9.

60. Mallouhi A, Rieger M, Czermak B, et al. Volume-rendered multidetector CT angiography: noninvasive follow-up of patients treated with renal artery stents. AJR Am J Roentgenol 2003;180(1):233–9.

CT Angiography of the Lower Extremities

W. Dennis Foley, MD*, Troy Stonely, MD

KEYWORDS
• CT angiography • Applications
• Lower extremity arterial disease • Evaluation

Lower extremity arterial disease is an increasingly common disease process reflecting longer life expectancy and increasing prevalence of atherosclerosis. Disease manifestations range from claudication to rest pain and tissue ischemia. Most patients present with claudication symptoms.[1] Clinical history and physical examination, if consistent with lower extremity arterial disease, are usually evaluated with a series of noninvasive tests aimed to demonstrate the level and severity of disease. However, the planning of intervention by percutaneous endovascular technique or by operation requires accurate mapping of the arterial inflow (aortoiliac) and arterial outflow (femoropopliteal and tibioperoneal) circulation (Fig. 1).

The advent of multidetector computed tomographic (CT) scanning and magnetic resonance (MR) angiography made possible the accurate mapping of disease for interventional planning by a noninvasive technique.[2–4] Computed tomographic angiography (CTA) and MR angiography have displaced intra-arterial digital subtraction angiography (DSA) as diagnostic angiographic techniques, although DSA may be used as a combined diagnostic/interventional approach in patients with focal disease clearly established by noninvasive testing, such as focal arterial bypass graft stenoses.[4–7]

This article provides an overview of injection/acquisition and display techniques for multidetector row CT scanning and demonstrates the utility of CTA in focal and diffuse arterial disease and follow-up of patients who have had intravascular stents and arterial bypass grafts.

Each section has a commentary on the appropriate role of noninvasive, nonangiographic diagnostic testing and the utility of a disease classification system in patient management decisions.

PREVALENCE, NATURAL HISTORY, AND CLINICAL PRESENTATION OF PERIPHERAL ARTERIAL OCCLUSIVE DISEASE

Lower extremity arterial occlusive disease is typically secondary to stenotic occlusive atherosclerotic disease, a process that usually begins after the age of 50 years and becomes progressively incapacitating.

The estimated prevalence of peripheral arterial disease (PAD) as defined by an ankle-brachial index (ABI) of 0.9 or less is 2.5% in subjects of age group 50 to 59 years and 14.5% in subjects older than 70 years.[8] The major risk factors for PAD are diabetes and smoking. The disease is common in elderly male patients and more common among African Americans than Caucasians.[9] Hypertension, dyslipidemia, elevated inflammatory markers such as C-reactive protein, and hyperhomocysteinemia predispose to PAD. About 40% to 60% of patients with PAD have coexistent coronary artery disease and cerebral artery disease. The extent of coronary artery disease correlates with the ABI. Autopsy studies have shown that patients who die from a myocardial infarction are twice as likely to have a significant stenosis in the iliac and carotid arteries compared with patients dying from other causes.

Mortality rates in patients with PAD average 2% per year, and the rates of nonfatal myocardial infarction, stroke, and vascular death are 5% to 7% per year.

Department of Radiology, Medical College of Wisconsin, 9200 West Wisconsin Avenue, Milwaukee, WI 53226, USA
* Corresponding author.
E-mail address: dfoley@mcw.edu

Radiol Clin N Am 48 (2010) 367–396
doi:10.1016/j.rcl.2010.02.008
0033-8389/10/$ – see front matter © 2010 Elsevier Inc. All rights reserved.

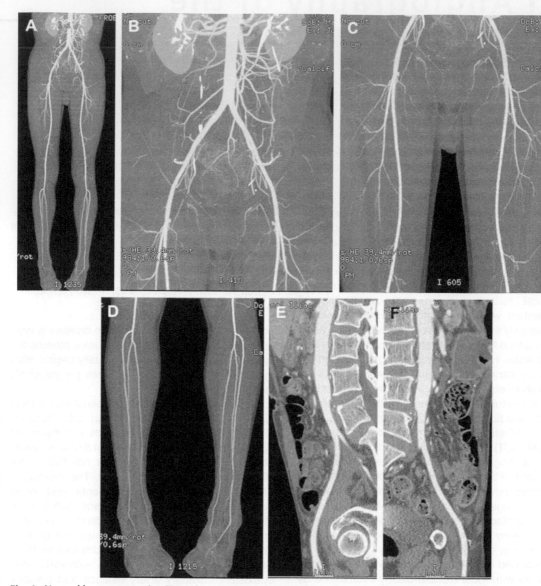

Fig. 1. Normal lower extremity CTA using maximum intensity projection (MIP) display and curved planar reformation (CPR). (*A*) Complete topographic MIP display of aortoiliac inflow and femoropopliteal and tibioperoneal outflow segments. (*B*) MIP display of normal aortoiliac inflow segment. (*C*) MIP display of femoral and above-knee popliteal segment. (*D*) MIP display of the distal popliteal and tibioperoneal segments. (*E*) CPR in lateral projection of the right aortoiliac arterial inflow segment. (*F*) CPR in lateral projection of left aortoiliac arterial inflow segment.

Only 25% of patients who initially present with intermittent claudication significantly deteriorate, and the overall intervention rate in patients with intermittent claudication approximates 5%.[10] Patients with mild PAD may develop symptoms of intermittent claudication only when they become physically very active. Few of the patients with claudication progress to chronic critical ischemia with rest pain and tissue loss. However, this is an uncommon clinical sequela, with the rate of major amputation in the claudicant population at 1 to 3 per 1000 during a 5-year period.[11–13] The best predictor of deterioration is an ABI of less than 0.5 and a hazard ratio of more than 2 compared with patients with an ABI greater than 0.5.

Depending on the level and severity of disease, patients with lower extremity arterial disease may present with buttock, thigh, or calf claudication, buttock and thigh claudication being secondary to aortoiliac disease, and calf claudication to femoropopliteal disease.

The primary treatment of critical limb ischemia is either revascularization or primary amputation. There is a 40% rate of limb loss within 6 months and a 20% mortality rate in patients in whom reconstruction is not possible or in whom attempts at reconstruction have failed. Amputations may be below or above the knee; approximately 50% of amputations are of either type.

Nonatherosclerotic stenotic occlusive disease is uncommon and secondary to entities such as arteritis, including Takayasu and Buerger disease. Takayasu disease most commonly affects the aortoiliac inflow circulation, whereas Burger disease affects the femoropopliteal or tibioperoneal outflow circulation. Takayasu arteritis and Burger disease most commonly affect early-adult–aged to middle-aged patients.

Aneurysmal disease of the lower extremities is uncommon, and preferential sites include the femoral and popliteal arteries. Abdominal aortic aneurysms are present in 60% of patients with popliteal aneurysms and 85% of patients with femoral artery aneurysms.[1,14] The inverse association is rare, reflecting the higher prevalence of abdominal aortic aneurysms; only 10% to 14% of patients with abdominal aortic aneurysms have either femoral or popliteal artery aneurysms. Patients with aneurysms may present with pulsatile swelling or clinical complications including rupture and thromboembolism. Rest pain in the foot secondary to thromboembolism from a popliteal artery aneurysm is an uncommon but real entity.[14]

Another cause of sudden severe distal ischemia with rest pain is arterial embolism, with the embolus arising from a cardiac source or prominent atherothrombotic thoracic or abdominal aortic disease. The clinical manifestations of peripheral arterial embolism are usually sudden onset of pain with accompanying pallor and paresthesia and possible paralysis. Other possible causes include thromboembolism from peripheral arterial aneurysm, whether femoral or popliteal; in situ thrombosis in patients with hypercoagulable states; or acute vessel dissection, particularly distal extension of a thoracoabdominal dissection into the iliac and femoral vessels.[15,16]

Uncommon causes of distal ischemia include posttraumatic arterial thrombosis, arteriovenous fistula, popliteal artery entrapment syndrome and adventitial cystic disease of the popliteal artery, thrombosis of a persistent sciatic artery, and fibrodysplastic disease of the iliac vessels.

CTA: INJECTION/ACQUISITION TECHNIQUE

The major technical advantage of CTA is rapid volume coverage speed with submillimeter isotropic resolution, both attributes best achieved with wide detector systems with a 64-channel count or greater.

The acquisition table speed of the CT system, dependent on vendor configuration, can be rapid. For helical CT scanning, the table speed is determined by the beam width, pitch, and scan rotation speed. Depending on the detector element aperture and the number of detector rows, beam width can vary between 4 and 8 cm (Box 1). For a nonhelical system operating in an incremental dynamic or

---

Box 1
TASC classification of aortoiliac lesions

Type A lesions

- Stenoses (unilateral or bilateral) of common iliac artery (CIA) or less than 3 cm of external iliac artery (EIA)

Type B lesions

- Stenoses (≤3 cm) of infrarenal aorta or stenoses (3–10 cm) of the EIA not involving the CFA
- Occlusion, unilateral CIA or EIA not involving the origin of the internal iliac or CFA

Type C lesions

- Stenoses unilateral EIA extending into CFA or bilateral EIA (3–10 cm) not extending into the CFA
- Occlusion, unilateral EIA occlusion involving the origins of internal iliac artery and/or CFA.
- Occlusion, unilateral calcified EIA with or without involving the origins of the internal iliac artery and/or CFA

Type D lesions

- Diffuse disease of aorta and both iliac arteries
- Stenoses, diffuse multiple involving unilateral CIA, EIA, and CFA
- Stenoses, iliac in patient with abdominal aortic aneurysm requiring surgical management
- Occlusions, unilateral occlusions of CIA and EIA or bilateral involving EIA
- Occlusion, infra renal aortal

CIA, common iliac artery; EIA, external iliac artery; CFA, common femoral artery; AAA, abdominal aortic aneurysm.
Adapted from Norgren L, Hiatt WR, Dormandy JA, et al. Inter-society consensus for the management of peripheral arterial disease (TASC II). Eur J Vasc Endovasc Surg 2007;33:S1–S75; with permission.

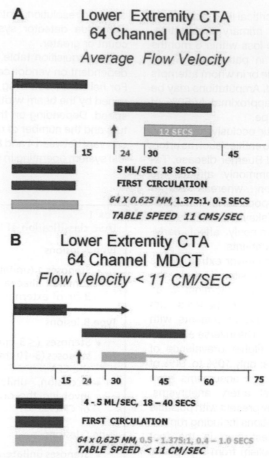

Fig. 2. Injection acquisition techniques for lower extremity CTA. (*A*) Standard injection acquisition technique presuming an arterial flow velocity measured by aortopopliteal transit time in the range of 10 to 15 cm/s. Time line is on the X axis. Injection interval is denoted by the blue bar, first circulation of the injected contrast bolus through the anatomic region of interest by the red bar, and acquisition interval by the green bar. Table speed (11 cm/s) is determined by beam width (64 channels × detector collimation of 0.625 mm = 40 mm), pitch (1.375:1), and rotation speed (0.5secs). Acquisition interval is determined by anatomic coverage (130 cm) divided by table speed (11 cm/s) and equals 12 seconds. The table speed is equivalent to the predetermined arterial flow velocity. Acquisition begins 6 seconds after arrival of the contrast bolus at the level of the suprarenal aorta, denoted as 24 seconds arrival time in this schematic. Injection interval is the combination of the delay time between arrival of the contrast bolus and the beginning of acquisition (6 seconds) and the acquisition interval (12 seconds). For an injection interval of 18 seconds, total contrast volume, assuming an injection rate of 5 mL/s, is 90 mL. (*B*) Injection acquisition technique for lower extremity CTA with adjustment of table speed related to measured flow velocities of less than 11 cm/s. Table speed is adjusted to be equivalent to the measured arterial flow velocity by decrease in pitch, increase in rotation time, and if necessary decrease in beam width. Acquisition interval is increased with the decrease in table speed, with a corresponding increase in injection interval. With the longer injection interval, the contrast load is adjusted by decreasing the injection rate.

step-and-shoot mode, a 16-cm detector width is available. Pitch, in conjunction with beam width, determines the table movement per 360° rotation; a pitch value greater than or lesser than 1 correspondingly moves the table greater or lesser than the beam width. Scan rotation speeds determine the number of 360° rotations per second; a faster scan rotation speed results in faster table movement in the z-axis. A wide beam width, high pitch value, and high scan rotation speed result

in fast table motion. The table speed may be decelerated by choosing a slower scan rotation speed, lower pitch value and, if necessary, narrower beam width.

Although adaptable table speed and submillimeter isotropic resolution are important attributes of a CT scanner for lower extremity arteriography, image quality is also dependent on adequate intraarterial iodine concentration, selection of kVp, and tube current selection.

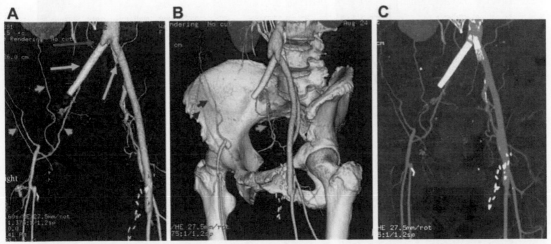

Fig. 3. Volume rendering with and without bone segmentation in a patient with aortoiliac disease. The patient has bilateral occluded common iliac endovascular stents and an occluded right limb of an aortobifemoral graft. (A) Volume rendered image in a frontal projection demonstrating bilateral occluded stents (*green arrows*) and occluded right limb of aortobifemoral graft (*red arrow*). Parietal collateral circulation via epigastric, circumflex iliac, and obturator arteries (*blue arrows*) is demonstrated. (B) Volume rendered image in the left anterior oblique projection without bone segmentation demonstrates the parietal collateral circulation (*dark blue arrows*) overlaying the right iliac bone and the internal iliac and obturator collateral circulation at the right pelvic sidewall (*light blue arrow*). (C) Maximum intensity projection display in a frontal projection provides slightly better clarity of small vessel detail but lacks the 3-dimensional perspective of the volume rendered display.

In general, intra-arterial iodine concentration of 300 to 350 mg/mL[3,17,18] in the imaged vessel results in good vessel opacity, distinction of contrast-enhanced lumen from calcified vessel wall, and accurate delineation of small caliber vessels of the order of 1.5 mm or greater. A kVp value of 120 or preferably less is recommended.[2] A lower kVp value more closely approximates the K edge of iodine and accentuates the photon attenuation and the perceived intravascular opacity. An intravascular iodine concentration of 300 to 350 mg/mL in

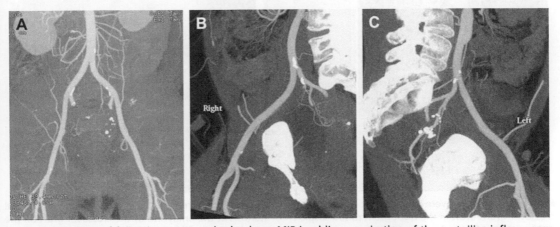

Fig. 4. Comparison of full-volume MIP and subvolume MIP in oblique projection of the aortoiliac inflow vasculature. (A) MIP display in frontal projection. Scattered calcific atherosclerotic plaque in the subrenal aorta and common iliac arteries. Superior and inferior mesenteric arterial branches overlay the distal aorta and proximal iliac arteries. (B) Subvolume MIP in oblique projection of the right iliac and proximal femoral extremity outflow vessels displays normal arterial patency without vessel overlay. (C) Subvolume MIP in oblique projection of the left iliac and proximal femoral extremity outflow vessels displays normal arterial patency without vessel overlay. The oblique projection obtained in (B) and (C) better displays the internal iliac artery vessel orifices and proximal segments.

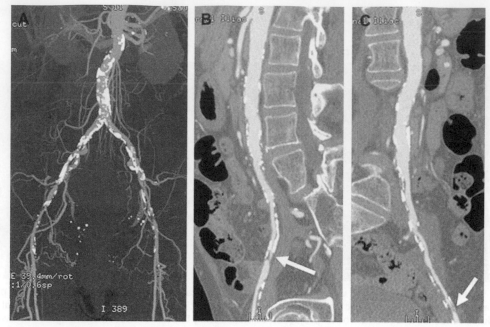

Fig. 5. Comparison of MIP and CPR display in a patient with calcific aortoiliac disease and iliac artery stenoses. (*A*) MIP display in frontal projection demonstrates diffuse infrarenal aortic and bilateral common and external iliac artery calcific atherosclerosis. The degree of underlying stenosis is uncertain. (*B*) CPR of infrarenal aorta and right common and external iliac arteries defines a tight stenosis in the proximal external iliac artery (*arrow*) with moderate but insignificant stenosis in the remaining segments. (*C*) CPR of the infrarenal aorta and left common and external iliac arteries demonstrates moderate diffuse iliac artery disease with a higher level of stenosis in the distal external iliac artery (*arrow*).

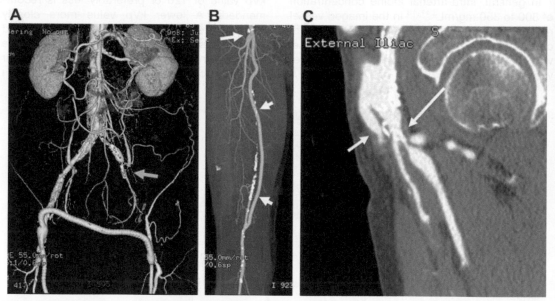

Fig. 6. Patient with severe bilateral iliac atherosclerosis, occluded left external iliac artery, and a femoro femoral crossover graft. Bruit in the right groin raised suspicion of stenosis at the onlay site of the crossover graft on the right common femoral artery. (*A*) Volume rendered image in frontal projection demonstrates bilateral calcific atherosclerotic disease of the iliac vessels with left external iliac artery occlusion (*green arrow*) The femoro femoral crossover graft is patent. Residual parietal and visceral arterial collateral circulation in the left pelvis was present before the placement of the femoro femoral crossover graft. (*B*) MIP display in frontal projection of the right femoral circulation demonstrates a patent femoral to above-knee popliteal arterial bypass graft (*short arrows*). Profunda artery (*long arrow*) is patent, but orifice is not clearly displayed. (*C*) CPR in lateral projection demonstrates a tight orifice stenosis of a proximal profunda femoral artery branch (*long arrow*). The proximal component of the femoropopliteal bypass graft (*short arrow*) is only partly included in the imaging plane.

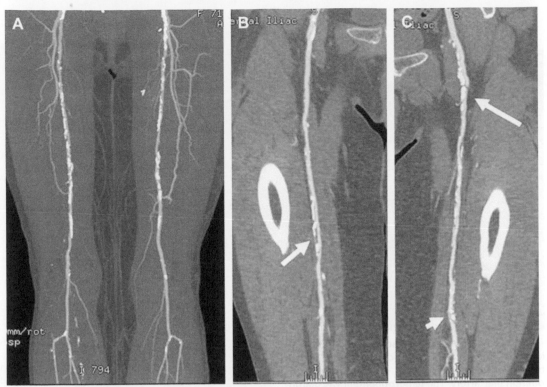

Fig. 7. Calcific atherosclerosis of the femoropopliteal arterial segments, with degree of stenosis best determined by CPR. (A) MIP display of femoropopliteal segments in frontal projection. Extensive calcific atherosclerosis, predominantly in the bilateral common femoral, proximal left superficial femoral and bilateral distal femoral, and proximal popliteal arteries, precludes an accurate assessment of the underlying degree of stenosis. (B) CPR of the right femoral artery in frontal projection defines residual lumen with a moderate degree of stenosis in the midsegment (arrow). (C) CPR of the left femoral artery in frontal projection demonstrates tight stenosis in the proximal superficial femoral artery (long arrow) and adductor regions (short arrow).

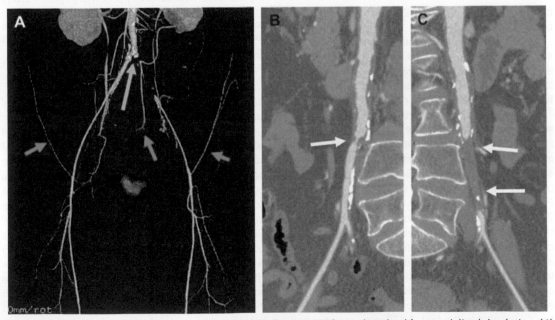

Fig. 8. Leriche Type I. Distal aortic and bilateral common iliac artery atherosclerosis with normal distal circulation. (A) Volume rendered image in frontal projection displays calcific atherosclerosis of the distal aorta and proximal right common iliac artery and occluded left common iliac artery (green arrow). Collateral circulation is via parietal circumflex iliac branches and the hemorrhoidal branch of a reconstituted inferior mesenteric artery (blue arrows). (B) CPR in lateral projection demonstrates a tight atherosclerotic stenosis at the orifice of the right common iliac artery (arrow). (C) CPR in lateral projection demonstrates thrombotic occlusion of the left common iliac artery (arrows).

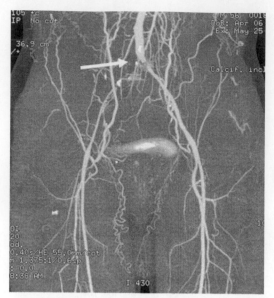

Fig. 9. Leriche Type II. Aortoiliac atherosclerosis with right common iliac artery occlusion and diffuse stenosis of the right external iliac artery and left common iliac artery. The femoropopliteal vasculature was normally patent. MIP display in frontal projection demonstrates right common iliac artery occlusion (*arrow*) and stenoses of the right external iliac and left common iliac arteries with profuse parietal and visceral collateral circulation to reconstitute normal caliber proximal femoral arteries.

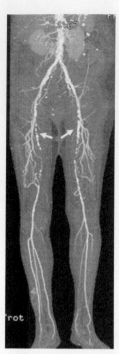

Fig. 10. Lariche Type III. Atherosclerosis with diffuse calcific disease of the iliac vessels and occluded bilateral superficial femoral arteries. MIP in frontal projection demonstrates patent iliac arteries with prominent calcific atherosclerosis, occluded calcified bilateral superficial femoral arteries (*arrows*), and prominent profunda collateral circulation reconstituting the distal femoral artery/proximal popliteal artery in the adductor canal. Normal patency of the reconstituted popliteal artery with 3-vessel tibioperoneal runoff to the ankle on the right and 2-vessel runoff to the ankle on the left.

conjunction with 100 to 120 kVp is considered optimal.

Adequate photon statistics and a low-noise imaging chain are important in providing adequate signal-to-noise and contrast-to-noise ratio. A lower kVp selection requires a higher tube current to maintain signal-to-noise ratio.

Two basic approaches are used for injection/acquisition for lower extremity arteriography. In most patients with PAD, the average flow velocity in the aortoiliac and femoropopliteal arterial segments varies between 5 and 10 cm/s, and in patients with poor cardiac output and significant PAD, average flow velocity may be as slow as 2 cm/s.[19] These arterial flow velocities are less than the table speed achievable in systems with beam width of 4 cm or greater. The most common approach for imaging the peripheral arterial circulation is to delay acquisition until the injected contrast bolus has been delivered to the peripheral arterial system with opacification from the level of the diaphragm to the feet. A 130-cm coverage can then be achieved, dependent on table speed, in 10 to 15 seconds. This approach requires preset contrast volume, with the beginning of acquisition delayed until the leading edge of the contrast

bolus has been distributed to the tibioperoneal circulation.[5,20]

An alternative approach is to measure arterial flow velocity by determining the travel time of contrast material from the supraceliac aorta to the popliteal arteries. This approach requires 2 mini bolus injections of contrast medium to produce aortic and popliteal artery time-attenuation curves to determine transit time and thus flow velocity.[19] On the time-attenuation curves, time to peak is considered to be the "arrival time." Table speed is then adjusted to arterial flow velocity, and acquisition is set to begin 6 seconds after arrival of the contrast material in the supraceliac aorta. With this approach, the contrast volume, with a preset injection rate, is mainly dependent on the acquisition time. A longer acquisition time, secondary to a slower flow velocity, requires a greater contrast volume. However, contrast volumes can be adjusted by decreasing injection rate in patients

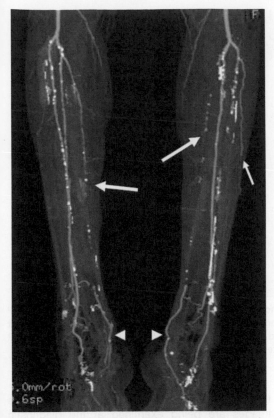

Fig. 11. Prominent tibioperoneal arterial vascular calcification in a patient with diabetes. Scattered calcific atherosclerotic plaque was present in the femoral and popliteal arteries, with insignificant stenosis on CPR display. Extensive bilateral tibioperoneal calcific atherosclerosis with occluded right and left posterior tibial arteries (*long arrows*) and left anterior tibial artery (*short arrow*). Collateral circulation from the peroneal arteries reconstitutes the plantar arch bilaterally (*arrowheads*). There is inflow into both dorsal pedal arteries via direct inflow on the right and collateral reconstitution on the left. Incomplete removal of bone in relation to the ankle and foot simulates bulk calcific atherosclerosis in these sites.

with slower flow velocity and longer acquisition times (**Fig. 2**).[19,21]

Patients with peripheral arterial occlusive disease may have coexistent renal impairment. Attention to patient hydration and use of only that volume of contrast material necessary to adequately opacify the peripheral arterial system are important aspects of CTA in lower extremity arterial disease.

IMAGE DISPLAY

The full range of image display techniques available for CT scanning are used in lower extremity CTA.

Volume rendering with a 3-dimensional perspective is useful for overall topographic display, particularly in demonstrating collateral circulation in the aortoiliac segment (**Fig. 3**). However, opacity settings may not provide an accurate rendering of vessel contours and relative degree of stenosis, and vessel wall calcification is not as clearly displayed as in a maximum intensity projection display. Volume rendering, without bone segmentation, is a powerful display technique in the preintervention evaluation because it allows bony landmarks and the accompanying soft tissue anatomy at sites of vascular disease to be displayed and appreciated by interventional radiologists and vascular surgeons (see **Fig. 3**).[5,22–24]

Maximum intensity projection (MIP) provides a more accurate rendition of vessel wall contour and vascular calcification than volume rendering and is useful in the topographic display of the outflow arterial circulation (femoropopliteal and tibioperoneal). However, in the abdomen and pelvis, a full-volume MIP suffers from overlay of abdominal visceral arteries, particularly intestinal over the aortoiliac inflow vessels. A subvolume slab MIP approach is best used in the abdominal pelvic segment (**Fig. 4**).[4]

Curved planar reformations (CPRs) using centerline tracking and edge detection provide a view of selected vessel segments that is rotatable in real time and allow the best projection angle to be selected for determining the degree of asymmetric vessel stenosis (**Fig. 5**). In addition, semicircumferential calcified plaque, which does not allow determination of underlying vessel lumen in an MIP display, is projected at the vessel edge in a CPR.[3,17] CPRs are useful for the display of the aortoiliac and femoropopliteal arterial segments. The abdominal aorta and right iliac vessel and subsequently the abdominal aorta and left iliac (ie, common and external iliac) vessel extending into the common femoral arteries are displayed separately. For each lower extremity, the common femoral, superficial femoral, and popliteal arteries are also displayed individually. A curved plane reformation of the iliac, common femoral, and profunda femoral arteries may be obtained, a technique that is of particular value in patients with superficial femoral artery disease in whom profunda plasty may be an important consideration for patient management (**Fig. 6**).[1]

Advances in CPR include a multipath approach in which each of the 3 tibioperoneal vessels, portrayed by CPR, can be displayed simultaneously in a rotatable format.

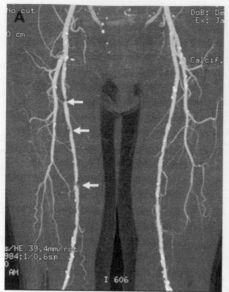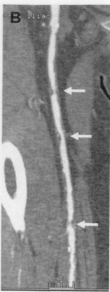

Fig. 12. Multifocal superficial femoral artery stenoses demonstrated by MIP and CPR display techniques. (*A*) MIP display of the common femoral, superficial femoral, and profunda femoral arteries. There are 3 significant right superficial femoral artery (SFA) focal stenoses (*arrows*) and a focal insignificant stenoses of the left SFA. (*B*) CPR display of the right SFA confirms multifocal high-grade stenoses in the proximal, mid, and distal SFA (*arrows*).

STENOSIS SIZING

Stenosis sizing is usually determined by visual observation or "eyeballing" rather than a computer-based technique. The combination of MIP, CPR, and axial plane imaging allows the experienced observer to categorize stenoses in the mild (0%–50%), moderate (50%–70%), and severe (>70%) category (Fig. 7).[25,26] Stenoses less than 50% are not considered as hemodynamically significant. Moderate and severe grades of stenoses are hemodynamically significant and compensated by development of collateral circulation. Of the 3 methods, the combination of projectional display using a rotatable CPR with correlative axial imaging of defined levels of stenosis achieves the best results.[26] The MIP technique, which is essentially a 2-dimensional projectional display, is unable to resolve the degree of stenosis at sites of circumferential calcified plaque. Only in patients with almost complete circumferential heavily calcified plaque is the curved planar reformation unable to demonstrate the residual contrast-enhanced lumen.[3,17]

Automated methods of stenosis sizing allow diameter and area reduction techniques to be used. Area reduction is intrinsically superior to diameter reduction because it provides a better estimate of flow reduction, particularly with asymmetric stenoses. For asymmetric stenoses, accurate determination of diameter reduction requires the right projection to be determined when the images are being examined at the diagnostic console.[26–30]

Standard methods of image evaluation and treatment planning have been derived from clinical trials using diameter reduction as the standard diagnostic criterion for degree of vessel stenosis. Future clinical trials related to vascular disease and its management may incorporate area reduction and length of stenosis in the patient evaluation strategy.[1,26]

CLINICAL DISEASE
Atherosclerosis

Atherosclerosis is segmental in distribution, predominantly affecting the aortoiliac inflow or the femoropopliteal or tibioperoneal segments of the outflow circulation.

In the Leriche classification of aortoiliac disease, Type I disease involves the distal aorta and common iliac arteries (Fig. 8), Type II disease involves distal aorta and complete iliac circulation (Fig. 9), and Type III disease involves the aortoiliac and femoropopliteal circulation (Fig. 10). Patients with aortoiliac disease commonly present with buttock or thigh claudication. Male patients with bilateral hypogastric artery stenoses/occlusion may present with a classic Leriche presentation of buttock claudication and impotence.

Box 2
Transatlantic intersociety consensus classification of femoral popliteal lesions

Type A lesions

- Stenosis 10 cm or less in length
- Occlusion 5 cm or less in length

Type B lesions

- Stenoses or occlusions, multiple, each 5 cm or less
- Stenosis or occlusion, single, 15 cm or less not involving the infrageniculate popliteal artery
- Stenoses or occlusions, single or multiple in the absence of continuous tibial vessels to improve inflow for a distal bypass
- Stenosis, single popliteal
- Occlusion, heavily calcified, 5 cm or less in length

Type C lesions

- Stenoses or occlusions, single or multiple, 15 cm or more with or without heavy calcification
- Stenoses or occlusions, recurrent after 2 endovascular interventions

Type D lesions

- Occlusions of common femoral artery (CFA) or superficial femoral artery, chronic, total (≥20 cm, involving the popliteal artery)
- Occlusion of popliteal artery and proximal trifurcation vessels, chronic, total

Adapted from Norgren L, Hiatt WR, Dormandy JA, et al. Inter-society consensus for the management of peripheral arterial disease (TASC II). Eur J Vasc Endovasc Surg 2007;33:S1–S75; with permission.

In patients with predominant femoral artery involvement, the initial and most significant site of disease is usually the distal superficial femoral artery in the adductor canal (see **Fig. 9**). These patients typically present with calf claudication because the flow-limiting lesion effects circulation in the popliteal artery and calf musculature with adequate circulation to the thigh musculature maintained by the profunda femoral and more proximal superficial femoral artery.

Atherosclerosis initially limited to the tibioperoneal arterial circulation is common in patients with diabetes who may have calf and foot claudication in addition to rest pain (**Fig. 11**).

The hemodynamic significance of disease depends on the degree and length of stenosis,

length of occlusion (if present), and the extent and adequacy of collateral flow. Patients with claudication may have stable symptoms over time because of the adequacy of collateral flow, and most patients can be managed medically and monitored by noninvasive, nonangiographic testing.

The commonly used noninvasive tests are determination of ABI, segmental arterial pressures, toe pressures, and common femoral artery pulsatility index. The ABI compares systemic arterial pressure in the distal posterior tibial and anterior tibial arteries to systolic arterial pressure in the brachial artery. This technique provides a quantitative assessment of perfusion pressure to the foot, in abnormal cases, without defining the level of stenosis or obstruction. An ABI of less than 0.9 defines PAD, with values of 0.9 to 0.4 associated with claudication and less than 0.4 associated with rest pain and potential tissue loss.[1,14] Calcified incompressible vessels, which are common in patients with diabetes, result in falsely-high ABIs. Segmental arterial pressures, obtained in proximal and distal thigh and proximal and distal calf are reasonably accurate in localizing the level of arterial disease in the iliac and common femoral arteries, superficial femoral arteries, and popliteal and tibioperoneal arteries, respectively. Toe pressures are a useful index of pedal perfusion pressure, particularly in patients with diabetes who may have especially high ABIs. Toe pressures are obtained using plethysmographic rather than ultrasonic recording techniques. The toe pressure is normally approximately 30 mm Hg less than the ankle pressure, and an abnormal toe to brachial index is less than 0.7. Femoral artery pulsatility index can identify unilateral iliac obstructive disease in the presence of a patent ipsilateral superficial femoral artery. A pulsatility index less than 4 in the presence of a patent ipsilateral superficial femoral artery predicts aortoiliac disease. However, the index does not distinguish stenosis from occlusion or the site, extent, or severity of stenosis. Thus, these nonimaging noninvasive tests may be useful in localizing segmental arterial disease, but not in determining extent or severity.

CTA

The major value of CTA is the preintervention evaluation of symptomatic patients with positive noninvasive test results who are deemed potential candidates for intervention. These studies are of particular value in patients with suspected aortoiliac or femoropopliteal arterial stenotic occlusive

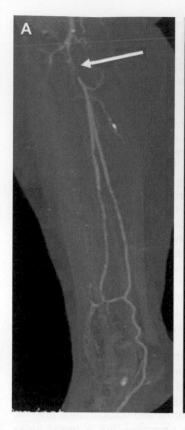

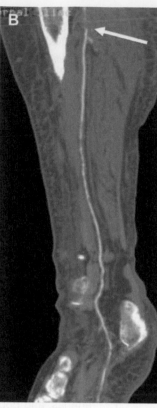

Fig. 13. Stenotic disease of the tibioperoneal trunk with occluded anterior tibial artery. (*A*) MIP display in lateral projection demonstrates a tight stenosis or occlusion of the tibioperoneal trunk (*arrow*). The anterior tibial artery is occluded. (*B*) CPR display seems to confirm focal occlusion of the tibioperoneal trunk (*arrow*). However, this is uncertain. The single vessel tracked by the CPR display is the posterior tibial artery with inflow into the plantar arch.

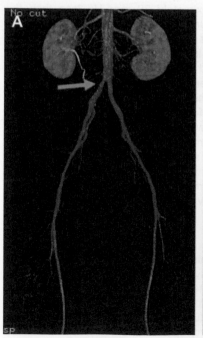

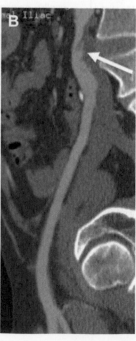

Fig. 14. A 35-year-old male patient with blue toe syndrome secondary to atheroembolism from a single right common iliac artery ulcerated plaque. (*A*) Volume rendered display of aortoiliac and proximal femoral arteries demonstrates mild narrowing of the proximal right common iliac artery (*arrow*). (*B*) CPR in lateral projection of the right iliac vasculature demonstrates an ulcerated plaque of the common iliac artery with a "collar button" appearance (*arrow*) The patient was treated with a covered stent and anticoagulation therapy.

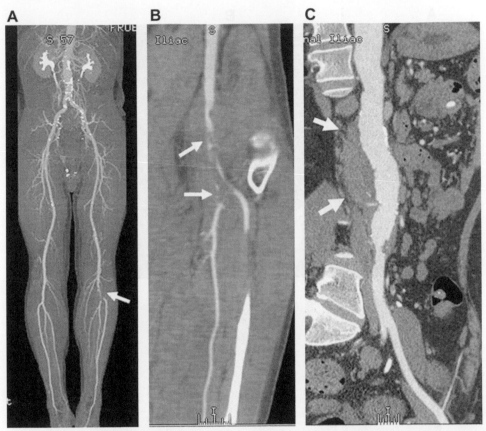

Fig. 15. Popliteal artery embolism originating from an infrarenal abdominal aortic aneurysm in a 50-year-old patient. (*A*) MIP display in frontal projection demonstrates subtotal occlusion of the distal popliteal artery with collateral circulation (*arrow*). Normal patency of the remaining aortoiliac, femoropopliteal, and tibioperoneal vessels. (*B*) CPR display of the distal left popliteal artery, tibioperoneal trunk, and peroneal artery demonstrating subtotal occlusion by an intraluminal filling defect (*arrows*). (*C*) CPR of infrarenal abdominal aorta and left iliac artery in lateral projection demonstrates an infrarenal abdominal aortic aneurysm (*arrows*) with prominent lining mural thrombus containing laminated calcification. Echocardiogram after popliteal artery embolectomy failed to reveal any cardiac source. The thrombus-lined abdominal aortic aneurysm was the presumed source.

disease, demonstrating the severity and length of stenosis and the length of occluded segment and providing critical information in decisions as to endovascular versus surgical bypass therapy (Fig. 12). These decisions are based on the TASC (Transatlantic Intersociety Consensus document on management of PAD), a series of recommendations by leading vascular interventional and surgical specialists in Europe and North America on the appropriate treatment strategy for various combinations of stenotic and occlusive disease differing in length of stenosis or occlusion, tandem lesions, and bilaterality (see Box 1; Box 2). The TASC format has 4 categories: A lesions are those with short-length stenoses or occlusions in which endovascular techniques in general produce excellent results; B lesions are suitable for an endovascular technique, which is preferred as the initial approach unless an open revascularization technique is required for other vascular disease in the same anatomic area; C lesions, longer than A or B lesions, are best treated with open revascularization with endovascular methods only used in patients at high risk for surgery; and D lesions are uniformly treated with surgical methods. Although endovascular interventional techniques will be preceded by diagnostic intra-arterial DSA to confirm the CTA findings, surgical management is usually performed without further invasive diagnostic testing and only with completion angiography in the operating room.[1]

CTA is less useful in patients with peripheral tibioperoneal atherosclerotic disease. This disease

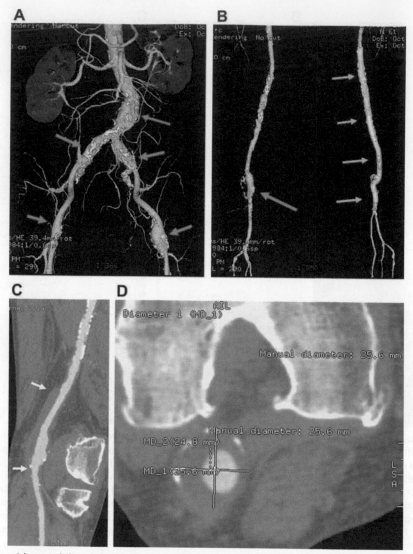

Fig. 16. Patient with aortobiliac, bilateral common femoral, and bilateral popliteal artery aneurysms. Prior endovascular stent grafting of the left popliteal artery. (*A*) Volume rendered display of aortoiliac and proximal femoral vasculature displays the aortic, iliac, and femoral aneurysms (*arrows*). (*B*) Volume rendered display of the distal femoral and popliteal artery circulation demonstrates a calcified midright popliteal artery aneurysm (*blue arrow*) and endovascular stenting of the distal left femoral and popliteal artery (*green arrows*). (*C*) CPR of the right popliteal artery demonstrates an extensive thrombus-filled aneurysm of the popliteal artery (*arrows*), lower margin at the level of the knee joint. (*D*) A 2.5-cm diameter aneurysm with prominent lining mural thrombus is demonstrated on the axial display.

occurs most frequently in patients with diabetes who have significant arterial vascular calcification, making the distinction of focal high-grade stenoses and occlusions difficult and obscuring long segments of the underlying arterial lumen because of the presence of calcified plaque. In small tibioperoneal vessels, CPR is useful but less so than observed in the aortoiliac and femoropopliteal segments (**Fig. 13**).[6,31–33]

In patients with diabetes or chronic renal disease and suspected predominant tibioperoneal arterial disease, MR angiography would be the preferred diagnostic angiographic method, unless contrast-enhanced MR angiography is contraindicated by the extent of renal impairment (estimated GFR<30).

ATHEROEMBOLISM

Atheroembolism may arise from focal atherothrombotic disease in the thoracoabdominal aorta or iliac vessels. Embolism may result in acute

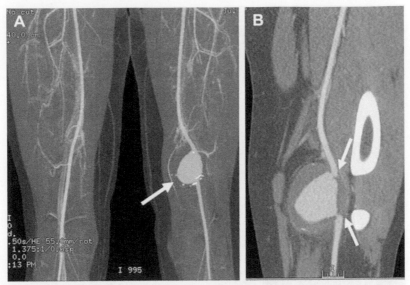

Fig. 17. Posttraumatic thrombus-filled pseudoaneurysm of the proximal popliteal artery in a 22-year-old woman. (*A*) MIP display of femoropopliteal and tibioperoneal circulation demonstrates a large saccular aneurysm of the proximal left popliteal artery (*arrow*). Normal caliber and patency of the distal left popliteal and tibioperoneal arteries. (*B*) CPR in lateral projection defines the wide aneurysm neck (*arrows*) and prominent lining mural thrombus.

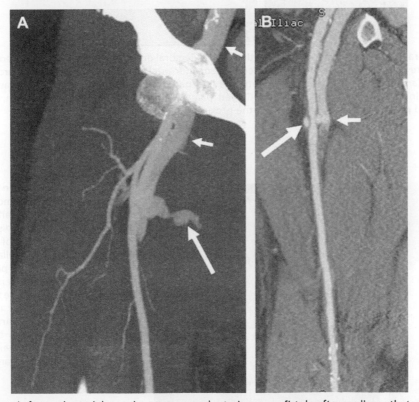

Fig. 18. Iatrogenic femoral arterial pseudoaneurysm and arteriovenous fistula after cardiac catheterization. Pseudoaneurysm established by color/spectral Doppler imaging. Arteriovenous fistula suspected. CTA performed before endovascular management. (*A*) Subvolume MIP in frontal projection demonstrates pseudoaneurysm medial to the proximal superficial femoral artery (*long arrow*) and an arteriovenous fistula with opacification of the proximal femoral vein (*short arrows*). (*B*) CPR in lateral projection clearly demonstrates the focal arterial injury, with pseudoaneurysm arising from the anterior wall (*long arrow*) and arteriovenous fistula from the posterior wall (*short arrow*).

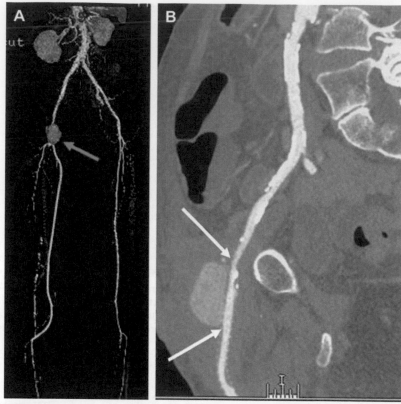

Fig. 19. Femoral artery pseudoaneurysm in a patient with a femoral distal arterial bypass graft. Preoperative arteriogram before surgical repair. (*A*) Volume rendered image in frontal projection demonstrates a prominent pseudoaneurysm (*arrow*) at the proximal anastomotic site of a patent femoral to distal arterial bypass graft. Distal implant site in the tibioperoneal trunk. (*B*) Curved planar reformation in lateral projection demonstrates a broad-based pseudoaneurysm contiguous to the proximal anastomotic site (*arrows*).

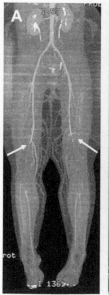
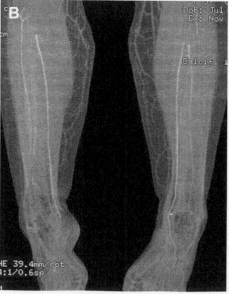

Fig. 20. Buerger disease in a 35-year-old woman with a heavy smoking history. Patient presented with calf claudication and low ABIs. (*A*) MIP display demonstrating focal occlusions of the popliteal arteries (*arrows*) with collateral circulation. Normal caliber and patency of the aortoiliac and proximal femoral vasculature. (*B*) MIP display of the tibioperoneal circulation demonstrates reconstitution of both posterior tibial arteries and an attenuated right anterior tibial and left peroneal artery. Prominent superficial veins noted in the subcutaneous adipose tissue.

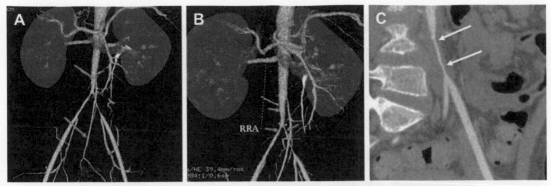

Fig. 21. Takayasu aortoarteritis in an 8-year-old boy with systemic symptoms and elevated erythrocyte sedimentation rate but no vascular symptoms. (A) Volume rendered image (VR) in frontal projection demonstrates circumferential smooth stenosis of the distal aorta and both common iliac arteries, more marked on the left. Note the enlarged inferior mesenteric artery (IMA) (arrows) and superior hemorrhoidal branch acting as visceral collateral circulation. (B) VR of aortoiliac circulation in a slight right anterior oblique (RAO) projection demonstrating the focal smoothly stenotic disease of the distal abdominal aorta and both common iliac arteries (arrows). The disease begins immediately distal to the orifice of the enlarged IMA. RRA, right renal artery. (C) Curved reformation of the distal aorta and left common, external iliac, and proximal internal iliac arteries. Note the prominent mural thickening of the left common iliac artery (arrows).

unilateral symptoms rather than bilateral symptoms.[34–36] An iliac arterial source by nature results in unilateral symptoms. The embolic events usually involve smaller-caliber peripheral arteries, with the classical clinical presentation of blue toe syndrome in otherwise asymptomatic patients. The atheroembolic source may be a focal ulcerative plaque in the thoracoabdominal aorta or iliac artery (Fig. 14).

CTA may be used with conventional coverage from diaphragm to feet with a negative study followed by a thoracic CT arteriogram. An alternative approach is to use CTA for a subtotal body angiogram encompassing the thoracoabdominal aorta and inflow and outflow circulation to the lower extremities.

Intravenous CTA is more efficacious than catheter-directed angiography because large area–

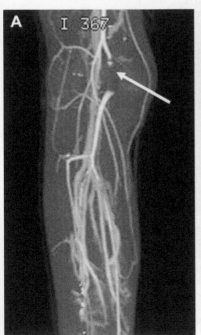
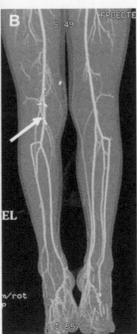

Fig. 22. Popliteal artery entrapment syndrome in an adolescent boy who presented with calf claudication. (A) MIP display in frontal projection demonstrates displaced and occluded popliteal artery immediately proximal to the level of the knee joint in the typical location of popliteal artery entrapment (arrow). Early venous opacification from calf musculature occurred with plantar flexion. (B) Postoperative study. MIP display in frontal projection. There is a patent short-segment venous bypass graft at the site of previously documented popliteal artery entrapment (arrow). Normal patency of the popliteal and tibioperoneal arterial circulation documented bilaterally. There is an anomalous high origin of the left posterior tibial artery.

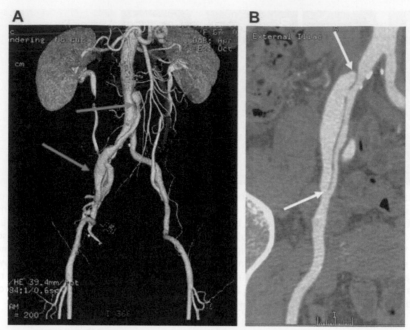

Fig. 23. Distal aortic and right common and external iliac artery dissection. Clinical presentation of sudden onset of abdominal pain in a 67-year-old woman. (*A*) Volume rendered image in frontal projection demonstrates an anterior false channel arising in the infrarenal aorta adjacent to the orifice of the inferior mesenteric artery, with the false lumen extending into the right common iliac and proximal external iliac artery (*arrows*). (*B*) CPR through distal aorta and right iliac system. The iliac component of the mural flap (*arrows*) involves common and proximal external iliac artery. Internal iliac artery arose from the posterior true lumen. Cause for dissection uncertain. Most likely cause would be aortic ulceration. There were no ischemic symptoms or physical findings in the right lower extremity. Patient remains under surveillance.

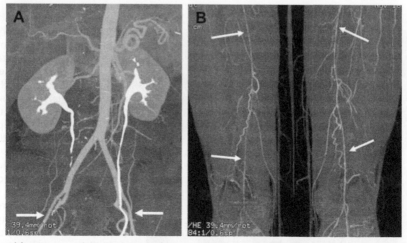

Fig. 24. 25-year-old woman with acute onset of lower extremity ischemia and rest pain. Absence of femoral and distal pulses. (*A*) MIP display in frontal projection of normal caliber abdominal aorta and bilateral common iliac arteries. Reduced caliber of bilateral external iliac arteries (*arrows*). (*B*) Diffuse narrowing of the superficial femoral and popliteal arteries (*arrows*) with normal caliber profunda femoral arterial branches in mid to distal thigh. There was minimal opacification of the tibioperoneal vessels. Clinical history after CTA revealed use of ergot-containing migraine medication in this human immunodeficiency virus–positive patient also taking ritonavir, a protease inhibitor that alters the metabolism of ergotamine. After discontinuation of migraine medication and institution of antiplatelet medication, there was spontaneous return to normal lower extremity arterial hemodynamics.

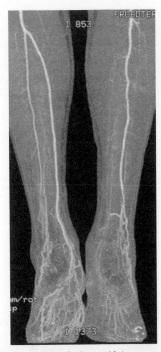

Fig. 25. CTA images of the calf in a candidate for fibular flap reconstruction with mandibular resection. MIP display in frontal projection demonstrates congenital absence of the right anterior tibial artery and of the left anterior tibial and posterior tibial arteries. Use of a distal fibular flap with accompanying distal peroneal artery considered inadvisable.

coverage angiography to evaluate for possible primary source can be combined with high-quality imaging of the peripheral arterial circulation to demonstrate sites of embolic obstruction. The intravenous technique is also less invasive and provides an angiographic roadmap to plan appropriate treatment.

Thromboembolic Peripheral Arterial Occlusion

Thomboemboli usually have a cardiac origin, left atrial or ventricular, although on occasion a paradoxic embolus may arise from the systemic venous circuit being transmitted through the heart via a patent foremen ovale or atrial septal defect. Thromboemboli are usually larger than atheroemboli and occlude more proximal vessels, most commonly the superficial femoral or popliteal arteries. As with atheroembolism, the disease process is usually unilateral, and the patient may be screened by echocardiography for a cardiac source. Alternatively, a gated thoracic aortic CT study encompassing the heart can be combined with a nongated aortoiliac and lower extremity arteriogram to evaluate for a cardiac source and

a systemic arterial source, most commonly an aortic aneurysm. CTA can demonstrate the site and extent of the peripheral arterial embolus, acting as a guide to surgical embolectomy (Fig. 15).

Peripheral Arterial Aneurysm

Aortoiliac arterial aneurysms may be combined with peripheral arterial occlusive disease or peripheral arterial aneurysms or both. Approximately 10% of patients with abdominal aortic aneurysms have femoral and/or popliteal artery aneurysms. A popliteal artery aneurysm is said to be present when the arterial diameter is greater than 7 mm, and a femoral artery aneurysm when the arterial diameter is greater than 10 mm.[14,37]

Peripheral arterial aneurysms may present as focal pulsatile masses. Alternatively, a patient may present with complications, most commonly acute thrombosis and occlusion of the arterial lumen, rupture or small vessel arterial embolic obstruction secondary to thromboembolism from the aneurysm.[38]

In evaluating patients with palpable popliteal artery aneurysms, it should be mandatory to image the aortoiliac segment as well as the femoropopliteal and tibioperoneal vasculature. Aneurysms are bilateral in 50% of patients (Fig. 16).[14,37,39,40] Patients with suspected popliteal artery aneurysm should have initial sonography as the definitive diagnostic test, allowing distinction of popliteal artery aneurysm from Baker cyst or cystic adventitial disease of the popliteal artery. If popliteal artery aneurysm is confirmed by sonography CTA is performed to define exact location, length of involvement, and extent of lining mural thrombus (Fig. 17). In addition, thromboembolic obstruction to the tibioperoneal and pedal circulation can be evaluated.

Femoral artery aneurysm caused by primary vessel disease is uncommon.[41] Most femoral artery aneurysms are secondary to trauma, not uncommonly iatrogenic, and secondary to femoral artery catheterization or surgical bypass grafting, including axillofemoral, aortofemoral, and femoro-popliteal bypasses (Figs. 18 and 19). Iatrogenic pseudoaneurysms of the femoral artery are best demonstrated by color/spectral Doppler study, which can define site of origin, aneurysm neck length, aneurysm sac dimensions, and extent of lining thrombus. Treatment can be instituted without defining the regional arterial circulation. However, if an angiographically assisted procedure using balloon occlusion of the upstream vasculature proximal to the pseudoaneurysm is to be used, then a preliminary CT angiogram

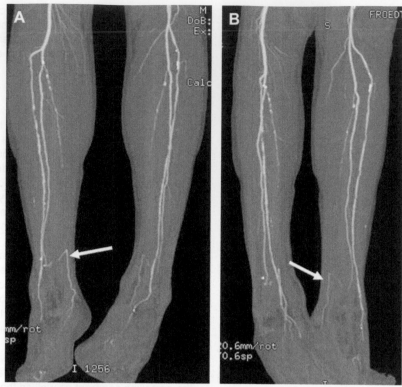

Fig. 26. Tibioperoneal arterial disease in a candidate for fibular flap reconstruction with mandibular resection. (*A*) MIP display in a left anterior oblique projection demonstrates occlusive disease of the right posterior tibial artery with reconstitution of the distal posterior tibial artery from a peroneal collateral (*arrow*). Proximal stenoses are noted in the anterior tibial artery, which is patent into the dorsal pedal branch. (*B*) Right anterior oblique MIP display demonstrates identical findings with attenuation and occlusion of the left posterior tibial artery and peroneal artery collateral to reconstitute the distal posterior tibial artery and plantar arch (*arrow*). Proximal stenoses are noted in the anterior tibial artery, which is patent into the dorsal pedal branch. Fibular harvesting with recruitment of the peroneal artery considered inadvisable.

may be appropriate to define presence of iliac and femoral native vessel disease.[42]

ARTERITIS

The most common types of arteritis affecting the peripheral arterial circulation are Buerger disease and Takayasu arteritis.

Buerger disease most commonly affects small and medium-sized arteries. Age of onset of disease is 40 to 45 years, with patients usually presenting with rest pain and associated tissue loss. There is a high association of the disease with smoking.

Typical sites of disease are the distal femoral and popliteal arteries and the proximal tibioperoneal vessels. Because the disease is slow in onset, patients typically have well-developed collateral circulation (**Fig. 20**).

The diagnosis of Buerger disease or inflammatory arteritis is based on clinical history, angiographic location of disease entity, and lack of coexistent atherosclerosis.[43] These patients typically have occlusive disease of medium size arteries (femoropopliteal), extending into the tibioperoneal circuit; therefore, arterial bypass graft is usually not an option because there is a lack of a viable distal landing zone and adequate distal extremity runoff. The angiographic appearance is one of abrupt vessel occlusion or focal high-grade concentric stenoses associated with well-established collateral circulation resulting in a "corkscrew appearance" on angiographic study.

Takayasu arteritis most commonly involves the thoracic aorta and brachiocephalic vessels with less-frequent involvement of the abdominal aorta and abdominal visceral arterial branches and the pulmonary arteries.[44] Abdominal aortic and iliac artery stenotic/occlusive disease with normal-caliber distal iliac and femoropopliteal/tibioperoneal vasculature in a young to middle-aged female patient is the usual clinical scenario of

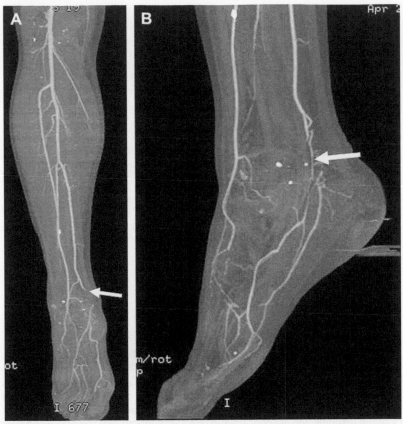

Fig. 27. CTA study of the right lower extremity in a soccer player who developed foot claudication after surgery to remove a ganglion related to the ankle joint. (*A*) MIP in frontal projection demonstrates focal occlusion of the distal posterior tibial artery (*arrow*), with collateral reconstitution of the plantar arch. Normal inflow into the dorsal pedal artery. Note the long tibioperoneal trunk bifurcating into the peroneal and posterior tibial arteries. (*B*) MIP display in lateral projection. Focal occlusion of the distal posterior tibial artery (*arrow*) with collateral reconstitution of the plantar arch. There is normal patency of the anterior tibial and dorsal pedal arteries.

this entity (Fig. 21). Takayasu disease is usually treated with corticosteroids and immunosuppression, in combination with endovascular stenting or surgical bypass graft as anatomically appropriate.

Giant cell arteritis is usually a predominant disease in young women. Characteristic angiographic features include symmetric bilateral stenoses and poststenotic aneurysmal dilatation associated with profuse collateral arterial blood supply.

Other forms of arteritis that may affect the peripheral circulation, although uncommon, include polyarteritis nodosa with small or medium-sized extremity vessel aneurysms, often in combination with visceral and renal artery aneurysms; Behcet disease, a vasculitis of small and large arteries often complicated by thrombosis requiring long-term anticoagulation; and Kawasaki disease, often manifesting in children and

involving coronary arteries and abdominal visceral arterial branches with multifocal aneurysm formation. Thrombosis of aneurysms may lead to focal occlusions.

In patients with arteritis, the underlying disease entity may be suspected before or after angiography. The clinical indications for performing arteriography in general are consistent with those used in patients with other forms of obstructive arterial disease and relate to peripheral ischemic symptoms, objective findings of tissue ischemia, or suspected peripheral arterial aneurysms.

POPLITEAL ARTERY ENTRAPMENT

Popliteal artery entrapment syndrome has 4 categories; the first 3 are based on delayed migration of the medial head of the gastrocnemius muscle in relation to formation of the popliteal artery

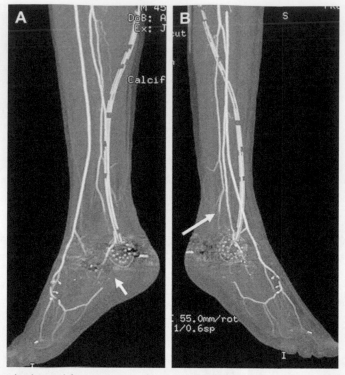

Fig. 28. Patient suffered calcaneal fracture and soft tissue injury with a subsequent free flap transfer. Postoperative study to evaluate distal arterial circulation. (*A*) MIP in lateral projection demonstrates surgical wound vacuum drain overlaying the distal posterior tibial artery. The proximal plantar arch is occluded (*arrow*). There is normal patency of the peroneal and anterior tibial arteries with inflow into the dorsal pedal vessel to the level of metatarsal arch. (*B*) MIP display in oblique projection. Site of posterior tibial artery occlusion (*arrow*) is depicted without overlaying wound vacuum drain. Gas locules are noted in the surgical bed.

from the primitive axial artery.[14,45–52] Delayed migration results in medial displacement of the popliteal artery around the medial border of the gastrocnemius, as is found in Type I disease, and in a lesser degree of displacement by an incompletely migrated medial head of the gastrocnemius in Type II disease. In Type III disease, the popliteal artery is displaced only by a portion of the medial head of the gastrocnemius muscle (**Fig. 22**).

The popliteal artery entrapment syndrome may be recognized on sonographic imaging and on compression and narrowing of the popliteal artery demonstrated with dorsiflexion of the foot. The same maneuver can be used during angiographic examination to demonstrate compression of the displaced popliteal artery with dorsiflexion.

In Type IV entrapment syndrome, the primitive axial artery persists as the distal popliteal artery and is deep to the popliteus muscle.

An entrapped popliteal artery may be treated by localized myomectomy or, in the presence of localized arterial wall damage, by a venous arterial bypass graft.

Cystic Adventitial Disease

In cystic adventitial disease, a mucoid cyst in the arterial adventica causes either concentric or eccentric smooth luminal narrowing of the popliteal artery.[53] Because the disease may present in younger patients and be initially demonstrated on sonography, MR angiography may be the preferred diagnostic imaging technique.[54] Angiographic studies demonstrate a characteristic smooth indentation of an undisplaced popliteal artery. The disease can be treated by aspiration of the cystic component or by ligation and arterial bypass.[55]

AORTOILIAC ARTERIAL DISSECTION

Iliac artery dissection is usually a distal extension of a thoracoabdominal aortic dissection, either Type A or Type B or an isolated aortoiliac

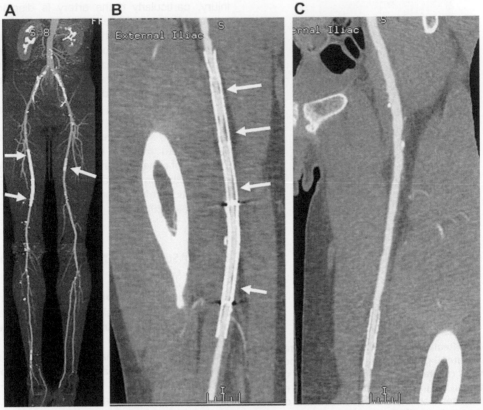

Fig. 29. Right femoropopliteal above-knee arterial stent and left distal femoral arterial stent. (*A*) MIP display in frontal projection demonstrates bilateral calcific atherosclerotic disease of the common and internal iliac arteries, right femoropopliteal stent (*arrows*), and left femoral stent (*arrow*). There was no significant iliac stenosis. Two-vessel tibioperoneal circulation to the level of the ankle is demonstrated. (*B*) CPR display demonstrates diffuse multifocal neointimal hyperplasia in the right femoropopliteal stent without significant luminal compromise (*arrows*). (*C*) CPR display demonstrates short segment distal left superficial femoral artery stent with minimal neointimal hyperplasia.

dissection. Aortic dissection may be primarily caused by cystic medial necrosis or penetrating aortic ulcer (Fig. 23). A congenital defect in the composition of the arterial wall, such as in Marfan syndrome or Ehler-Danlos syndrome, may also lead to aneurysm and dissection with involvement of the iliac arteries.[56–61] Marfan syndrome and Ehler-Danlos syndrome are secondary to disorder in the formation of collagen. The most serious manifestation of Marfan syndrome is with the Louis Dietz variant, which is often combined with skeletal anomalies. The most significant form of Ehrler-Danlos syndrome is Type IV, the arterial ecchymotic type.

ERGOTISIM

Ergotisim is a vasospastic disease that is most common in patients receiving medication for migraine and in those with access to illicit drugs, including lysergic acid diethylamide. Ergotisim results in a diffuse vasospasm of the aortoiliac and distal arterial circulation, a condition that is reversible on removal of the ergot medication (Fig. 24).

PLASTIC SURGERY

The advent of noninvasive CTA has allowed plastic surgeons to visualize pertinent arterial anatomy before either performing pedicle flaps to the lower extremity or using a fibular graft in patients having radical neck surgery for cancer of the floor of the mouth requiring mandibulectomy and fibular reconstruction.[62] Examples of vessels used as pedicle for musculocutaneous flaps are the inferior branch of the lateral circumflex femoral artery in the thigh and the anterior perforating branch of the peroneal artery in the calf.[63]

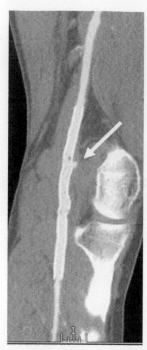

Fig. 30. Popliteal artery stent with focal stent fracture. (A) CPR in lateral projection demonstrates a focal out pouching of contrast medium on the anterior surface of the stent at the junction of the proximal and middle third of the stent (*arrow*). Small adjacent focus of neo-intimal hyperplasia. The patient is at risk for subsequent enlarging aneurysm. Stent fracture is possibly related to repetitive angular stress from knee flexion/extension.

In patients having a fibular graft for mandibular replacement, CTA is used to detect any variant arterial anatomy of the tibioperoneal vessels, which might preclude the use of a fibular graft, and proximal arterial disease, which may complicate the removal of the peroneal artery in conjunction with its fibular graft (Figs. 25 and 26).[62,64,65] Examples of variant arterial anatomy that could result in foot ischemia if the peroneal artery was harvested with the fibular graft include absence or hypoplasia of the anterior or posterior tibial arteries, with blood supply to the dorsal pedal and plantar arch vessels dependent on peroneal artery collaterals.

In young to middle-aged patients, intravenous angiography can be used for definitive analysis of the distal crural and pedal circulation when there is localized vessel occlusion secondary to trauma or embolism (Fig. 27).

ORTHOPEDIC APPLICATIONS

Patients with acute lower extremity fractures or fracture dislocations may have coexistent arterial injury, particularly if the artery is displaced or impressed by a displaced bone fragment. The arterial injury may result in thrombosis, pseudoaneurysm, or arteriovenous fistula. These vascular injuries are best evaluated at the time of initial presentation, before fracture reduction. Intravenous CTA has replaced intra-arterial DSA as the technique of choice in suspected posttraumatic arterial injury.[65–67]

In patients who have had internal or external fixation with metallic hardware, arterial vessel integrity, of either the femoropopliteal or tibioperoneal circuits, may still be established by CTA using thin section reformation or curved planar techniques (Fig. 28).

ENDOVASCULAR STENTS AND ARTERIAL BYPASS GRAFTS

Endovascular stents vary in diameter, metallic composition, strut thickness, and the presence of metallic markers. Various stent types are used in the iliac and femoral arterial circulation. Stents are subject to neointimal hyperplasia with superimposed thrombosis and in-stent stenosis or occlusion.[68–72]

Patients with stents may be evaluated by noninvasive imaging tests in a serial manner. If in-stent stenosis is suspected, a combined diagnostic and therapeutic intra-arterial DSA approach is usually used.

CTA is useful in patients with multiple unilateral or bilateral iliac and femoral artery stents who have persistent symptoms because noninvasive testing may be inconclusive in the presence of multiple stents.

In-stent luminal narrowing requires high spatial resolution in conjunction with adequate arterial luminal attenuation to be detected on CTA (Figs. 29 and 30). The major technical factors limiting accurate assessment of in-stent restenosis are blooming and beam hardening artifacts.[73–78]

An array of arterial bypass grafts are used in patients with arterial occlusive disease, including aortobiiliac and aortobifemoral grafts, axillofemoral and femoral femoro grafts, femoropopliteal (above and below knee) and femoral distal arterial bypass grafts (Fig. 31). Proximal grafts anastomosed to the femoral artery are almost uniformly prosthetic in nature. Femoropopliteal grafts are preferably venous, either in situ saphenous or reverse saphenous bypass grafts. In patients without adequate length or caliber of saphenous veins for venous bypass grafts, a prosthetic or composite prosthetic/venous bypass graft can be used.

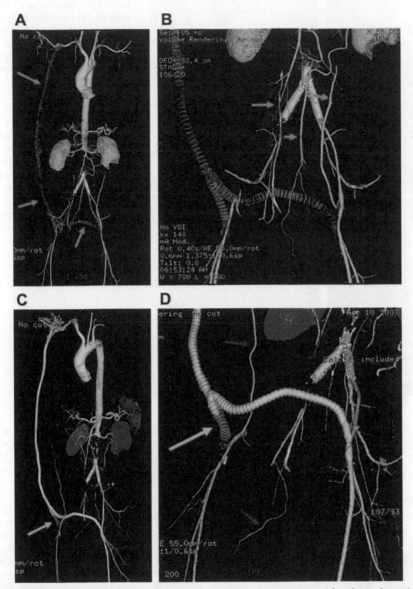

Fig. 31. Axillofemoral and femoro femoral bypass graft occlusion in a patient with subrenal aortic occlusion and occluded bilateral common iliac artery stents. (*A*) Thoracoabdominal aortic and extremity study documents occlusion of the right axillofemoral and femoro femoral bypass graft (*arrows*). (*B*) Localized image of low abdomen and pelvis demonstrates occluded grafts and epigastric parietal and mesenteric/hemorrhoidal visceral collateral circulation (*arrows*) to reconstitute distal left iliac and proximal femoral vasculature. (*C*) Replacement axillofemoral and femoro femoral bypass graft reevaluated with thoracoabdominal aortic and extremity study. Axillofemoral graft is patent into a femoro femoral crossover graft, but distal component attached to the right femoral artery is occluded (*arrow*). (*D*) Pelvic and upper thigh image better demonstrates the occluded distal component of the axillofemoral graft (*green arrow*) and collateral circulation to the right lower extremity (*blue arrows*).

Ultrasound surveillance is commonly used in patients with femoropopliteal or femoral distal arterial bypass grafts. Diagnostic criteria include waveform characteristics and peak systolic flow velocity. Soon after implantation, a venous bypass graft has low-resistance arterial flow waveforms, reflecting vasodilatation of the arterial system distal to the bypass graft. Subsequently, as arterial tone in the lower extremity returns to normal, a typical triphasic flow pattern is noted within the bypass graft. Criteria for significant stenosis include a doubling of the peak systolic flow velocity along the course of the graft or a decrease in peak systolic flow velocity to less than 50 cm/s.

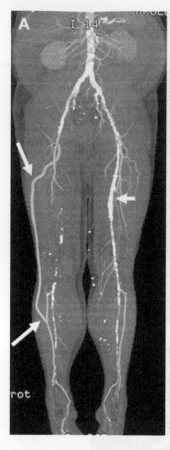

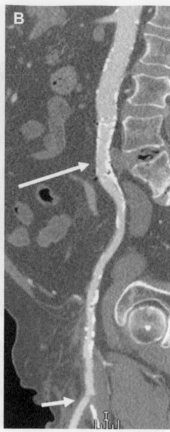

Fig. 32. Patent right femoral anterior tibial arterial bypass graft and proximal common iliac artery stent. (*A*) MIP display in frontal projection demonstrates a patent right-sided bypass graft with distal implant into the proximal anterior tibial artery (*arrows*). Peroneal and posterior tibial arteries are occluded bilaterally. Collateral circulation in distal calf opacifies the distal posterior tibial arteries and plantar arch. There is an angiographic stent in the midleft superficial femoral artery (*short arrow*). (*B*) CPR in lateral projection demonstrates normal patency of a right common iliac artery stent (*arrow*) and normal patency of diseased external iliac and common femoral artery. Proximal anastomotic site of the femoral anterior tibial artery bypass graft is demonstrated (*short arrow*).

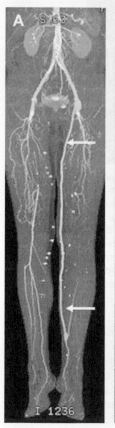

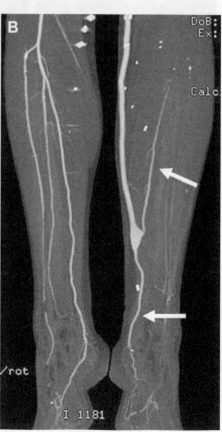

Fig. 33. Left femoral to posterior tibial artery bypass graft with antegrade and retrograde opacification from the distal implant site. Previous aortobifemoral graft. (*A*) MIP display in frontal projection demonstrates a left femoral posterior tibial artery prosthetic bypass graft implanted into the midposterior tibial artery (*arrows*). There is prominent left profunda arterial circulation. There is an occluded right superficial femoral artery with prominent profunda collateral circulation to reconstitute the popliteal artery and 3-vessel tibioperoneal runoff to the ankle. (*B*) MIP display in frontal projection of the left calf circulation. Prosthetic arterial bypass graft is attached to mid to distal posterior tibial artery. Posterior tibial artery is opacified proximal and distal to the implant site (*arrows*), with inflow into the plantar arch.

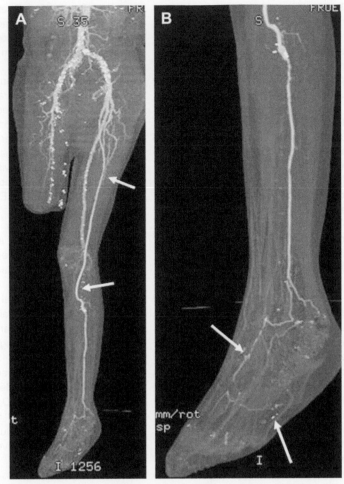

Fig. 34. Amputee with a patent below-knee long arterial bypass graft to the viable contralateral extremity. (*A*) MIP in frontal projection demonstrates a right above-knee amputation and a left femoral to peroneal distal arterial bypass graft (*arrows*) with single-vessel runoff to the ankle and foot. The left popliteal artery is occluded in distal thigh. (*B*) MIP display in lateral projection demonstrates a patent peroneal artery to supramalleolar level with collateral flow to the dorsal pedal and plantar arch circulation (*arrows*).

CTA can be used in patients with peripheral arterial bypass grafts when there is a nondiagnostic or equivocal ultrasonographic study or conflicting results of ultrasonography and ABI measurements.

CTA can be used to evaluate patients with aortoiliac, aortofemoral, or axillofemoral bypass grafts who re-present with extremity symptoms and have abnormal noninvasive, nonangiographic imaging test results (**Figs. 32–34**).

SUMMARY

CTA has become the imaging technique of choice in the evaluation of the lower extremity arterial system for a wide and diverse range of applications. Understanding and applying the principles

of injection/acquisition and display with interpretation targeted at appropriate clinical practice is the key to successful application of the modality.

REFERENCES

1. Norgren L, Hiatt WR, Dormandy JA, et al. Intersociety consensus for the management of peripheral arterial disease (TASC II). Eur J Vasc Endovasc Surg 2007;33:S1–70.
2. Hiatt MD, Fleischmann D, Hellinger JC, et al. Angiographic imaging of the lower extremities with multidetector CT. Radiol Clin North Am 2005;43:1119–27.
3. Rubin GD, Schmidt AJ, Logan LJ, et al. Multidetector row CT angiography of lower extremity arterial inflow and runoff: initial experience. Radiology 2001;221(1):146–58.

4. Chin AS, Rubin GD. CT angiography of peripheral arterial occlusive disease. Tech Vasc Interv Radiol 2006;9:143–9.

5. Fleischmann D, Lammer J. Peripheral CT angiography for interventional treatment planning. Eur Radiol 2006;16(Suppl 7):M58–64.

6. Bui TD, Gelfand D, Whipple S, et al. Comparison of CT and catheter arteriography for evaluation of peripheral arterial disease. Vasc Endovascular Surg 2005;39(6):481–90.

7. Heuschmid M, Kneger A, Beierlein W, et al. Assessment of peripheral arterial occlusive disease: comparison of multislice-CT angiography (MS-CTA) and intraarterial digital subfraction angiography (IA-DSA). Eur J Med Res 2003;8(9):389–96.

8. Selvin E, Erlinger TP. Prevalence of and risk factors for peripheral arterial disease in the United States: results from the National Health and Nutrition Examination Survey, 1999–2000. Circulation 2004;110(6):738–43.

9. Criqui MH, Vargas V, Denenberg JO, et al. Ethnicity and peripheral arterial disease: the San Diego Population Study. Circulation 2005;112(17):2703–7.

10. McDermott MM, Criqui MH, Greenland P, et al. Leg strength in peripheral arterial disease: associations with disease severity and lower-extremity performance. J Vasc Surg 2004;39(3):523–30.

11. Widmer L, Biland L. Risk profile and occlusive peripheral arterial disease. Proceedings of the 13th International Congress of Angiology. Athens (Greece), June 9–14, 1985. p. 28.

12. Kannel WB, Skinner JJ Jr, Schwartz MJ, et al. Intermittent claudication. Incidence in the Framingham Study. Circulation 1970;41(5):875–83.

13. Dormandy JA, Charbonnel B, Eckland DJ, et al. Secondary prevention of macrovasacular events in patients with type 2 diabetes in the PROactive Sstudy (PROspective pioglitAzone clinical trial in macrovascular events): a randomized controlled trial. Lancet 2005;366(9493):1279–89.

14. Wright LB, Matchett WJ, Cruz CP, et al. Popliteal artery disease: diagnosis and treatment. Radiographics 2004;24:467–79.

15. Aldrich HR, Girardi L, Bush HL Jr, et al. Recurrent systemic embolizations caused by aortic thrombi. Ann Thorac Surg 1994;57:466–8.

16. Ota H, Takase K, Igarashi K, et al. MDCT compared with digital subtraction angiography for assessment of lower extremity arterial occlusive disease: importance of reviewing cross-sectional images. AJR Am J Roentgenol 2004;182(1):201–9.

17. Ofer A, Nitecki SS, Linn S, et al. Multidetector CT angiography of peripheral vascular disease: a prospective comparison with intraarterial digital subtraction angiography. AJR Am J Roentgenol 2003;180(3):719–24.

18. Martin ML, Tay KH, Flak B, et al. Multidetector CT angiography of the aortoiliac system and lower extremities: a prospective comparison with digital subtraction angiography. Am J Roentgenol 2003;180(4):1085–91.

19. Fleischmann D, Rubin GD. Quantification of intravenously administered contrast medium transit through the peripheral arteries: implications for CT angiography. Radiology 2005;236:1076–82.

20. Meyer BC, Oldenburg A, Frericks BB, et al. Quantitative and qualitative evaluation of the influence of different table feeds on visualization of peripheral arteries in CT angiography of aortoiliac and lower extremity arteries. Eur Radiol 2008;18:1546–55.

21. Fleischmann D, Rubin GD, Bankier AA, et al. Improved uniformity of aortic enhancement with customized contrast medium injection protocols at CT angiography. Radiology 2000;214(2):363–71.

22. Willimann JK, Mayer D, Banyai M, et al. Evaluation of peripheral arterial bypass grafts with multi-detector row CT angiography: comparison with duplex US and digital subtraction angiography. Radiology 2003;229(2):465–74.

23. Lookstein RA. Impact of CT angiography on endovascular therapy. Mt Sinai J Med 2003;70(6):367–74.

24. Laswed T, Rizzo E, Guntern D, et al. Assessment of occlusive arterial disease of abdominal aorta and lower extremities arteries: value of multidetector CT angiography using an adaptive acquisition method. Eur Radiol 2008;18:263–72.

25. Catalano C, Fraioli F, Laghi A, et al. Infrarenal aortic and lower-extremity arterial disease: diagnostic performance of multi-detector row CT angiography. Radiology 2004;231:555–63.

26. Schernthaner R, Stadler A, Lomoschitz F, et al. Multidetector CT angiography in the assessment of peripheral arterial occlusive disease: accuracy in detecting the severity, number, and length of stenoses. Eur Radiol 2008;18:665–71.

27. Kanitsar A. Advanced visualization techniques for vessel investigation [Master Thesis]. Vienna, 2001; University of Technology.

28. Kanitsar A, Fleischmann D, Wegenkittl R, et al. CPR-curved planar reformation. IEEE visualization. Boston: IEEE Computer Society; 2002. p. 37–44.

29. Kanistar A, Wegenkittl R, Felkel P, et al. Computed tomography angiography: a case study of peripheral vessel investigation. San Diego (CA): IEEE Visualization; 2001. p. 477–80.

30. Kanitsar A, Wegenkittl R, Felkel P, et al. Automated vessel detection at lower extremity multislice CTA. Eur Radiol 2001;11(S1):236.

31. Thomsen HS. How to avoid nephrogenic systemic fibrosis: current guidelines in Europe and the United

States. Radiol Clin North Am 2009;47(5):871–5, vii. Review.

32. Rodriguez JA, Navarro FJ, Fernandez R, et al. [Gadolinium-induced systemic fibrosis in advanced kidney failure] [review]. Nefrologia 2009;29(4):358–63 [in Spanish].

33. Altun E, Semelka RC, Cakit C. Nephrogenic systemic fibrosis and management of high-risk patients [review]. Acad Radiol 2009;16(7):897–905.

34. Auer J, Aschi G, Berent R, et al. Systemic embolism from a large descending aortic thrombus. Int J Cardiol 2003;89:305–7.

35. Berneder S, van Ingen G, Eigel P. Arch thrombus formation in an apparently normal aorta as a source for recurrent peripheral embolization. Thorac Cardiovasc Surg 2006;54:548–9.

36. Thaler DE, Saver JL. Cryptogenic stroke and patent foramen ovale. Curr Opin Cardiol 2008;23(6):537–44 Review.

37. Diwan A, Sarkar R, Stanleyu JC, et al. Incidence of femoral and popliteal artery aneurysms in patients with abdominal aortic aneurysms. J Vasc Surg 2000;31:863–9.

38. Graham LM. Femoral and popliteal aneurysms. In: Rutherford RB, editor. Vascular surgery. 5th edition. Philadelphia: Saunders; 2000. p. 1345–68.

39. Crawford ES, Debakey ME. Popliteal artery arteriosclerotic aneruysm. Circulation 1965;32:515–6.

40. Friesen G, Ivins JC, James JM. Popliteal aneurysms. Surgery 1962;51:90–8.

41. Sharma S, Nalachandran S. Isolated common femoral artery aneurysm: a case report. Cases J 2009;2:7552.

42. Lopera JE, Trimmer CK, Josephs SG, et al. Multidetector CT angiography of infrainguinal arterial bypass. Radiographics 2008;28:529–49.

43. Puechal X, Feissinger JN. Thromboangiitis obliterans or Buerger's disease. Rheumatology (Oxford) 2007;46(2):192–9.

44. Chung WJ, Kim HC, Ho Y, et al. Patterns of aortic involvement in Takayasu arteritis and its clinical implications: evaluation with spiral computed tomography angiography. J Vasc Surg 2007;45:906–14.

45. Stuart TP. Note on a variation in the course of the popliteal artery. J Anat Physiol 1879;13:162.

46. Love JW, Whelan TJ. Popliteal artery entrapment syndrome. Am J Surg 1965;109:620–4.

47. Fowl RJ, Kempczinski RF. Popliteal artery entrapment. 5th edition. In: Rutherford RB, editor. Vascular surgery. Philadelphia: Saunders; 2000. p. 1087–93.

48. Bouroutos J, Daskalakis E. Muscular abnormalities affecting the popliteal vessels. Br J Surg 1981;68: 501–6.

49. Gibson MH, Mills JG, Johnson GE, et al. Popliteal entrapment syndrome. Ann Surg 1977;185: 341–8.

50. Levien IJ, Veller MG. Popliteal artery entrapment syndrome: more common than previously recognized. J Vasc Surg 1999;30:587–98.

51. Collins PS, McDonald PT, Lim RC. Popliteal artery entrapment: an evolving syndrome. J Vasc Surg 1989;10:484–90.

52. Turnipseed WD. Popliteal entrapment syndrome. J Vasc Surg 2002;35:910–5.

53. Atkins HJ, Key JA. A case of myoxomatous tumor arising in the adventitia of the left external iliac artery. Br J Surg 1947;34:426.

54. Van Isenghem BW, Gryspeerdt SS, Baekelandt MB. Claudication type lower limb pain in an athlete without atherosclerotic risk factors: a case of cystic adventitial disease of the popliteal artery. JBIR-BTR 2003;86(5):272–5.

55. Deutsch AL, Hyde J, Miller SM, et al. Cystic adventitial degeneration of the popliteal artery: CT demonstration and directed percutaneous therapy. AJR Am J Roentgenol 1985;145:117–8.

56. Tonnessen BH, Sternbergh WC 3rd, Mannava K, et al. Endovascular repair of an iliac artery aneurysm in a patient with Ehlers-Danlos syndrome type IV. J Vasc Surg 2007;45(1):177–9.

57. de Paiva Magahlhaes E, Fernandes SR, Zanardi VA, et al. Ehlers-Danlos syndrome type IV and multiple aortic aneurysms – a case report. Angiology 2001; 52(3):223–8.

58. Meldon S, Brady W, Young JS. Presentation of Ehlers-Danlos syndrome: iliac artery pseudoaneurysm rupture. Ann Emerg Med 1996;28(2):231–4 Review.

59. Mattar SG, Kumar AG, Lumsden AB. Vascular complications in Ehlers-Danlos syndrome. Am Surg 1994;60(11):827–31.

60. Safioleas MC, Kakisis D, Evangelidakis EL, et al. Thromboendarterectomy of the right common iliac artery in a patient with Marfan's syndrome and restoration. Int Angiol 2001;20(3):241–3.

61. Hatrick AG, Malcolm PN, Burnand KG, et al. A superficial femoral artery aneurysm in a patient with Marfan's syndrome. Eur J Vasc Endovasc Surg 1998;15(5):459–60.

62. Jin KN, Lee W, Yin YH, et al. Preoperative evaluation of lower extremity arteries for free fibula transfer using MDCT angiography. J Comput Assist Tomogr 2007;31(5):820–5.

63. Rad AN, Singh NK, Rosson GD. Peroneal artery perforator-based propeller flap reconstruction of the lateral distal lower extremity after tumor extirpation: case report and literature review. Wiley-Liss, Inc. Microsurgery 2008;28:663–70.

64. Oxford L, Ducic Y. Use of fibula-free tissue transfer with preoperative 2-vessel runoff to the lower extremity. Arch Facial Plast Surg 2005;7:261–4.

65. Chow LC, Napoli A, Klein M, et al. Vascular mapping of the leg with multi-detector row CT angiography

prior to free-flap transplantation. Radiology 2005; 237(1):353–60.

66. Hsu CS, Hellinger JC, Rubin GD, et al. CT angiography in pediatric extremity trauma: preoperative evaluation prior to reconstructive surgery. Hand (N Y) 2008;3(2):139–45.

67. Chang H, Heo C, Jeong J, et al. Unilateral buttock reconstruction using contralateral inferior gluteal artery perforator flap with the aid of multi-detector CT. J Plast Reconstr Aesthet Surg 2008;61(12):1534–8.

68. Parakevas KI, Baker DM, Pompella A, et al. Does diabetes mellitus play a role in restenosis and patency rates following lower extremity peripheral arterial critical overview. Ann Vasc Surg 2008; 22(3):481–91.

69. Powell RJ, Fillinger M, Walsh DB, et al. Predicting outcome of angioplasty and selective stenting of multisegment iliac artery occlusive disease. J Vasc Surg 2000;32(3):564–9.

70. Donas KP, Schwindt A, Schonefeld T, et al. Below-knee bare nitinol stent placement in high-risk patients with critical limb ischemia and unlimited supraceliac treatment of choice. Eur J Vasc Endovasc Surg 2009;37(6):688–93.

71. Weisinger B, Heller S, Schmehl J, et al. Percutaneous vascular interventions in the superficial femoral artery. A review. Minerva Cardioangiol 2006;54(1):83–93.

72. Comerota AJ. Endovascular and surgical revascularization for patients with intermittent claudication [review]. Am J Cardiol 2001; 87(12A):34D–43D.

73. Blum MB, Schmook M, Schernthaner R, et al. Quantification and detectability of in-stent stenosis with CT angiography and MR angiography in arterial stents. AJR Am J Roentgenol 2007;189(5): 1238–42.

74. Choi HS, Choi BW, Choe KO, et al. Pitfalls, artifacts, and remedies in multi-detector row CT coronary angiography. Radiographics 2004;24(3):787–800 Review.

75. Musicant SE, Giswold ME, Olson CJ, et al. Postoperative duplex scan surveillance of axillofemoral bypass grafts. J Vasc Surg 2003;37(1):54–61.

76. von Jessen F, Rordam P, Sillesen HH, et al. [Postoperative duplex ultrasonic surveillance of infrainguinal arterial reconstructions] [review]. Ugeskr Laeger 1992;154(20):1402–6 [in Danish].

77. Nielsen TG, von Jessen F, Schroeder TV. [Earlier experiences with duplex scanning of femoropopliteal and crural vein bypass]. Ugeskr Laeger 1993; 155(2):881–4 [in Danish].

78. Disselhoff B, Buth J, Jakimowicz J. Early detection of stenosis of femoro-distal grafts. A surveillance study using colour-duplex scanning. Eur J Vasc Surg 1989;3(1):43–8.

Upper Extremity Computed Tomographic Angiography: State of the Art Technique and Applications in 2010

Jeffrey C. Hellinger, MD[a],*, Monica Epelman, MD[b],
Geoffrey D. Rubin, MD[c]

KEYWORDS

- Upper extremity • Computed tomographic angiography
- Arterial occlusive disease • Venous occlusive disease
- Trauma • Vascular masses • Vascular mapping
- Hemodialysis access

Computed tomographic (CT) angiography can be performed on all currently available multidetector-row CT (MDCT) scanners (4- through 320-channels) to assess the upper extremity (UE) vasculature in a wide spectrum of clinical presentations. Based upon the clinical indications, four upper extremity CT angiogram (CTA) protocols are recommended: Aortic Arch with Upper Extremity Runoff, Upper Extremity Runoff, Upper Extremity Indirect CT Venography (CTV), and Upper Extremity Direct CTV (Table 1). Clinical success of these protocols depends upon thorough understanding of UE normal and abnormal anatomy (cardiovascular and non-cardiovascular), UE pathology and pathophysiology, and UE CTA (UECTA) technical principles. While practical knowledge of UECTA acquisition parameters and contrast medium administration strategies is paramount for efficient and effective utilization, technically, the cardiovascular imager should also be familiar with methodologies for patient preparation and post-processed image display, interpretation, and quantitative analysis. In the first part of this review, key UE arterial and venous anatomy is presented followed by a detailed overview of upper extremity CTA technical considerations and strategies. In the second part, clinical applications are discussed and illustrated.

VASCULAR ANATOMY

Arterial System

Inflow

Main inflow arterial segments are the aortic arch, brachiocephalic artery, and right and left subclavian artery (Fig. 1). With conventional left aortic arch anatomy, the brachiocephalic artery is the first artery off the aortic arch, giving rise to the right subclavian artery. The left subclavian artery arises directly from the aortic arch just distal to the left common carotid artery. The subclavian arteries are divided into 3 segments, each of which can exhibit specific pathology. The major subclavian artery branches are the vertebral artery, internal

[a] Cardiovascular Imaging and 3D Imaging Laboratory, Department of Radiology, The Children's Hospital of Philadelphia, University of Pennsylvania School of Medicine, South 34th Street & Civic Center Boulevard, Philadelphia, PA 19104, USA
[b] Neonatal Imaging, Department of Radiology, The Children's Hospital of Philadelphia, University of Pennsylvania School of Medicine, South 34th Street & Civic Center Boulevard, Philadelphia, PA 19104, USA
[c] Cardiovascular Imaging, Department of Radiology, Stanford University Medical Center, Stanford University School of Medicine, 300 Pasteur Drive, Palo Alto, Stanford, CA 94304, USA
* Corresponding author.
E-mail address: jeffrey.hellinger@yahoo.com

Radiol Clin N Am 48 (2010) 397–421
doi:10.1016/j.rcl.2010.02.022
0033-8389/10/$ – see front matter © 2010 Elsevier Inc. All rights reserved.

Table 1
UECTA protocols

Protocol	Coverage	Distance (mm)	Reference Level[a]	Application
Aortic arch with runoff	Arterial inflow and outflow	700–1000	Aortic arch	Arterial occlusive disease Arterial bypass grafts and stents Vasculitis Trauma Vascular masses Vascular mapping Hemodialysis access
UE runoff	Targeted arterial outflow	300–600	First slice of acquisition	Trauma Follow-up vasculitis Vascular masses Vascular mapping
Indirect venogram	Peripheral and central veins	400–700	None (60–70 delay)[b]	Venoocclusive disease
	Targeted	700–1000	Aortic arch	Venous stents
	Complete			Vascular masses
				Venous mapping
Direct venogram	Peripheral and central veins	400–700	None (60–70 delay)[b]	Venoocclusive disease
	Targeted	700–1000	SVC	Venous stents
	Complete			Venous mapping

[a] Reference level is defined as the targeted vascular segment when utilizing either a timing bolus or automated triggering to synchronize the image acquisition with the delivery of contrast medium.
[b] Indirect and direct venography are performed with an empiric 60–70 sec delay. Alternatively, to optimize venous enhancement, arterial phase synchronization is made to the aortic arch (indirect CTV) or SVC (direct CTV) and images are acquired after a 50–60 sec delay.

mammary artery, thyrocervical trunk, costocervical trunk, and dorsal scapular artery, all of which can provide important routes of collateral flow.

Outflow

The main outflow arteries to the hand include the axillary, brachial, radial, ulnar, and interosseous arteries (see **Fig. 1**). The axillary artery extends from the lateral margin of the first rib to the inferior margin of the teres major. Important branches for potential collateral flow are the superior thoracic, thoracoacromial, and lateral thoracic arteries and the subscapular and humeral circumflex arteries. The brachial artery extends from the lateral border of the teres major to the antecubital fossa, where it divides into radial and ulnar arteries. Major brachial arterial branches for collateral flow are the brachial profunda, superior ulnar collateral, and inferior ulnar collateral arteries (**Fig. 2**). Distally, the brachial profunda divides into the radial collateral and middle collateral arteries (see **Fig. 2**). In

the forearm, the radial, ulnar, and interosseous arteries extend to the wrist, with the interosseous artery arising from the ulnar artery. The radial recurrent, interosseous recurrent, anterior ulnar recurrent, and posterior ulnar recurrent arteries form collateral networks around the elbow with communications to the second and third order brachial collateral branches (see **Fig. 2**). The radial and ulnar arteries may have aberrant, high origins, arising from axillary or brachial arteries.

Hand

In the hand, the interosseous arteries feed into palmar (volar interosseous) and dorsal (volar and dorsal interosseous) carpal arches, whereas the ulnar and radial arteries run off into the superficial and deep palmar arches, respectively (see **Fig. 1**). The carpal and palmar arterial arches supply and, by nature of their anatomy, provide collateral blood flow into the arborizing metacarpal and digital arteries (**Fig. 3**). Other regions of collateral

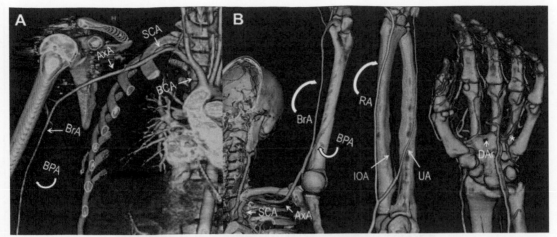

Fig. 1. Normal UE arterial inflow and outflow anatomy. (*A*) A volume rendered (VR) image obtained in a 12-year-old patient who sustained penetrating trauma to the right UE and underwent a CTA for decreased pulses. The arm was scanned along the patient's side. (*B*) A 3-station VR runoff obtained in a 40-year-old patient who underwent left UECTA for preoperative vascular mapping. The arm was scanned in an abducted position, raised above the patient's head. Arterial anatomy is normal for both patients. In (*B*), note the robust enhancement to the tufts of the fingers, with early venous drainage. An intact palmar arch system is demonstrated with communication between the deep and superficial systems (*asterisk*). AxA, axillary artery; BCA, brachiocephalic artery; BPA, brachial profunda artery; BrA, brachial artery; DAr, deep arch; IOA, interosseous arteries; RA, radial artery; SCA, subclavian artery; UA, ulnar artery.

flow include perforating arteries between the dorsal metacarpal arteries (dorsal carpal arch) and the deep and superficial palmar arches; at the common digital arteries; and at the distal phalangeal tufts where there are connections between the dorsal and palmar digital arteries.

Venous System

The UE venous system consists of peripheral veins in the hand, wrist, forearm, upper arm, and shoulder, and central ipsilateral thorax veins draining into the superior vena cava (SVC). It is defined by superficial and deep veins, linked by perforating veins and venous networks (plexi). Valves in superficial, deep, and perforating veins function to keep blood flowing antegrade and prevent blood flowing from the deep to superficial veins.

The superficial veins (Fig. 4) are located subcutaneously within the superficial fascia. They are the principal means for venous drainage in the hand, forearm, and upper arm, coursing as single structures. Infrequently, accessory veins are present. All superficial venous drainage ultimately transitions into the axillary deep vein.

In the hand, superficial veins include the dorsal digital veins, dorsal metacarpal veins, the dorsal venous network (DVN), palmar digital veins, and the palmar venous plexus. The cephalic and

basilic veins form as cephalad extensions from the radial and ulnar aspects of the DVN, respectively, and serve as dominant superficial venous drainage routes along the lateral and medial aspects of the forearm and upper arm, respectively. They are united by the median cubital vein, which arises from the cephalic vein, just proximal to the elbow and courses obliquely in the antecubital fossa, to drain into the basilic vein. In the forearm, the median antecubital vein drains the palmar venous network from the hand and ascends to drain most commonly into either the median cubital vein or the basilic vein just below the elbow. Alternatively, the median antecubital may divide into the median basilic and median cephalic veins. In the upper arm, the basilic vein perforates the deep fascia at the midarm level, coursing medial to the brachial artery until the inferior border of the teres major where it joins with the medial brachial vein to form the axillary vein. The cephalic crosses the deep fascia at the axilla with drainage into the axillary vein.

The deep veins (Figs. 5 and 6) are located intramuscularly, deep to the superficial fascia, accompanying the extremity arteries (venae comitans). In the hand, forearm, and upper arm, the deep veins are duplicated; within the axilla and thorax, the major deep veins occur as single structures. In the hand, deep veins include the common and

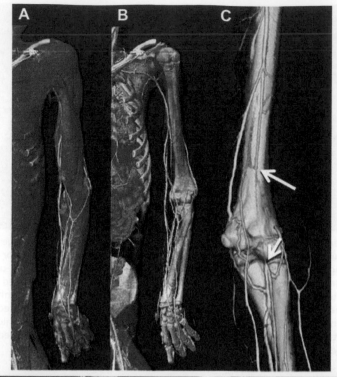

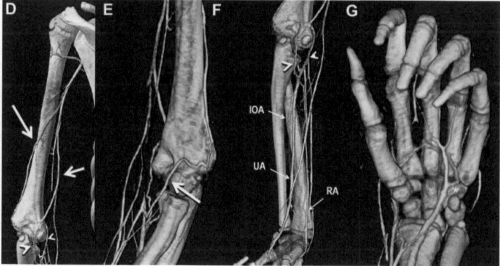

Fig. 2. Vascular mapping for Volkmann's contracture. Complete left UECTA was performed in a 10-year-old female with low-dose technique and the affected extremity alongside the patient. VR images (*A, B*) demonstrate flexion deformities at the elbow and wrist with increased collateral flow at the elbow. A magnified VR display confirms distal brachial artery occlusion (*C, long arrow*) with reconstitution in the proximal forearm (*C, short arrow*). Targeted VR images emphasize 2 major routes of collateral flow at the elbow (*D–F*). One is the radial collateral artery (*D, long arrow*) feeding into the radial recurrent artery (*E, long arrow*) to reconstitute radial artery flow. The other route consists of the ulnar collateral arteries (*D, short arrow*) feeding into the ulnar recurrent arteries (*D, F; arrowheads*). Flow is preserved into the hand with communication between the deep and superficial palmar arches (*G, asterisk*). IOA, interosseous arteries; RA, radial artery; UA, ulnar artery.

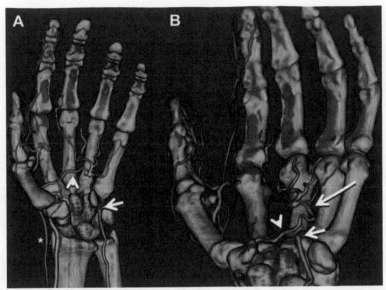

Fig. 3. Hypothenar hammer syndrome. Volume rendered frontal and oblique projections of the left hand in a patient with repetitive work-related motion demonstrate ulnar artery occlusion (*short arrow*) at the edge of the hook of the hamate. An intact deep arch (*arrow head*) reconstitutes flow into the superficial palmar arch (*long arrow*) with asymmetric delayed arterial flow in the ulnar digital distribution. Third to fifth digital artery enhancement is seen faintly for the proximal interphalangeal joints only. Enhancement in the radial distribution is seen well to the tufts of the thumb and second finger with early venous drainage, including enhancement of the cephalic vein (*asterisk*).

metacarpal palmar veins, the superficial and deep palmar venous arches, and the carpal venous plexus. In the forearm, the major deep veins are the paired radial, ulnar, and interosseous veins; in the upper arm, the paired brachial veins and the single axillary vein are the major deep venous

routes. The axillary vein crosses into the costoclavicular space, transitioning to the subclavian vein. The subclavian vein joins with the internal jugular vein to form the brachiocephalic vein. The right and left brachiocephalic veins unite to form the SVC, which then drains into the right atrium.

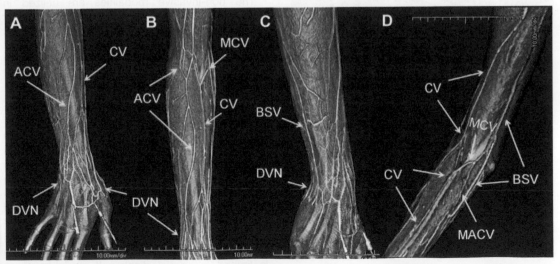

Fig. 4. Superficial veins: hand and forearm. Direct right UE CT venography VR images demonstrate normal superficial veins in the hand and forearm. Note the venous catheters in the dorsal veins of the hand (*A*). A second catheter was necessary as the first did not provide adequate flow. ACV, accessory cephalic vein; BSV, basilic vein; CV, cephalic vein; DVN, dorsal venous network; MACV, median antecubital vein; MCV, median cubital vein.

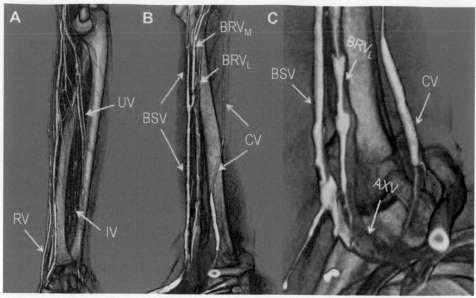

Fig. 5. Peripheral deep and superficial veins: upper arm. Direct right UE CT venography VR images demonstrate normal superficial and deep veins in the upper arm. AXV, axillary vein; BSV, basilic vein; BRV, brachial vein (L, lateral; M, medial) CV, cephalic vein; IV, interosseous vein; RV, radial vein; UV, ulnar vein.

IMAGING CONSIDERATIONS

Diagnostic catheter angiography (CA) is accepted as the gold standard for evaluating the UE arterial and venous systems. However, with state of the art capabilities of vascular ultrasound (VUS), magnetic resonance imaging (MRI) and

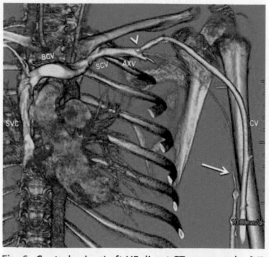

Fig. 6. Central veins. Left UE direct CT venography (VR display) demonstrates brachial vein occlusion (*arrow*) with dominant drainage via the cephalic vein (CV). The cephalic-axillary vein junction (*arrowhead*) and the central veins are widely patent. AXV, axillary vein; BCV, brachiocephalic vein; SCV, subclavian vein; SVC, superior vena cavae.

angiography (MRA), MDCT angiography, and Positron Emission Tomography (PET) - CTA, diagnostic catheter angiography is currently reserved for when these non-invasive imaging modalities do not answer all clinical questions or they lead to discordant information. CA may also be utilized as a primary diagnostic modality when direct hemodynamic analysis is required for treatment planning or when there is intent to perform endovascular intervention in one combined procedure.

The non-invasive modalities are utilized in a complementary manner, emphasizing their benefits. For many diagnostic scenarios, evaluation frequently begins with radiography. UE radiographs are useful for localizing phleboliths and other calcifications, hardware, foreign bodies, and soft tissue gas; assessing bone mineralization; and evaluating associated primary (ie, fracture) and secondary osseous abnormalities (ie, osteomyelitis related to arterial occlusive disease). VUS is utilized as a first line arterial and venous screening and surveillance modality for most pediatric and adult patients, providing cost and workflow efficiency. Flow hemodynamics are evaluated along with morphology of the vessel lumen and wall. However, VUS is operator dependent, does not fully evaluate UE arterial inflow and central thoracic venous anatomy, and is limited in spatial display. If available, three dimensional (3D) VUS is recommended to improve UE spatial displays and minimize operator dependence.

Based upon the results of VUS, the clinical presentation, suspected pathology, co-morbid patient risk factors, and modality availability, MRI - MRA or CTA are subsequently obtained. MRI-MRA is advantageous as it does not require the use of electromagnetic radiation or iodinated CM, affords dynamic 3D acquisitions with multiple vascular phases, and can directly assess arterial and venous hemodynamics. However, it has a relatively long exam time (particularly for complete UE coverage), has a narrow bore (conventional closed system), and is limited by the presence ferrous metallic and implantable devices. The narrow bore may preclude large body habitus patients and those with claustrophobia. Despite its inherent radiation and contrast medium dependence, volumetric 3D CT arteriography and venography offer advantages over MRI including a short exam time, greater availability, higher spatial resolution (essential for small vessel imaging in the hand), greater routine vessel wall characterization, reliable depiction of and imaging in the presence of calcium and ferrous metallic devices, and its comprehensive evaluation of non-cardiovascular structures. In addition, UECTA can be performed safely in patients with non-MRI compatible implantable devices, large body habitus, or claustrophobia. CTA is also advocated over MRA in renal failure patients, provided they are on hemo- or peritoneal dialysis, as gadolinium is contraindicated (for the risk of nephrogenic systemic sclerosis), whereas iodinated CM can still be administered. While CTA involves the use of ionizing radiation, it is noteworthy that the radiosensitivity of extremity tissue is very low and therefore the sequelae of radiation exposure from CT distal to the axilla is negligible. PET-CTA is utilized on a select basis. The main applications are vasculitis and atherosclerosis whereby increased radiotracer activity, corresponding to inflammation, is fused with the UE arterial anatomy.

CTA TECHNIQUE
Patient Preparation

All external metallic objects should be removed from the expected scan coverage as they can limit photon exposure and degrade image quality. At a minimum this includes the chest and affected extremity. When the arm is scanned in an abducted position, portions of the neck and head are included and regions should be pre-screened for metallic objects. When the arm is scanned at the side of the body, the abdomen and pelvis require screening.

For CT arteriography and indirect venography, an 18–20 gauge (g) peripheral intravenous catheter (PIVC) is placed in a contralateral UE vein, as high density inflowing contrast material in an ipsilateral vein will cause streak artifact and degrade vascular assessment. The antecubital location is the preferred access site since high flow rates are necessary. If this is not a feasible location, other options include the forearm or hand, with the likely need to decrease the CM injection rate. If these secondary sites are not accessible, considerations include a contralateral external jugular vein or a centrally placed venous catheter which can accommodate power injection.

The exceptions for these rules are UE direct CTV and pediatric UECTA. For direct CTV, a 20–24 g PIVC is placed in an ipsilateral hand or peripheral forearm vein. For most pediatric imaging, the PIVC is 20–22 g, with 24 g reserved for younger patients (ie, neonates, infants, young children) who have small caliber veins. In many instances, a hand vein may be the only accessible access site in these patients.

The final preparation is positioning the patient on the CT table. The first choice is to position patients supine and head first into the scanner with the affected extremity extended above the patient's head, isocenter in the gantry with the palm ventral and the fingers spread apart (Fig. 7). The contralateral arm is placed at the patient's side. Pillows, blankets, or both are utilized as needed to support the patient's head and body, and assure that the center of gantry is at the mid axillary line level. Tape is applied to secure positioning of the forearm and hand and assist the patient in not moving the UE. A modified swimmer's or prone position may be required to ensure isocenter positioning.

If the affected extremity cannot be raised above the patient's head, the exam is performed with the UE adjacent to the patient's body, accepting that there is increased noise and streak artifacts (See Fig. 1; Fig. 8). The patient is placed supine or prone on the table with isocenter positioning of the UE to be imaged. This most often requires shifting of the patient's body to the contralateral side. To reduce artifacts in this position, the contralateral UE may be raised out of the field of view.

Bilateral exams are acquired by scanning both arms together (targeted runoff for forearm or hand coverage, Fig. 7) or by scanning each arm individually (16–320 channel scanners). Functional UECTA is performed for thoracic inlet and outlet syndromes, with neutral and challenged CTA acquisitions. In the neutral phase, the affected extremity is placed at the patient's side. In the challenged phase, the arm is abducted with extension and the patient's head is turned ipsilateral, simulating the Adson maneuver.

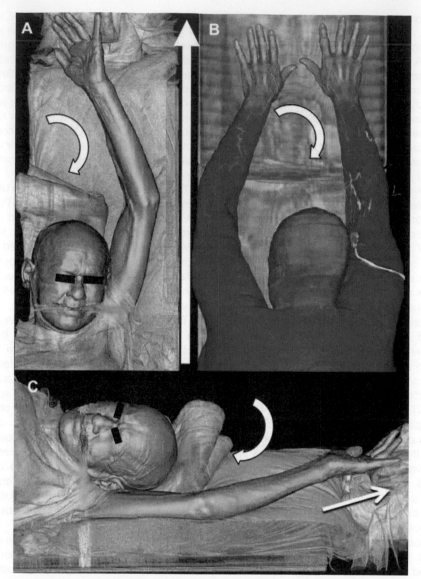

Fig. 7. Patient positioning: arm(s) raised. Patient positioning is important for achieving high UECTA image quality. The first consideration is to place the affected UE(s) above the patient's head on the gantry table (*A*, *B*), as close to isocenter as possible. For a unilateral examination, although this is most readily facilitated with the patient supine (*A*), a modified swimmer's position is often necessary (*C*). Alternatively, scanning can occur with the patient prone. Prone positioning often provides more patient comfort with a bilateral UE examination (*B*). In all instances, pillows, blankets, or both (*curved arrows*) are used to support the patient's head and body and also raise the UE height so that it is at the same level as the midaxillary line. Tape is used to secure forearm and hand positioning (*short straight arrow*). Scans proceed in a caudocranial direction for an arteriogram (*long straight arrow*) and craniocaudad direction for a venogram.

Acquisition

Protocol series

UECTA protocols may have up to five acquisition series. The first series is a required low dose anterior-posterior scout topogram. To prescribe precise coverage and field of view, a lateral view may also be obtained. The second series is an optional non-contrast acquisition (NCA) with 0.5–2.5 mm thick sections. Coverage may be identical to the planned angiographic acquisition or may target a selected region in the chest or UE. The primary objective of the NCA is to identify high density material which may limit radiographic image quality and interpretation or may itself be obscured by the CM. NCA images help to assess

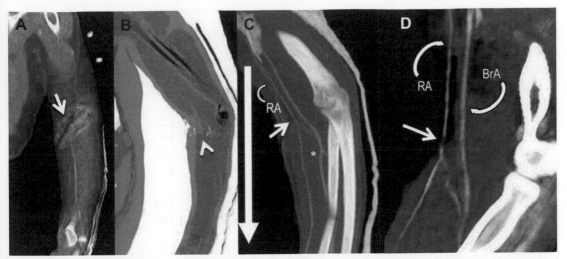

Fig. 8. Patient positioning: arms down. If arm abduction is not feasible, UECTA proceeds with the affected extremity placed along the patient's side. In the case shown, a 35-year-old man sustained a stab wound to the left antecubital fossa and had diminished distal pulses. As the patient could not raise his arm, the left UECTA runoff was performed from the shoulder through to the hand, with the patient supine and the affected UE at the patient's side To minimize noise, the contralateral UE was raised above the patient's head (not shown). Imaging proceeded in a craniocaudad direction (*long arrow*). VR (*A*) and MinIP (*B*) images demonstrate a left antecubital laceration (*A, arrow*) with foci of air (*B, arrowhead*), respectively. MIP (*C*) and VR (*D*) angiographic images demonstrate high origin of the radial artery (RA) with focal vasospasm (*arrows*) at the level of injury, but without luminal interruption or contrast extravasation. The brachial artery (BrA) is normal, dividing into ulnar and interosseous arteries (*C, asterisk*).

calcifications, endovascular stents and stent-grafts, surgical clips, surgical grafts, catheters, bone fragments (ie, trauma), residual intravenous contrast, active bleeding, and hematomas. With dual-energy MDCT scanners, a virtual NCA is possible, limiting the amount of patient radiation exposure.[1] The third series is a low dose timing acquisition, which is essential for precise synchronization of the image acquisition with either arterial or venous enhancement or both. The arrival time is determined with bolus tracking software or alternatively, as a separate timing bolus acquisition. By nature of an UECTA, all protocols require the fourth series, in which the contrast enhanced angiographic images are acquired. For slow acquisitions (table speed ≤30 mm/sec), breath-holding is required when scanning through the chest. In the setting of suspected cardiogenic UE thromboembolism, prospective or retrospective ECG-gated cardiac CTA can be combined with routine non-ECG gated imaging through the upper chest and the UE runoff vasculature. The fifth series is an optional delayed post-contrast acquisition. The delayed acquisition is useful in the setting of suspected vasculitis, vascular masses, and hemorrhage. It can also be used to acquire a venous phase (indirect venogram) after the arterial phase. When monitoring the exam, if the

acquisition gets ahead of the contrast bolus, an immediate delayed phase can be obtained.

UE CT angiogram
Coverage In the aortic arch with upper extremity runoff protocol, the complete inflow and outflow UE vascular tree is evaluated. When the arm is abducted, coverage begins just below the aortic arch and extends in a caudocranial direction through the fingers, yielding a scan distance of 700 to 1000 mm for an adult (see Fig. 7). If the arm is placed at the patient's side, coverage begins at the thoracic inlet and extends through the fingers in a craniocaudad direction (see Fig. 1). In the upper extremity runoff protocol, outflow segments are targeted. Coverage begins at the shoulder or elbow and extends through to the fingers, in a caudocranial or craniocaudad direction, depending on the UE position, for a scan length of 300 to 600 mm (see Fig. 8). For the upper extremity indirect and direct CTV protocols, peripheral and central veins are evaluated to the cavoatrial junction. The arm may be raised (see Fig. 5) or placed at the patient's side (see Fig. 6), with the scan direction often prescribed coinciding with venous flow. Depending on the clinical indications, coverage may extend to peripheral veins at either the elbow (400–700 mm scan distance) or the hand

Table 2
UECTA acquisition and reconstruction parameters

MDCT Scanner	Detector Configuration (Channels × mm)	Pitch	Gantry Rotation Time (s)	Table Speed (mm/s)	Scan Time (s)	Slice Thickness (mm)	RI (mm)	Number of Images
4-Channel								
GE	4 × 2.5	1.5	0.5	30	30	2.5	1.5	600
Philips	4 × 2.5	1.5	0.5	30	30	2.5	1.5	600
Siemens	4 × 2.5	1.5	0.5	30	30	2.5	1.5	600
Toshiba	4 × 2.0	1.5	0.5	24	37.5	2	1.0	900
8-Channel								
GE	8 × 1.25	1.35	0.5	27	33	1.25	0.8	1125
Toshiba	8 × 1.0	1.438	0.5	23	39	1.0	0.8	1125
GE	8 × 2.5	1.35	0.5	54	17	2.5	1.5	600
Toshiba	8 × 2.0	1.438	0.5	46	19.5	2.0	1.0	900
16-Channel								
GE	16 × 0.625	1.375	0.5	27.5	33	0.625	0.5	1800
Philips	16 × 0.75	1.2	0.5	29	31	0.75	0.5	1800
Siemens	16 × 0.75	1.2	0.5	29	31	0.75	0.5	1800
Toshiba	16 × 0.5	1.438	0.5	23	39	0.5	0.4	2250
GE	16 × 1.25	1.375	0.5	55	16	1.25	0.8	1125
Philips	16 × 1.5	1.5	0.5	72	12.5	1.5	0.8	1125
Siemens	16 × 1.5	1.5	0.5	72	12.5	1.5	0.8	1125
Toshiba	16 × 1.0	1.438	0.5	46	19.5	1.0	0.8	1125

Scan times are for an average Z-axis coverage of 900 mm. Acquisition parameters (detector configuration, pitch, gantry rotation speed) reflect single source helical scanning. Reconstruction parameters: slice thickness and reconstruction interval (RI).

(700–1000 mm scan distance). The delayed acquisition may be programmed to cover the entire UE arterial tree or only the outflow. If the series is used because contrast did not adequately opacify the forearm and hand arteries on the first acquisition, the scan should begin just above the elbow.

Acquisition Parameters

Tables 2–4 list UECTA helical acquisition (detector configuration, pitch, gantry speed) and reconstruction (slice thickness, reconstruction interval) parameters using three generations of MDCT scanners respectively. Based on the type of MDCT scanner, parameter selection reflects a balance between the desired spatial resolution, scan coverage, scan duration, and the acceptable minimum radiation exposure. With 4–16 channel MDCT scanners (see Table 2), protocol design emphasizes coverage with the fastest possible speed which will match UE physiologic flow and accommodate a reasonable breathhold, while providing acceptable image

quality for advanced visualization. These goals are most readily achieved with a 16-channel system to the point that routine protocols may be too rapid and new strategies are required to avoid "getting ahead" of the contrast bolus. Beginning with 20–64 channel systems (see Table 3), protocol design transitions to acquisitions with improved spatial resolution and image quality at reduced radiation exposure, while utilizing principles to avoid "getting ahead" of the contrast bolus. These goals are further emphasized with the latest state of the art 128-, 160-, 256-, and 320-channel systems (Table 4), whereby low dose scanning is routinely possible without sacrificing image quality. However, it is even more critical to employ strategies to compensate for the faster inherent table speed.

Regarding radiation exposure, a tube voltage of 80 kV is recommended for patients up to 80 kg. Between 80–120 kg and greater than 120 kg, 100 kV and 120 kV are recommended, respectively. Use of a lower voltage will increase iodine attenuation as the photons will be closer to the k-edge of

Table 3
UECTA acquisition and reconstruction parameters

MDCT Scanner	Detector Configuration (Channels × mm)	Pitch	Gantry Rotation Time (s)	Table Speed (mm/s)	Scan Time (s)	Slice Thickness (mm)	RI (mm)	Number of Images
20-Channel								
Siemens	20 × 0.6	1.2	0.5	29	31	0.75	0.5	1800
Siemens	16 × 1.2	1.5	0.33	87	10	1.5	0.8	1125
32-Channel								
GE	32 × 0.625	0.984	0.7	28	32	0.625	0.5	1800
Toshiba	32 × 0.5	0.844	0.5	27	33	0.5	0.4	2250
GE	32 × 1.25	1.375	0.35	157	6	1.25	0.8	1125
Toshiba	32 × 1.0	1.5	0.4	120	7.5	1.0	0.8	1125
40-Channel								
Philips	40 × 0.625	0.6	0.5	30	30	0.75	0.5	1800
Siemens	2 × 20 × 0.6	1.2	0.5	29	31	0.75	0.5	1800
Philips	32 × 1.25	1.5	0.4	150	6	1.5	0.8	1125
Siemens	16 × 1.2	1.5	0.33	87	10	1.5	0.8	1125
64-Channel								
GE	64 × 0.625	0.516	0.7	30	30	0.625	0.5	1800
Philips	64 × 0.625	0.5	0.75	27	34	0.75	0.5	1800
Siemens	2 × 32 × 0.6	0.7	0.5	27	33.5	0.75	0.5	1800
	(2) 2 × 32 × 0.6[a]	0.7	0.5	27	33.5	0.75	0.5	1800
Toshiba	64 × 0.5	0.5	0.6	27	33	0.5	0.4	2250
GE	32 × 1.25	1.375	0.35	157	6	1.25	0.8	1125
Philips	32 × 1.25	1.5	0.4	150	6	1.5	0.8	1125
Siemens	24 × 1.2	1.5	0.33	131	7	1.5	0.8	1125
	(2) 24 × 1.2[a]	3	0.33	262	3.5	1.5	0.8	1125
Toshiba	32 × 1.0	1.5	0.4	120	7.5	1.0	0.8	1125

Scan times are for an average Z-axis coverage of 900 mm. Acquisition parameters (detector configuration, pitch, gantry rotation speed) reflect helical scanning. Reconstruction parameters: slice thickness and reconstruction interval (RI).

[a] Dual source.

iodine (33.2 keV).[2] This reaches a maximum effect at 80 kVp. With reduced voltage, however, noise will increase. When available, the use of automated tube current modulation is recommended with the goal of utilizing the lowest possible amperage that will generate acceptable diagnostic quality images per body weight. Recommended reference amperage values for patients <20 kg, 21–40 kg, 41–60 kg, 61–80, 81–100, 101–120, and >120 kg are 15 mAs, 25 mAs, 45 mAs, 65 mAs, 85 mAs, 110 mAs, and 150 mAs, respectively.

With 4-row systems, to scan the complete UE tree in a reasonable duration, a 4 × 2.0 mm or 4 × 2.5 mm detector configuration is necessary (see Table 2). 2.0–2.5 mm images are reconstructed at 1.0–1.5 mm increments, yielding an effective slice thickness of 3.0 mm. These "standard resolution" acquisitions with up to 1000 images are adequate to depict the vascular tree through to the hand. However, when visualization of the palmar and digital arteries is essential for diagnosis and management, "higher spatial resolution" imaging with a 4 × 1 mm or 4 × 1.25 mm configuration may be necessary. The scan duration would be twice as long, such that if this configuration is applied during an Aortic Arch with Upper Extremity Runoff, there will be an increased risk for venous

Table 4
UECTA acquisition and reconstruction parameters

MDCT Scanner	Detector Configuration (Channels × mm)	Pitch	Gantry Rotation Time (s)	Table Speed (mm/s)	Scan Time (s)	Slice Thickness (mm)	RI (mm)	Number of Images
128-Channel								
Siemens	2 × 64 × 0.6	0.4	0.5	30.7	29	0.75	0.5	1800
	(2) 2 × 64 × 0.6[a]	0.4	0.5	30.7	29	0.75	0.5	1800
Siemens	32 × 1.2	1.5	0.33	174.5	5	1.5	0.8	1125
	(2) 32 x 1.2[a]	3.5	0.33	407	2.2	1.5	0.8	1125
160-Channel								
Toshiba	160 × 0.5[b]	0.5	0.75	53	17	0.5	0.4	2250
Toshiba	80 × 1.0[b]	1.5	0.4	300	3	1.0	0.8	1125
256-Channel								
Philips	(2) 64 × 0.625[a]	0.5	0.75	27	34	0.625	0.5	1800
	(2) 128 × 0.625[a]	0.5	0.75	53	17	0.625	0.5	1800
Philips	(2) 64 × 1.25[a]	1.5	0.27	444	2	1.25	0.8	1125
Toshiba	160 × 0.5[b]	0.5	0.75	53	17	0.5	0.4	2250
Toshiba	80 × 1.0[b]	1.5	0.4	300	3	1.0	0.8	1125

Scan times are for an average Z-axis coverage of 900 mm. Acquisition parameters (detector configuration, pitch, gantry rotation speed) reflect helical scanning. Reconstruction parameters: slice thickness and reconstruction interval (RI).
[a] Dual source.
[b] Helical mode - Pending US Food and Drug Administration clearance.

contamination. As a result, depending upon the exam indications, higher spatial resolution techniques, using a 4-row system, are more commonly reserved for Upper Extremity Runoff protocols.

With an 8-row system, the complete vascular tree is imaged with higher spatial resolution techniques (8 × 1.0, 8 × 1.25 mm) in a duration comparable to 4 × 2.0 and 4 × 2.5 mm acquisitions (see Table 2). Vascular enhancement from the mid chest through the fingers is optimized, while the palmar arch and digital arteries are depicted with reliable detail. This technique also improves visualization of small vessels off the subclavian, axillary, brachial, and proximal radial and ulnar arteries. Datasets are reconstructed every 0.8 mm into 1.0–1.25 mm thick images, yielding up to 1250 images. Coverage of the thoracic and abdominal aorta can be combined with an UECTA using "standard resolution" (8 × 2.0 mm, 8 × 2.5 mm) or higher spatial resolution modes and the fastest gantry speed and maximum pitch. With increased coverage and longer scan durations, however, the risk for venous contamination may increase.

With 16-row systems (see Table 2), a complete UECTA is now possible with a near isotropic resolution mode. Isotropic exams are acquired with submillimeter collimations (16 × 0.5 mm, 16 × 0.625 mm, 16 × 0.75 mm), further improving visualization of small vessels. Datasets (reconstructed into 0.5–0.75 mm sections at 0.4–0.5 mm increments) are generated in durations similar to 4 × 2.0–2.5 mm and 8 × 1.0–1.25 mm acquisitions. Challenges using the near-isotropic mode include 1) the potential for increased noise and the subsequent need for increasing the tube current, and 2) the increased number of images. For a volume coverage of 1000 mm, up to 2500 images may be generated for a 16-channel angiogram reconstructed at 0.4–0.5 mm increments. To reduce excessive noise, the original (near-isotropic) dataset can be reconstructed into thicker images (1.0–1.5 mm) at less overlap (0.6–0.8 mm). Alternatively, under select clinical applications, at the discretion of the monitoring imager, the exam can be acquired using a higher spatial resolution mode (16 × 1.0 mm, 16 × 1.25 mm or 16 × 1.5 mm).

For most clinical applications with a 16-channel system, the higher spatial resolution mode does provide adequate detail to reliably depict upper extremity vasculature. The table speed with this mode is often too fast for contrast medium transit in the upper extremity vascular tree, which as alluded to above, can potentially yield an acquisition that "out-runs" the bolus. One solution is to slow the table speed either by using submillimeter collimation, a lower pitch, decreased gantry rotation speed, or a combination of these strategies. A second solution is to lengthen the delay prior to initiating the scan. With a 16-channel system, the increased table speed can be utilized to scan the complete UE vasculature and thoracic and abdominal aorta with a higher spatial resolution technique.

With 20–320-row systems (see Tables 3 and 4), both isotropic and higher spatial resolution helical modes are also standard options. As with 16-channel scanners, the submillimeter acquisitions can be reconstructed into isotropic resolution (0.5–0.75 mm × 0.4–0.5 mm) and higher spatial resolution datasets (1.0–1.5 mm × 0.8 mm). For both modes, the table speed is substantially faster than with 16-channel systems, directly proportional to the number of detector-rows and the collimation coverage per gantry rotation. To optimize vascular enhancement through to the digital vessels and avoid the greater potential for "out-running the bolus," it is even more essential to slow the acquisition speed or prescribe an appropriate scan delay. For detector arrays between that are between 12–40 mm, slowing the table speed to a uniform rate is readily possible by utilizing submillimeter collimation (isotropic resolution), reduced pitch, and reduced gantry speed. With an 80 mm detector array and all higher spatial resolution modes up to a 40 mm detector array, extending the delay is the recommended strategy. To take advantage of radiation reduction using a 20–320 - row scanner, it is recommended to select parameters which will generate the fastest scan possible for the desired spatial resolution (eg, highest pitch, fastest gantry rotation speed). In this case, as in imaging pediatric patients, extending the scan delay may be the only option. These principles are further discussed in the article by Hellinger and colleagues elsewhere in this issue. When using a 20–320- row scanner, based upon the scan length and duration, an isotropic or a higher spatial resolution technique can be prescribed for a whole body CTA, imaging the UE, complete aorta, and lower extremity vasculature.

CM Delivery

UECTA enhancement should reach at least a minimum of 300–350 HU, while indirect UECTV enhancement should be in the range of 150–250 HU. Optimizing enhancement for these protocols is dependent on synchronized delivery of contrast medium with an minimum iodine dose of 400–600 mg Iodine per kilogram (1.3–2.0 ml/kg for 300 mg Iodine/ml concentration) and for most patients (30–100 kg), an iodine flux of 0.9–1.5 g Iodine per second (3–5 ml/sec for 300 mg Iodine/ml concentration). Direct CTV achieves enhancement on the order of 500–1200 HU, depending on the degree of contrast dilution (75–90% mixture). The iodine dose is similar, but is delivered at a lower iodine flux. For all acquisitions, injection protocols can be tailored to the specific patient, by adjusting the CM concentration (300–370 mg Iodine per milliliter), injection rate (1.5–6 ml/sec), injection volume, and/or injection duration based upon a patient's body weight, cardiac function, the scan distance, speed of the scanner, and the anticipated image noise.

Strategies for CM administration

Synchronization Determining contrast medium transit time with automated bolus tracking software or a test bolus injection is a prerequisite for optimized enhancement given the variable time for CM to travel from the site of injection through the UE vasculature. This step is a mandatory for arterial phase imaging and recommended, but optional for venous phase imaging. With the test bolus technique, the time to peak enhancement is determined at a reference level in serial axial images and then pre-selected as the minimum diagnostic delay (contrast medium transit time). With automated tracking, reference vessel attenuation is monitored in near real-time. Once a predetermined threshold opacification (120–150 HU) is attained at the reference level, the scan is triggered. In comparison to a test-bolus injection, the actual time required to trigger the scan is longer with automated triggering secondary to inherent interscan and image reconstruction delays, in addition to the diagnostic delay. Depending upon the scanner, the minimum additional scan delay may range between 2 and 8 seconds. For indirect and direct CTV, if a timing acquisition is obtained, the diagnostic delay is extended to approximately 50–60 seconds. If the indirect CTV is obtained as a delayed phase, 20–30 seconds is applied as the delay following the arterial phase. If indirect or direct CTV are acquired without a timing acquisition, the recommended empiric delay is 60–70 seconds. Suggested reference levels for the UE protocols are listed in Table 1. The aortic arch (Aortic Arch with Runoff, Indirect CTV) and SVC (Direct CTV) are recommended as routine reference levels given their reliable size and ease of identification by the scanning technologist. For the Upper Extremity Runoff protocol, the first slice of the acquisition is the reference level.

Injection parameters Extrapolating from lower extremity CT arteriography CM principles, UE inflow and outflow arterial enhancement is optimized when the table speed does not exceed 30 mm/sec.[3] For complete UE coverage, this translates to scan durations of approximately 25–35 seconds (700–1000 mm coverage), while for targeted runoff coverage, 10 to 20 seconds (300–600 mm distance). Accordingly, UE injection protocols are designed based upon slow (≤30 mm/sec table speed) and fast (>30 mm/sec) acquisitions, with variable injection rates and CM volumes dependent on the body weight, cardiac function, and CM concentration. For all applications, if the desired injection rate exceeds the tolerable limit for the accessed vein, to maintain iodine dose at a reduced injection rate, the iodine concentration, the injection duration, or both should be increased. If the injection duration is increased, the diagnostic delay should be increased by the same amount.

Slow acquisitions (≤30 mm/sec) occur with 4-channel standard resolution; 8-channel higher spatial resolution; and 16-256 channel isotropic resolution modes having a detector width of not more than 40 mm (see Tables 2–4). For adolescent and adult patients, the scan duration for complete coverage (700–1000 mm) is typically 25 seconds or greater; the injection duration is set to equal the scan duration (Table 5). A biphasic injection protocol is utilized, as it achieves more uniform enhancement. In the first phase, 20% of the total volume is administered at a higher rate (3.5–6 ml/sec) over a short duration (ie, 5–7 seconds). In the second phase, the remaining volume is infused at a slower injection rate (2.5–5 ml/s) for the remainder of the exam. If automated triggering is used, the injection duration is extended to account for the inherent delay. When the scan duration is less than 25 seconds (ie, targeted runoff; patient weight <40 kg), the injection duration is also set to equal the scan duration, however a uniphasic injection is used. The injection rate in this instance is determined by dividing the CM volume by the scan (injection) duration.

Fast acquisitions occur with 8-channel standard resolution; 16–128 channel high spatial resolution; and all 160–320 channel 80 mm detector array modes (see Tables 2–4), yielding table speeds of 46–444 mm/sec when the volume coverage averages 900 mm. For both an Aortic Arch with Upper Extremity Runoff and an Upper Extremity Runoff protocol, if the injection duration is set to equal the scan duration, an insufficient iodine dose may be delivered and the scan acquisition will be too fast for the required transit time through the upper extremity vascular tree. A variable portion of the injected contrast may not have any meaningful contribution to the angiographic acquisition, unless there is a delayed phase. The key strategy to prevent the acquisition from "outrunning" the contrast bolus is to use predetermined injection duration according to an anticipated scan duration when the extremity is scanned at 25–30 mm/sec. A uniphasic or biphasic protocol is utilized based upon the anticipated injection duration. The diagnostic scan delay is increased such that the true scan duration and the pre-determined injection duration end simultaneously (Table 6). The scan delay can be extended by 5 seconds, such that scan will end after the infusion of contrast, increasing the probability that contrast medium will reach the digital arteries. To attain the required iodine dose, the injection rate and concentration are varied according to the body weight. One potential pitfall with this approach is venous opacification in the inflow and outflow regions, potentially obscuring arterial depiction.

Injection parameters for indirect CTV, whether obtained as a primary or delayed acquisition, follow those of an UE CT arteriogram, as the goal is to get contrast rapidly into the UE vascular system. The key is to apply an appropriate delay so that the acquisition is optimized with the majority of contrast in the veins. With direct CTV, low injection rates (1.5–3 ml/s) for a 75–90% diluted contrast mixture, are applied over 50–70 seconds to optimize uniform enhancement using first venous pass and recirculation phases.

Saline flush As with other CTA protocols, saline flush with a dual-chamber injector is recommended immediately following CM infusion. The saline injection improves contrast use and reduces perivenous streak artifacts; 20 to 40 mL (>20 kg) is injected at a rate equal to the CM injection rate. If a biphasic CM protocol is used, the saline injection rate defaults to the second injection rate.

Image Analysis

Aortic arch with upper extremity runoff and complete CTV protocols yield some of the largest non–ECG-gated vascular CTA examinations. As mentioned earlier, the UE CT angiogram alone may have up to 2500 images (2–3 gigabytes worth of data). Optional noncontrast and delayed imaging further add to potential data overload.

Table 5
UECTA injection protocols: MDCT table speed ≤30 mm/s

Weight (kg)	Scan Delay (s)	Average Iodine Dose (g)	Iodine Flux (g at g/s)	300 mg I/mL CM		350 mg I/mL CM		370 mg I/mL CM	
				Volume (mL)	Injection (mL at mL/s)	Volume (mL)	Injection (mL at mL/s)	Volume (mL)	Injection (mL at mL/s)
41–50	t_{CMT}+2–8[a]	22.5	4.5 at 1.1 / 20 at 1.0	75	15 at 3.0 / 60 at 2.4	64	13 at 2.6 / 51 at 2.0	61	12 at 2.4 / 49 at 1.9
51–60	t_{CMT}+2–8[a]	27.5	5.5 at 1.1 / 22 at 1.0	92	18 at 3.7 / 74 at 3.0	79	16 at 3.2 / 63 at 2.5	74	15 at 3.0 / 59 at 2.4
61–70	t_{CMT}+2–8[a]	32.5	6.5 at 1.3 / 26 at 1.1	108	22 at 4.3 / 87 at 3.8	93	19 at 3.7 / 74 at 3.2	88	18 at 3.5 / 70 at 3.1
71–80	t_{CMT}+2–8[a]	37.5	7.5 at 1.5 / 30 at 1.3	125	25 at 5.0 / 100 at 4.0	107	21 at 4.3 / 86 at 3.4	101	20 at 4.0 / 81 at 3.2
81–90	t_{CMT}+2–8[a]	42.5	8.5 at 1.7 / 34 at 1.5	142	28 at 5.7 / 114 at 4.6	121	24 at 4.9 / 97 at 3.9	115	23 at 4.6 / 92 at 3.7
91–100	t_{CMT}+2–8[a]	47.5	9.5 at 1.9 / 38 at 1.7	158	32 at 6.3 / 126 at 5.1	136	27 at 5.4 / 109 at 4.7	128	26 at 5.1 / 102 at 4.1
101–110	t_{CMT}+2–8[a]	52.5	11 at 2.1 / 42 at 1.8	175	35 at 6.4 / 140 at 5.7	150	30 at 5.5 / 120 at 4.9	142	28 at 5.1 / 114 at 4.7
111–120	t_{CMT}+2–8[a]	57.5	12 at 2.3 / 46 at 2.0	192	38 at 6.9 / 154 at 6.3	164	33 at 6 / 131 at 5.3	155	31 at 5.6 / 124 at 5.1

Injection protocols are for an average Z-axis coverage of 900 mm and a table speed of ≤30 mm/s for patients weighing between 41 and 120 kg. The injection duration is programmed to equal the scan duration. The delay is determined by automated triggering or a timing bolus.

Abbreviations: CM, contrast medium; t_{CMT}, contrast medium transit time.

[a] When automated triggering is used, the overall scan delay and injection duration are increased by a value equivalent to the inherent delay (ie, 2–8 seconds). The iodine dose (~500 mg I/kg) and flux are optimized with flexible injection rates and contrast medium volume and concentration. A biphasic injection is utilized with 20% of the contrast volume administered over the first 5–7 seconds and 80% delivered during the remainder of the acquisition. For all injections, saline flush follows the second phase of contrast.

Table 6
UECTA injection protocols: MDCT table speed >30 mm/s

Scan Time (s)	Scan Delay (s)	Iodine Dose (g)	Iodine Flux (g at g/s)	300 mg I/mL CM		350 mg I/mL CM		370 mg I/mL CM	
				Volume (mL)	Biphasic Injection (mL at mL/s)	Volume (mL)	Biphasic Injection (mL at mL/s)	Volume (mL)	Biphasic Injection (mL at mL/s)
30	t_{CMT}	35	7 at 1.4 / 28 at 1.1	117	23 at 4.7 / 93 at 3.7	100	20 at 4.0 / 80 at 3.2	95	19 at 3.8 / 76 at 3.0
20	t_{CMT}+10[a]	35	7 at 1.4 / 28 at 1.1	117	23 at 4.7 / 93 at 3.7	100	20 at 4.0 / 80 at 3.2	95	19 at 3.8 / 76 at 3.0
15	t_{CMT}+15[a]	35	7 at 1.4 / 28 at 1.1	117	23 at 4.7 / 93 at 3.7	100	20 at 4.0 / 80 at 3.2	95	19 at 3.8 / 76 at 3.0
10	t_{CMT}+20[a]	35	7 at 1.4 / 28 at 1.1	117	23 at 4.7 / 93 at 3.7	100	20 at 4.0 / 80 at 3.2	95	19 at 3.8 / 76 at 3.0
5	t_{CMT}+25[a]	35	7 at 1.4 / 28 at 1.1	117	23 at 4.7 / 93 at 3.7	100	20 at 4.0 / 80 at 3.2	95	19 at 3.8 / 76 at 3.0
2	t_{CMT}+28[a]	35	7 at 1.4 / 28 at 1.1	117	23 at 4.7 / 93 at 3.7	100	20 at 4.0 / 80 at 3.2	95	19 at 3.8 / 76 at 3.0

Injection parameters are for a 70 kg patient, scanned over an average distance of 900 mm with a table speed of >30 mm. A biphasic protocol with an injection duration of 30 seconds is utilized to achieve enhancement through the digital arteries, as would be performed had the table speed equaled 30 mm/s. Contrast medium transit time (CMT) is established with automated triggering or bolus timing.

High concentration contrast medium (CM) allows for reduced injection rates and volumes. Saline flush follows the second phase of contrast medium injection.

[a] A diagnostic delay is added to the beginning of the scan duration, so that the delivery of contrast medium and the scan duration end together. When automated triggering is used to determine CMT, the overall scan delay and injection duration are increased by a value equivalent to the inherent delay for automated triggering.

Table 7
Advanced visualization techniques

	Display	Principle Use	Advantages	Disadvantages
MPR	2D	Structural detail Quantitative analysis	Slice through dataset in coronal, sagittal, and oblique projections Real-time multiplanar interrogation Simplify image interpretation	Limited spatial perception
CPR	2D	Structural detail Centerline display Simplify MPR	Single anatomic display Longitudinal cross-sectional anatomic display	Operator dependent
Ray-Sum	2D	Structural overview	Slice through dataset in axial, coronal, sagittal, and oblique projections Real-time multiplanar interrogation Radiograph-like display	Loss of structural detail with increased slab thickness
MIP	2D	Structural overview Angiographic display	Slice through dataset in axial, coronal, sagittal, and oblique projections Real-time multiplanar interrogation Improved depiction - small caliber vessels - poorly enhanced vessels Communicate findings	Anatomic overlap (vessels, bone viscera) with increased slab thickness Visualization degraded by high-density structures (ie, bone, calcium, stents, coils) Loss of structural detail with increased slab thickness Limited grading of stent lumens
MinIP	2D	Structural Overview Tracheobronchial Airway Lung air trapping Soft tissue air	Slice through dataset in axial, coronal, sagittal, and oblique projections Real-time multiplanar interrogation Depict low density structures Communicate findings	Anatomic overlap Loss of structural detail with increased slab thickness
VR	3D	Structural overview Angiographic display	Slice through dataset in axial, coronal, sagittal, and oblique projections Real-time multiplanar interrogation Depict structural relationships Accurate spatial perception Communicate findings	Opacity-transfer function dependent Anatomic overlap Loss of structural detail with increased slab thickness

Abbreviations: 2D, two-dimensional; 3D, three-dimensional; MPR, multiplanar reformation; CPR, curved planar reformation; MIP, maximum intensity projection; MinIP, minimum intensity projection; VR, volume rendered.

Review, display, and interpretation of these large CTA datasets are most efficient and accurate when using a combination of the advanced workstation imaging techniques (Table 7) and the source images. Whether seeking an angiographic (overview) display with 3D volume rendered (VR) or maximum intensity projection (MIP) techniques (see Fig. 8), or an analysis of the UE vessel lumen and wall with multiplanar (MPR) or curved planar (CPR) reformations (Fig. 9), the advanced techniques are used in complementary fashion for their advantages, while minimizing their disadvantages (see Table 7). Minimum intensity projection (MinIP) and Ray-Sum (see Table 7) have limited applications in UE display, but can be used to generate maps of abnormal air collections (see Fig. 8) and radiographic-like images (Fig. 10), respectively. Source images are reviewed in a targeted manner to assess image quality, confirm findings, and exclude artifacts. This review may proceed with the original transverse sections, batch thin-section coronal and sagittal reformations, or both. The quality of all UECTA postprocessed images is directly dependent on the dataset's spatial resolution and degree of contrast-to-noise ratio.

With contemporary technology, the entire UEC-TA examination is transferred to a picture archiving and communication system (PACS) for viewing and storage; the thin-section isotropic or high-resolution angiographic series, and possibly the noncontrast series, are sent to an imaging workstation. The workstation may be a thin client server system or a stand-alone single unit, with both potentially integrated into PACS. The time for transfer will reflect the size of the UE examination, the network bandwidth speed, and use of compression software.

The workstation should be used for real time interactive UECTA display and interpretation, applying the range of advanced visualization techniques and tool functions. Additionally, protocol-driven static post-processed VR, MIP, and CPR images along with batch MPRs, may be generated for use along with the source images on PACS or the workstation.

With both approaches, VR and MIP displays require pre-rendering editing or sliding thin-slabs to remove bone and other anatomical structures which may obscure vascular visualization. Given the variable anatomy over the long coverage, it is recommended to analyze the inflow and outflow arteries and peripheral and central veins with an anatomical, segmental station approach, using interactive rotation and magnification. The longitudinal cross-sectional CPR tracings can also be created and analyzed with a station approach. 90 degree orthogonal views are recommended as generating each CPR view is operator and software dependent. For all techniques, it is essential to use flexible angiographic window and level

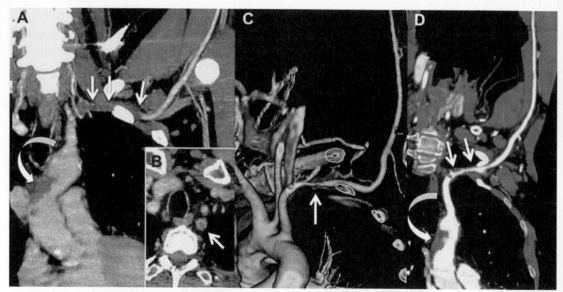

Fig. 9. Acute arterial occlusive disease. A 60-year-old man presented with acute left UE ischemia. Initial screening non–ECG-gated left UECTA demonstrates complex aortic arch atheroma (A, MPR; curved arrow) with complete occlusion (A, straight arrows) of the postostial subclavian artery (SCA) beginning at the transition between vertical and horizontal segments. The axial image in (B) confirms central filling defect in the SCA (arrow). A follow-up study 3 months later shows interval partial SCA recanalization (C, VR; D, CPR; arrows) without significant change in the aortic arch atheroma (D, curved arrow).

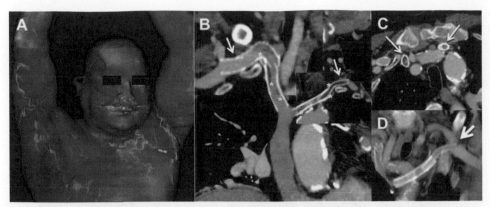

Fig. 10. Chronic venous occlusive disease. A surface VR image in a 75-year-old man with chronic central VOD shows well-developed bilateral chest and upper arm collateral veins (*A*). A composite MPR coronal display demonstrates overlapping bare stents extending from the bilateral central axillary veins (*arrows*) to the confluence of the brachiocephalic veins (*B*). Moderate right and moderate to marked left in-stent restenosis from neointimal hyperplasia (*B, asterisks*), accounts for the collateral veins. Findings are confirmed on a transverse slice through the stents (*C, arrows*). A Ray-Sum image through the left stents shows mild buckling of the most peripheral stent as it crosses the costoclavicular space (*D, arrow*).

settings, including a wide window setting to account for vascular calcification, high contrast attenuation, and noise.

Non-UE cardiovascular and noncardiovascular anatomy, included in the scan range, requires evaluation. Review may detect relevant contributory (ie, cervical ribs in the case of suspected thoracic outlet syndrome) and incidental findings. Depending on the UE positioning, additional cardiovascular territories to review include the heart, pulmonary vasculature, thoracic and abdominal aorta, supra- and abdominal aortic branch arteries, cervicocerebral vasculature, IVC, and mesenteric, portal, and visceral veins. In addition to the ipsilateral appendicular musculoskeletal system, imaged noncardiovascular anatomy may include the airway, lungs, pleura, mediastinum, axilla, chest wall, axial skeleton, neck, head, and abdominal-pelvic viscera. Review of the non-UE cardiovascular anatomy proceeds in a manner similar to that outlined for the UE vasculature. Review of the noncardiovascular structures is facilitated by generating 3- to 5-mm-thick axial reconstructions. Alternatively, thin-section coronal and sagittal reformations can be used.

CLINICAL APPLICATIONS
Arterial Occlusive Disease

CTA is widely used in current clinical algorithms to evaluate acute and chronic symptomatic UE arterial occlusive disease (AOD) (see Figs. 9 and 11). It is an ideal modality for this application, given the ability to rapidly assess the vessel lumen and wall, while generating robust 3D angiographic reconstructions of the complete UE arterial system from the inflow segments through to the digital arteries. Dynamic imaging can be performed (ie, thoracic outlet syndrome) and alternative nonvascular diagnoses can be made (ie, cervical spine degenerative disc disease). CTA can also be applied to screen asymptomatic patients. Earlier diagnosis can guide medical management and endovascular treatments before developing limb ischemia, potentially changing the disease course and improving patient outcome. Similarly, CTA is used for stent and surgical graft surveillance.

Acute UE AOD (see Fig. 9) occurs when there is abrupt hemodynamically significant stenosis and/or occlusion without development of sufficient collaterals, impairing UE blood flow and tissue perfusion. Symptoms include pain, pallor, pulselessness, paresthesias, poikilothermia, and paralysis. Prompt diagnosis and intervention is imperative to maintaining hand viability. Acute UE AOD may result from primary thrombosis, thromboembolism, and trauma. Primary UE thrombosis typically is the sequela from a ruptured plaque (ie, chronic peripheral arterial disease, PAD) or from in situ aneurysm thrombosis. When UE arterial thromboembolism occurs, emboli arise upstream, typically from the heart, atherosclerotic lesions, aneurysms, or regions of intimal irregularity (ie, chronic repetitive trauma). Stents and grafts can occlude acutely as a result of in situ thrombosis, emboli, or inflow and outflow flow disturbances.

In chronic UE AOD (see Fig. 11), luminal stenosis, occlusion, or both compromise blood flow over an extended period of time, often with progressive worsening. Collateral arterial networks

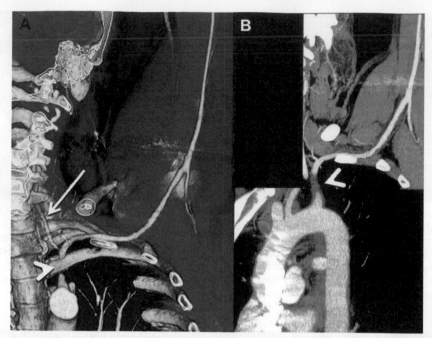

Fig. 11. Chronic arterial occlusive disease. A 45-year-old woman with progressive worsening of left UE exertional claudication, underwent a left UECTA to evaluate for potential subclavian steal syndrome. VR (*A*) and composite MPR-CPR (*B*) displays, show short segment occlusion of the distal vertical segment of the left subclavian artery (*arrowhead*) with reconstituted flow beginning at the left vertebral artery (*arrow*), confirming the suspected diagnosis.

and microcirculation changes develop with sufficient degree to reconstitute blood flow and restore local tissue perfusion. The most common cause of chronic UE AOD in adults is peripheral atherosclerotic disease (native and postsurgical or endovascular). Other causes of chronic UE AOD include vasculitis, radiation arteritis, repetitive compression, or microtrauma (ie, thoracic outlet syndrome; hypothenar hammer syndrome; see **Fig. 3**), and recurrent thromboembolism. Vasculitis and thoracic outlet syndrome are common causes in pediatric patients.

With regards to vasculitis, Takayasu arteritis and giant cell arteritis involve large inflow and medium size proximal outflow UE arteries. Thromboangiitis obliterans (Buerger disease) and Behcet disease can involve medium and small size arteries in addition to UE veins. Causes of UE small-vessel vasculitis include rheumatoid arthritis, Sjögren syndrome, Wegener granulomatosis, polyarteritis nodosa, scleroderma, systemic lupus erythematosus, polymyositis, dermatomyositis, and mixed connective tissue disorders.

Clinically, patients with chronic UE AOD have variable symptoms, depending on the cause, severity, and duration of disease. Symptoms may range from paresthesias, digital pallor, and cold intolerance to intermittent claudication (ie,

impaired functional activity) to rest pain, nonhealing ulcers, gangrene, and tissue loss (ie, threatened UE). If pathology is related to repetitive compression, symptoms may only be elicited with specific motion or activity. Patients with UE vasculitis typically present with constitutional symptoms (ie, fever, myalgias, arthralgias, and malaise), along with ischemia. Medium and small arterial involvement may lead to secondary Raynaud vasospastic phenomenon.

When preparing for the UE CTA in the setting of AOD, it is recommend to screen for PAD risk factors, including tobacco use, hypertension, diabetes mellitus, hyperlipidemia, coronary atherosclerotic disease, and carotid atherosclerotic disease.[4] Assessment of cardiomegaly and arrhythmias is made to determine the likelihood of cardiogenic emboli and the need for imaging of the heart with or without ECG-gating. If the CTA is performed for suspected vasculitis, elevated cellular inflammatory markers should be reviewed, including erythrocyte sedimentation rate, C-reactive protein, antineutrophilic cytoplasmic antibodies (ANCA), and antiendothelial cell antibodies.[5]

CTA findings for acute UE AOD include single or tandem central arterial filling defects, abrupt arterial cutoff, or both. This may occur in either the inflow or outflow territories, depending on the etiology. Grafts and stents typically show a "cast" of thrombus. Distal tissue enhancement is diminished and collateral pathways are absent. In chronic UE AOD, lesions are characterized with regards to the number, type (ie, stenosis vs occlusion), location, length, and etiology. It is recommended to report lesions with quantitative and qualitative descriptions as follows: less than 25% (minimal stenosis), 25–49% (mild stenosis), 50–69% (moderate stenosis); 70–99% (severe stenosis); occluded. For both acute and chronic AOD, all UE CTA findings factor into endovascular and surgical treatment planning, including endovascular access and device selections, surgical approach and graft selections, and technical considerations.

Specific PAD analysis includes plaque composition, degree of calcifications, presence of plaque ulcerations (including penetrating ulcers), and the nature of eccentric lesions. Stents and grafts are evaluated for integrity, patency, neointimal hyperplasia, and in situ thrombus. Secondary evaluation assesses end organ sequelae, including skin ulcers, tissue loss, and muscle atrophy.

Specific vasculitis analysis includes recognition of vessel wall thickening with or without adjacent inflammatory changes. Exclusion of concomitant proximal or alternative disease is crucial. Stenoses may be short and long segment or focal; occlusions may be focal or tandem. Aneurysms and pseudoaneurysms may also be found. In thromboangiitis obliterans, corkscrew collateral arteries are often present. If palmar or digital arteries show poor or absent enhancement during the first pass, an immediate delayed acquisition should be acquired. Venous enhancement on delayed phase with persistent, diffuse poorly enhanced arteries in the hand indicates small-vessel disease.

Venous Occlusive Disease

UE venous occlusive disease (VOD) most commonly involves the deep system. Causes may be primary or secondary. Primary thrombosis occurs spontaneously or in the setting of intrinsic thrombophilia, extrinsic compression (ie, Paget-Schroetter syndrome), or both. Causes of thrombophilia include mutations of factor V Leiden and prothrombin and deficiencies of antithrombin, protein C, and protein S.[6] Secondary thrombosis occurs as a result of extrinsic factors that increase the inherent thrombotic state, including intravenous devices, malignancy, oral contraceptives, surgery, pregnancy, puerperium, and prolonged immobilization.

Patients with UE VOD may present with extremity enlargement, pain, heaviness, skin discoloration, or a combination thereof. Physical findings include UE edema, erythema, and prominent ipsilateral veins with or without a palpable cord. With complete venous obstruction, arterial flow may be compromised, leading to arterial ischemia with or without gangrene.

Prompt recognition of UE deep venous thrombosis (DVT) is essential. Altough venous ultrasound is the primary diagnostic imaging modality, in select clinical settings, including pre-intervention mapping and surveillance, both indirect (Fig. 10) and direct (Fig. 6) UE CTV can be utilized to identify the presence of thrombus, estimate its burden, determine whether thrombus is occlusive or non-occlusive, and demonstrate chronic stenoses and occlusions. In addition, alternative diagnoses are readily provided. Acute venous thrombosis manifests on CTV as a central venous filling defect, associated with expanded vein caliber, soft tissue stranding, and edema. Chronic venous thrombosis may appear as mural thickening, webs, or attenuated caliber from negative remodeling and recanalization. Primary and secondary risk factors can be identified with both techniques. Direct UE CTV is most useful to assess for pulmonary embolism during a single acquisition. With an indirect UE CTV, two acquisitions are necessary–the CT pulmonary arteriogram followed by the delayed indirect CT venogram.

Trauma

CTA is useful and effective for assessing UE trauma, including exposure injuries and blunt and penetrating trauma.[7] In most medical centers, CT scanners are in close proximity to the emergency room, are readily available, and are conducive to managing critical trauma patients. CT provides a complete 1-stop shop for cardiovascular and noncardiovascular multiorgan system evaluations. In contrast to CA, CTA can more reliably define vascular injuries in relation to skeletal fractures and soft-tissue injuries.

CTA exposure referrals comprise radiation (radiation arteritis), caustic agents, polyvinylchloride (acro-osteolysis), electrical current (electrical injuries), and extreme temperatures (thermal injury) injuries. The common end point for these injuries is vascular inflammation and fibrosis. Referrals for blunt trauma include musculoskeletal injuries, repetitive vibration tool exposure, or repetitive work (hypothenar hammer syndrome) or athletic-related motions (thoracic outlet-inlet syndromes). Penetrating injuries consist of gunshot wounds and piercing objects including iatrogenic catheters. Blunt and penetrating trauma may cause injury to arteries, veins, or both. Many arterial injuries require endovascular or surgical treatment, whereas most venous injuries can be treated conservatively.

Patients with radiation exposure or repetitive vibration tool, work, or athletic blunt trauma may present with either subacute to chronic ischemia with or without secondary Raynaud phenomenon. All other trauma patients typically present emergently. Prompt recognition of UE arterial injury, uncontrolled venous injury, or both is important for limb survival. Initial UE evaluation and a wrist-brachial index triages patients into those with definite vascular injury, possible vascular injury, and proximity injury only.

Signs of UE vascular injury include active hemorrhage, expanding pulsatile hematoma, hemodynamic instability, and limb ischemia. These patients are brought emergently to either the endovascular suite or the operating room for control and repair of the vascular injury. CTA may be required to provide a vascular map and aid vascular and soft-tissue reconstructions. Patients with possible UE vascular injury are usually hemodynamically stable with nonthreatened limbs. However, patients may have decreased or absent distal pulses (see Figs. 1 and 8), a bruit, a decreased wrist-brachial index, a nonpulsatile expanding hematoma, or a pulsatile mass (Fig. 12), necessitating imaging to exclude vascular injury. CTA is performed in this group for diagnosis and treatment planning. Proximity injuries are traumatic wounds near a vascular structure. Patients are hemodynamically stable, with intact vascular supply and without expanding hematomas. The wrist-brachial index is normal

and extremities are viable. These patients are observed for delayed signs of UE vascular injury. CTA and other imaging are not initially required.

When the UE is the only area of injury, a targeted extremity runoff protocol is sufficient. Imaging begins 1 vascular territory above the injury and continues to the digits. When UE imaging is combined with other body regions, scan coverage is extended. In both situations, a delayed acquisition may be required to further define vascular injury. CTA readily depicts posttraumatic UE vascular compression, vasospasm, intimal tears, lacerations, occlusions, pseudoaneurysms, and arteriovenous fistulas. CTA pitfalls for imaging UE trauma include metallic streak artifacts (ie, hardware, bullets), nonenhanced segments, and early asymmetric venous enhancement. With nonenhanced segments, it is difficult to distinguish vasospasm from traumatic occlusion. Early asymmetric venous enhancement may reflect hyperemia or a traumatic arteriovenous fistula.

Vascular Masses

UE vascular masses include aneurysms, pseudoaneurysms (see Fig. 12), congenital lesions (ie, hemangiomas, vascular malformations, Fig. 13), benign and malignant tumors, and tumorlike conditions. As with other modalities, CTA primary objectives are to characterize the location, size, extent, and composition of the mass and map out the vascular supply to the mass. Noncardiovascular structures are evaluated for exclusion of local and distant organ involvement. Following surgical or

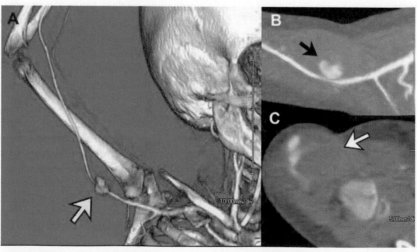

Fig. 12. Iatrogenic pseudoaneurysm. A 2-year-old girl developed a pulsatile mass with diminished distal pulses following an attempted right UE PICC line placement. CTA confirmed a suspected pseudoaneurysm (*A, B; arrows*) with adjacent hematoma (*C, arrow*). The runoff was patent without distal embolization (not shown).

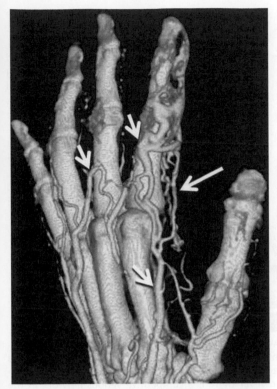

Imaging is most commonly required before vascularized tissue transfer reconstructions, whether the extremity is to be the donor or recipient site. Clinically, UECTA has been shown to be useful to plan surgical procedures, ensure flap viability, and prevent ischemia.[9] CTA objectives include assessing patency and caliber of the target arteries and veins, evaluating patency of and communication between potential collateral pathways, and screening for normal variant origins, atherosclerotic disease, perivascular fibrosis, radiation arteritis, and other vascular abnormalities (see **Figs. 1** and **2**).

When the UE is being considered as the procurement site, the radius or ulna may be used as composite free grafts. Imaging begins at the subclavian artery level as the radial or ulnar artery may arise aberrantly from as high as the axillary artery. Imaging extends to the digits for assessment of the palmar arches. For UE recipient reconstructions (pedicle or free flaps), CTA coverage is applied in a more targeted fashion such that imaging often begins 1 vascular territory above the wound. In most instances, coverage extends through to the digital arteries.

Fig. 13. Arteriovenous malformation. VR display demonstrates a high-flow arteriovenous malformation centered at the second digit. Primary arterial supply is from the radialis indices (*long arrow*) and other recruited arteries from the radial artery deep branch and deep arch. Venous outflow spreads along the dorsal surface of the finger and hand (*short arrows*) to the DVN.

endovascular treatment of vascular masses, CTA can assess residual and recurrent disease, and postoperative complications. The CTA protocol is tailored to the location and the type of suspected or known vascular mass. In most instances, a targeted extremity runoff protocol is sufficient. Imaging begins 1 vascular territory above the mass and continues through the digital arteries. A delayed phase may be required to further define the mass, particularly if the mass is a venous or venolymphatic malformation.

Vascular Mapping: Surgical Reconstruction

Options for surgical reconstructions of extremity wounds include direct wound closure, skin grafting, local tissue transfer, and free tissue transfer ("free flap").[8] Depending on the complexity of the wound, the planned surgical reconstruction, and the presence of underlying vascular disease, imaging may be required to map out the arteries and veins.

Hemodialysis Access

Options for hemodialysis vascular access include temporary or permanent central venous catheter insertion and arteriovenous fistula (AVF) or graft (AVG) surgical shunt creation. Dialysis Outcome Quality Initiative (K/DOQI) guidelines recommend autogenous AVF as the first choice since they achieve better long term patency rates, have fewer complications, and have lower costs.[10–11] Most surgical AVF and AVG are placed in the UE.

Vascular mapping is a useful adjunct to achieving and maintaining a well-functioning permanent central line, AVF or AVG. Along with VUS and nongadolinium-based MR imaging and MRA sequences, CTA with a delayed venous phase can be performed to define the caliber and patency of central veins, potential shunt arteries and veins, and native palmar arches. Small luminal diameters, arterial and venous stenoses and occlusions, and incomplete palmar arches detected by CTA factor into creating an AVF or AVG and selecting the planned site. Recognition of venous side branches on the delayed phase is also essential, as flow through side branches can contribute to AVF nonmaturation. Depending on the anticipated AVF or AVG access site, diameter measurements to report include at least the peripheral and central cephalic vein, basilic vein, axillary vein, radial artery, brachial artery, and axillary artery.

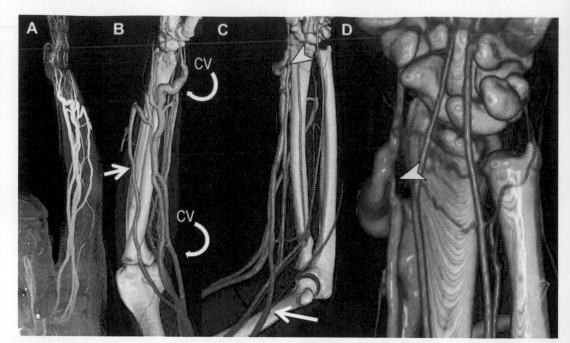

Fig. 14. Hemodialysis access: radial artery-cephalic vein AVF. A 14-year-old boy with a 6-month-old left radial-cephalic AVF had diminished pressure and flow with recent hemodialysis. A full MIP display of the left UE shows continuous venous outflow to the central veins without stenosis. Targeted VR displays (*B, C*) demonstrate dominant, patent cephalic venous outflow (*curved arrows*), however there is a competitive venous network in the forearm (*B, short arrow*) draining into the basilic-brachial system in the upper arm (*D, long arrow*). Note the paired cephalic veins (CV) beginning in the midforearm. Cephalic venous flow is further diminished by an acquired arterial inflow 50% stenosis (*C, D; arrowhead*). AVF, arteriovenous fistula.

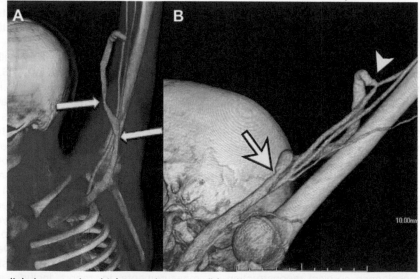

Fig. 15. Hemodialysis access: brachial artery-(transposed) basilic vein AVF. A 14-year-old girl with a 3-year-old left arm brachial-basilic vein AVF had elevated venous pressures with recent hemodialysis. VR displays (*A, B*) demonstrate nonflow, limiting, postanastomotic irregularity (*arrowhead*) with 2 tandem midbasilic outflow vein 50% stenoses. Central veins were patent (not shown). AVF, arteriovenous fistula.

CTA can also be used to assess dysfunctional AVF and AVG and aid in planning endovascular and surgical interventions, particularly when the graft is calcified or when there are stents, coils, or surgical clips along the shunt pathway (**Figs. 14 and 15**). Hemodynamically significant stenoses and occlusions typically occur in the shunt's arterial inflow or venous outflow. However, whether the shunt is at the wrist, forearm, or upper arm, the aortic arch with upper extremity runoff protocol is recommended to assess distal arterial flow and exclude steal, embolization, or both. AVF should also be assessed for venous outflow side branches. Rarely, AVG and AVF puncture site pseudoaneurysms may be seen.

As iodinated CM is used, the CTA is coordinated with the patient's hemodialysis schedule. For evaluation of dysfunctional AVG or AVF, targeted noncontrast images are useful to define the location of grafts, surgical clips, and embolization coils. Unenhanced images are not routinely required for vascular mapping.

SUMMARY

Diagnostic CTA is applicable in a wide spectrum of UE vascular disorders for pediatric and adult patients. Acquiring the images with robust detail at low risk and radiation exposure levels begins with patient preparation and requires selection of appropriate angiographic options and CM strategies based on the suspected or known UE vascular disease, the MDCT scanner, and the patient's physiologic parameters. Advanced workstation visualization is necessary for efficient interrogation of these datasets, particularly for endovascular and surgical planning and surveillance. Continued innovations in CT technology, CM delivery, and workstations will lead to further advancements in UECTA and subsequent modification of protocols.

REFERENCES

1. Sommer WH, Graser A, Becker CR, et al. Image quality of virtual noncontrast images derived from dual-energy CT angiography after endovascular aneurysm repair. J Vasc Interv Radiol 2010;21(3):315–21.
2. Huda W, Ogden KM, Khorasani MR. Effect of dose metrics and radiation risk models when optimizing CT x-ray tube voltage. Phys Med Biol 2008;53(17):4719–32.
3. Fleischmann D, Rubin GD. Quantification of intravenously administered contrast medium transit through the peripheral arteries: implications for CT angiography. Radiology 2005;236(3):1076–82.
4. Selvin E, Erlinger TP. Prevalence of and risk factors for peripheral arterial disease in the US: results from the National Health and Nutrition Examination Survey, 1999–2000. Circulation 2004;110(6):738–43.
5. Falk RJ, Jennette JC. ANCA small-vessel vasculitis. J Am Soc Nephrol 1997;8(2):314–22.
6. Martinelli I, Battaglioli T, Bucciarelli P, et al. Risk factors and recurrence rate of primary deep vein thrombosis of the upper extremities. Circulation 2004;110(5):566–70.
7. Peng PD, Spain DA, Tataria M, et al. CT angiography effectively evaluates extremity vascular trauma. Am Surg 2008;74(2):103–7.
8. Willcox TM, Smith AA. Upper limb free flap reconstruction after tumor resection. Semin Surg Oncol 2000;19(3):246–54.
9. Klein MB, Karanas YL, Chow LC, et al. Early experience with computed tomographic angiography in microsurgical reconstruction. Plast Reconstr Surg 2003;112(2):498–503.
10. NKF-DOQI clinical practice guidelines for vascular access. National Kidney Foundation-Dialysis Outcomes Quality Initiative. Am J Kidney Dis 1997;30(4 Suppl 3):S150–91.
11. III. NKF-K/DOQI Clinical Practice Guidelines for Vascular Access: update 2000. Am J Kidney Dis 2001;37(1 Suppl 1):S137–81.

CT Angiography in Trauma

Jennifer W. Uyeda, MD*, Stephan W. Anderson, MD,
Osamu Sakai, MD, PhD, Jorge A. Soto, MD

KEYWORDS

• Angiography • Trauma • Multidetector • CT

CT has become the primary imaging modality used in patients who suffer significant trauma. With the advent of the multidetector CT (MDCT) technology, high-resolution images with shorter acquisition times are now routine and the quality of multiplanar and 3-D reformations has revolutionized the evaluation of trauma victims. These technologic advances, in particular the shorter image acquisition times, enable complex, multiphasic imaging studies of the entire body specifically aimed at determining the integrity of the vasculature.

Rapid assessment and diagnosis of traumatic arterial injuries are critical in the evaluation of acutely injured patients because these injuries contribute considerably to the morbidity and mortality of major trauma. CT angiograms (CTAs) of the head and neck, chest, pelvis, and extremities have become common imaging methods in busy trauma centers. Although digital subtraction angiography (DSA) historically was the preferred method for evaluating patients with possible vascular injuries, it has been largely replaced by CTA due to its speed, noninvasive nature, accuracy, and widespread availability. Rapid acquisition of submillimeter isotropic data sets allows for accurate assessment of vascular injury extending from the head and neck to the torso and extremities. This article reviews the current use of MDCT angiography in trauma with attention to technique and protocol considerations, illustrates findings of many commonly encountered injuries, and discusses the clinical implications of vascular trauma throughout the body.

TECHNIQUE

The diagnostic quality of a CTA examination depends on many factors, but careful attention to technique and adequate patient preparation are always necessary, especially in the setting of trauma when multiple events often happen simultaneously and every second may be critical.

The importance of proper patient positioning cannot be underestimated. Patients are typically placed supine on a CT table. In the majority of cases (chest, abdomen, pelvis, or lower-extremity imaging), placing both arms above the head is the preferred position for image acquisition. For upper-extremity CTA, the injured extremity is ideally raised above the head to decrease beam-hardening artifact from the torso and secured with adhesive tape to decrease artifact from patient motion. In the rare scenario where there is suspicion for bilateral upper-extremity vascular lesions, both arms should be raised. An alternative positioning is to place patients prone with 1 or both extremities raised over the head, the so-called superman position. If a patient's clinical condition does not allow an injured extremity to be raised over the head, both arms are secured by the patient's side. This is also the preferred positioning for CTA of the head and neck. For lower-extremity CTA, the legs are secured to the table and both limbs are included in the field of view. Inclusion of the contralateral extremity in trauma CTA may be useful as a reference during interpretation of findings in the injured side.

The protocols used at the authors' institution were designed for 64-row scanners but can be used with other generations of MD scanners with only minor modifications. In all cases, an 18- or 20-gauge intravenous catheter is placed in a superficial vein in the antecubital fossa (ideal), the forearm, or the dorsum of the hand (less optimal). For upper-extremity CTA, venous access

Boston Medical Center, 820 Harrison Avenue, FGH Building, 3rd Floor, Boston, MA 02118, USA
* Corresponding author.
E-mail address: Jennifer.Uyeda@bmc.org

Radiol Clin N Am 48 (2010) 423–438
doi:10.1016/j.rcl.2010.02.003
0033-8389/10/$ – see front matter. Published by Elsevier Inc.

should be placed in the arm contralateral to the injury. This is an important, but often forgotten, technical point. For the extremities, the acquisition typically includes the joint proximal to and the joint distal to the injured segments.

Using 64-row CT scanner, images are acquired at 0.625-mm detector collimation, with a pitch of 0.984 and gantry rotation time of 0.5 seconds. This results in a table speed of 8 cm per second (64–slice LightSpeed VCT, GE Healthcare, Milwaukee, WI, USA). Thicker axial slices (1.25–3.75 mm) and 2-D and 3-D reconstructions are reconstructed from the original data set and are used for study interpretation.

The speed of 64-row CT scanner allows for rapid acquisition of multistation examinations, using a single bolus of intravenous contrast material. Complex multiphasic studies are planned on whole-body (head to toe) CT digital radiographs (scout views).

The total contrast load necessary for the CTA varies with the type of scanner available and the number and sequence of regions of the body that are imaged. Contrast agents with higher concentrations of iodine (350 to 370 mgl/mL) and high injection rates (at least 4–5 mL/s) are preferred and are always followed by a 30 to 50 mL saline chaser, also injected at a rate of 4 to 5 mL per second. At the authors' institution, 100 to 120 mL of contrast medium is used for a standard chest/abdomen/pelvis study with a 64-row scanner. When CTA is integrated into a whole-body trauma scan to include head and neck, torso, and extremities, this single bolus of 100 to 120 mL of intravenous contrast material is used for the multiphasic torso and extremity imaging. In cases of isolated extremity angiography in which no torso imaging is required, 60 mL of intravenous contrast are used.

Three methods are commonly used to time the beginning of acquisition after the contrast bolus injection: standard delay, automated bolus tracking, and test injection. The standard delay method is simple and quick and the authors have found it robust when used in the trauma population, especially when the protocol includes imaging of multiple body parts (Table 1). A standard delay of 30 seconds for initiation of the routine thoracic scan is used in the majority of patients. A different standard delay technique is used when the chest CTA is integrated into a whole-body scan that includes head and neck, pelvis, extremities, chest, and abdomen, in that order. In these circumstances, typical standard delays used are 20 seconds for the head and neck, 23 seconds for the pelvis, 25 to 27 seconds for the upper extremities and proximal lower

Table 1 Standard delay and contrast bolus in trauma CTA		
	Standard Delay (Seconds)	Contrast Bolus (mL)
Routine torso scan		100–120
Chest	30	
Abdomen and pelvis[a]	70	
Isolated extremity angiography	Standard delay/test bolus	60
Whole-body scan		100–120
Head and Neck	20	
Pelvis	23	
Upper or proximal lower extremity	25–27	
Distal lower extremity	27–30	
Chest	~30[b]	
Abdomen and pelvis[a]	70	

[a] Delayed-phase image acquisition may be acquired at 5 to 7 minutes.
[b] Immediately follows CTA of other regions.

extremities, and 27 to 30 seconds for the distal lower extremities. Thoracic acquisition immediately follows pelvis or extremity imaging.

Test injection and bolus tracking methods are more precise (albeit slightly more cumbersome) and should always be used when the study is limited to the extremities, in the elderly population, and in patients whose cardiovascular system is compromised. If the more distal arteries of the extremity are imaged, the test injection method is preferred, because bolus tracking requires precise placement of the region-of-interest (ROI) cursor in the artery of interest. This is not always practical or feasible using a precontrast image.

For the test injection method for extremity CTA, circulation time to the affected area is determined in a vessel immediately proximal to the region of suspected injury. An appropriate artery—such as the brachial artery for a proximal upper-extremity trauma—is selected as the target for placement of the ROI measurement. A 20-mL injection of intravenous contrast material is injected at 4 to 5 mL per second followed by a 30-mL saline chaser, using a dual-syringe power injector. Contrast material arrival time is determined from a time attenuation curve generated from 12 to 14 low radiation dose CT images. The first image is acquired 5 seconds after the beginning of the injection and the remaining 11 to 13 images are acquired every 2 seconds thereafter. The time to peak arterial enhancement is measured from the time attenuation curve. CTA acquisition then begins 5 seconds after calculated time to peak enhancement to allow angiographic imaging during a relative plateau of sustained enhancement.

Because the trauma population often involves young, otherwise healthy, patients, radiation dose is of concern. Given that CTA is inherently a high-contrast examination, it is possible to use relatively lower radiation dose for a diagnostic examination. Most CT equipment vendors have developed various types of attenuation-based dose modulation features to optimize radiation dose. One such feature is the noise index which, in conjunction with the section thickness and pitch value selected, provides the desired signal-to-noise ratio by adjusting the tube current for each section, based on the total attenuation of the tissues at that specific location. Although the use of a noise index is specific to GE Healthcare CT scanners, other manufacturers offer methods of attenuation-based dose modulation. In the setting of trauma, CTA protocols are set with a noise index that is higher than that typically used for regular CT examinations. Given the inherently high contrast afforded by CTA, the authors use a noise index of 29 whereas portal venous phase abdominal and pelvic imaging is acquired using a noise index of 19.

CTA images are interpreted at a Picture Archiving and Communication System or independent workstation with interactive postprocessing capabilities. In addition to the axial images, orthogonal plane (sagittal and coronal) reformations are routinely generated. 3-D reformations, especially using volume-rendering applications, are most useful for illustrating abnormalities and to guide therapy performed by interventional radiologists or vascular surgeons. The optimal methods for 3-D reformations for trauma imaging are similar to other clinical applications of CTA.

CTA OF THE CHEST

Thoracic injuries account for 25% of trauma-related deaths in the United States and the thorax is the third most commonly injured body part in trauma.[1] MDCT angiography has rapidly become the imaging modality of choice in evaluating a wide variety of potentially life-threatening acute traumatic injuries of the aorta and other large vessels.[2–5] CTA provides high-resolution axial,

multiplanar, and 3-D data sets, which enable rapid diagnosis and characterization of thoracic vascular injuries with a high sensitivity and accuracy, dictating appropriate management and leading to earlier treatment.[1,6]

In patients who sustain polytrauma, the main purpose of thoracic CT is evaluation of the thoracic aorta and brachiocephalic arteries. Images of the chest should be acquired at the peak of aortic enhancement in order to maximize the detection of the often subtle direct signs of aortic trauma. A standard delay technique of 30 seconds after bolus injection of 100 to 120 mL of intravenous contrast material affords optimal image quality in the majority of patients. As discussed previously, in patients requiring CTA of other areas of the body, for instance the extremities, the extremities are imaged initially, followed immediately by image acquisition of the thorax.

An additional consideration in CTA of the chest is the use of cardiac gating. At the authors' institution, this technique is used on a limited basis for problem solving in cases in which there is a questionable finding on the routine admission trauma CT. In these cases, circulation timing is determined by using bolus triggering software or the test injection method. Cardiac gating limits motion blurring of the ascending aorta and aortic arch so that questionable or subtle aortic injuries may be better evaluated.

Imaging Findings and Clinical Implications

Acute traumatic injuries of the thoracic aorta are highly lethal.[1,2,7,8] It is estimated that 85% to 90% of the patients who suffer acute aortic trauma expire prior to reaching the hospital and 50% to 75% of the survivors die within 1 week without proper treatment.[1,2] A significant force is needed to tear the aorta and injuries to the aorta are usually the result of high speed trauma, such as motor vehicle collisions. The most likely location for aortic injuries is the aortic isthmus (Fig. 1), the proximal descending aorta at the level of the ligamentum arteriosum, where the relatively mobile aortic arch connects to the fixed descending aorta and where more than 90% of injuries occur.[2,7–9] Other locations for aortic injuries are the aortic arch (4%), aortic root (3%), and aortic hiatus at the diaphragm (0.3%).[1,8]

A periaortic or mediastinal hematoma may be detected on good-quality chest radiographs when there is mediastinal widening, left apical pleural capping (an extrapleural accumulation of blood), or paratracheal stripe thickening.[2,8,10] Other indirect signs are less useful. The sensitivity of chest

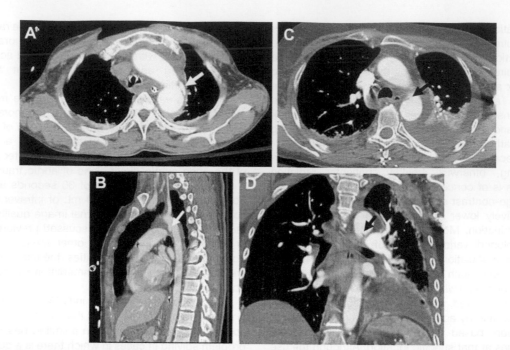

Fig. 1. Traumatic pseudoaneurysms are seen distal to the origin of the left subclavian artery at the aortic isthmus in 2 patients involved in motor vehicle collisions, the most common location for thoracic aortic injuries (*A, B*). Axial (*A*) and sagittal (*B*) CTA images in 2 different patients show saccular outpouchings of the aorta consistent with traumatic pseudoaneurysms (*arrows*). Note the associated mediastinal hematoma in both patients. Intimal disruption without pseudoaneurysm formation in a patient who sustained a traumatic injury to the aorta distal to the origin of the left subclavian artery is seen in the axial (*C*) and coronal (*D*).

radiographs for detecting aortic injuries may be as high as 90% but the specificity is extremely low, approximately 5%.[1,5] Therefore, the threshold for obtaining a chest CTA after an abnormal or nonconclusive radiograph should be very low.

Aortic injuries can be divided into those isolated to the intima (or possibly the intima and a portion of the media) and those that disrupt the intima, media, and possibly the adventitia. On CT, isolated intimal disruptions often demonstrate a small area of intimal irregularity, typically at the level of the ligamentum arteriosum (Fig. 1A, B). Often, these injuries are managed conservatively with close clinical and imaging follow-up. Acute traumatic aortic dissection can be seen occasionally and is characterized on CTA by an intimomedial flap separating the true and false lumina.[11,12]

An aortic rupture is most commonly seen distal to the left subclavian artery, on the anteromedial wall. Aortic rupture may involve the intima, media, and the adventitial layer and is classically seen on CT as a sleeve of contrast-enhanced blood accumulating abnormally in the subadventitial layer.[11] Emergent surgical intervention has been the mainstay of treatment. Endovascular stent graft placement has become an alternative option

associated with decreased morbidity and mortality.[2,13,14]

A pseudoaneurysm is an aortic rupture contained solely by the adventitia or periaortic tissues and is characteristically seen as a saccular outpouching (Fig. 1C, D). The risk of pseudoaneurysm rupture is high.[15] As with aortic rupture, surgery has been the treatment of choice; however, surgery may be associated with significant morbidity and mortality.[15] Endovascular interventions have recently evolved and are associated with lower morbidity and mortality.[2,15,16] Criteria for endovascular repair include accurate localization of the injury, distal vascular access of sufficient size, and limited tortuosity of the vessel.[17] Severe angulation of the aortic arch may cause technical difficulties limiting the possibility of successfully deploying a stent graft in some patients.[17] For pseudoaneurysms, the size of the neck determines whether or not stent grafts or catheter-directed delivery of coils is used.[15] Accurate characterization of thoracic vascular injuries by CTA assists in determining which injuries are amendable to endovascular treatment, surgical treatment, or conservative therapy.

Chronic pseudoaneurysms after previous traumatic injury may demonstrate calcification and thrombus within the wall. The risk of rupture of pseudoaneurysms is high and, thus, direct therapy with surgery or endovascular methods is recommended.[15,17]

Injuries to the proximal carotid and subclavian arteries can be assessed on CTA of the chest. They can occur in isolation or may be associated with aortic injuries (Fig. 2). Subclavian and innominate artery injuries are associated with seat belt injuries and sternal fractures.[18,19] Innominate artery injuries account for 9% of all major blunt intrathoracic arterial injuries.[19] Treatment varies with the type of injury and options include conservative management, endovascular intervention, or surgery. Occasionally, CTA may demonstrate injuries to other large thoracic vessels, such as the pulmonary artery, internal mammary, and intercostal arteries. One additional major benefit of CT is the concurrent assessment of other traumatic thoracic injuries, for example, a flail chest or large hemo/pneumothorax that may alter patient management.

CTA OF THE ABDOMEN

The main purpose of the abdominal CT examination in trauma patients is to detect injuries to and bleeding arising from the solid organs, hollow viscera, and mesentery, but the major abdominal vessels can also be evaluated.[20–23] Currently, specific CTA (arterial phase) images are not routinely obtained as part of the abdominal CT protocol at most large trauma centers. The upper abdominal aorta and its branches, however, are often scanned in a late arterial phase because

the lower images of the chest CT extend into the upper abdomen. Many types of injuries of the abdominal aorta and branches can be detected with CT, thereby reserving DSA for confirmation and, especially, for guiding therapy of these injuries.[22,24–26]

Imaging Findings and Clinical Implications

Retroperitoneal arteries, including the abdominal aorta, renal artery, proximal celiac axis, and superior mesenteric artery, are easily assessed with CTA of the abdomen (Fig. 3).[24,25,27] Abdominal aortic injury accounts for only 5% of all aortic injuries because the abdominal aorta is a protected structure located in the retroperitoneum.[24,25,28] Injury involves the infrarenal aorta in 98% of cases but the abdominal aortic branches are also susceptible to injury (Fig. 4).[24] The types of injuries occurring in the abdominal aorta are similar to those of the thoracic aorta.[24,28]

CT findings of arterial injuries of the major solid organs (liver, spleen, and kidneys) are similar, although the significance and therapy varies between the various organs (Fig. 5). Active arterial hemorrhage is seen as high attenuating regions representing extravasated contrast material and this can manifest as local extravasation into a parenchymal hematoma or as a jet spreading freely into the abdomen.[26,29–31] Pseudoaneurysms are seen as focal, rounded regions equal in attenuation to the aorta or surrounding arterial structures on an arterial phase image.

Multiphasic acquisitions are helpful for differentiating active extravasation from contained injuries, such as pseudoaneurysms. Obtaining delayed images in addition to the standard portal

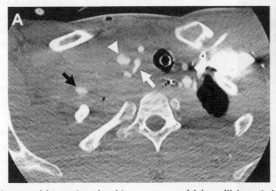
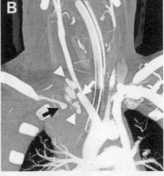

Fig. 2. A 19-year-old man involved in a motor vehicle collision. Axial arterial phase image (*A*) depicts a traumatic avulsion of the proximal right subclavian artery (*white arrow*), which reconstitutes distally (*black arrow*). Active contrast extravasation (*white arrowhead*) is seen representing active hemorrhage. Oblique MIP image (*B*) demonstrates foci of active contrast extravasation (*white arrowheads*) with the injured proximal subclavian artery (*white arrow*) and distal reconstitution (*black arrow*). This patient was taken emergently to the operating room for repair.

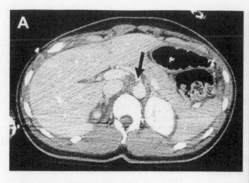

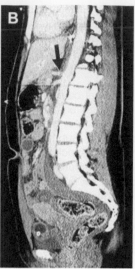

Fig. 3. Traumatic injury to the celiac axis. In a patient involved in a motor vehicle collision, axial (A) and sagittal (B) images reveal an intraluminal filling defect consistent with an acute intimal injury involving the proximal celiac axis (arrows).

venous phase is determined by an onsite radiologist. On delayed phases, foci of extravasated blood are typically larger, and the relative hyperattenuation persists throughout the various phases of image acquisition, whereas pseudoaneurysms are identical in size and shape and the attenuation is similar to the aorta in all phases, washing out on later phases of image acquisition (see **Fig. 5**).[20] This differentiation has important therapeutic implications. Active bleeding requires urgent endovascular or surgical management whereas

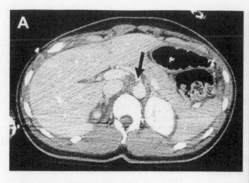

Fig. 4. Traumatic infrarenal aortic dissection in a patient involved in a high-speed motor vehicle collision. Arterial image demonstrates an intimomedial flap within the lumen (arrow) consistent with a dissection.

pseudoaneurysms or arteriovenous fistulas may be treated in a semiurgent manner.

The spleen is the most commonly injured solid abdominal organ. Traumatic injuries involving the spleen can result in active arterial hemorrhage as well as contained vascular injuries, such as pseudoaneurysms and arteriovenous fistula. This distinction can be made with multiphasic acquisitions (as described previously).[32] Hepatic vascular injuries can manifest as hepatic artery pseudoaneurysms, which may subsequently be treated with coil occlusion or embolisation.[33] Arterioportal fistulas are more common after penetrating injuries and manifest on CT as geographic areas of hyperenhancement seen in the liver parenchyma.[23] Active extravasation from the hepatic artery or branches is a potentially life-threatening injury when associated with hemodynamic instability. When present, this finding is a strong predictor of failure of nonsurgical treatment.[29,34] Arterial avulsion, dissection, and thrombosis are particularly important in the kidney, where they can occur as a result of acceleration-deceleration injuries (**Fig. 6**).[35–37] The one absolute indication for surgical treatment in renal injury is life-threatening arterial bleeding whereas other injuries may be managed nonemergently or conservatively.[35]

CTA OF THE PELVIS

Patients who suffer major blunt pelvic trauma and sustain displaced fractures have a high risk of major pelvic vascular injuries, with significant

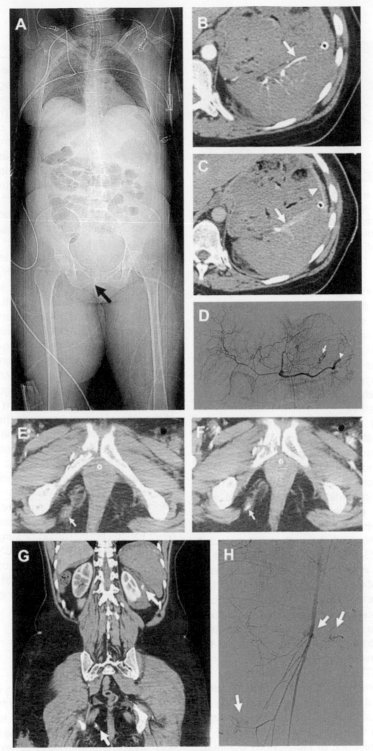

Fig. 5. A 47-year-old female pedestrian struck by an automobile. Scout (*A*) image demonstrates a pelvic ring fracture (*arrow*), a finding used to triage patients to receive pelvic CTA. Axial arterial (*B*) and delayed (*C*) CT images demonstrate active splenic hemorrhage (*arrows*) extending laterally on the delayed phase (*arrowhead*), which was confirmed with DSA and treated with embolization (*D*) (*arrow*). Occlusion of the distal splenic artery on angiography (*D*) (*arrowhead*) is also noted. Axial arterial (*E*) and venous (*F*) CT images show a focal area of active arterial hemorrhage in the pelvis (*arrow*), which enlarged over time, consistent with active hemorrhage. Coronal (*G*) CT image demonstrates pelvic and splenic arterial hemorrhage (*arrows*). Conventional angiogram of the pelvis and right lower extremity (*H*) shows multiple regions of contrast extravasation (*arrows*) in the pelvis and proximal lower extremity; these were subsequently embolized.

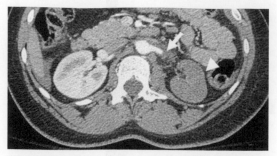

Fig. 6. Traumatic injury to the left renal artery in a patient in a high-speed motor vehicle collision. Axial image demonstrates occlusion of the left renal artery (*arrow*) with resulting lack of enhancement of the left kidney (*arrowhead*).

mortality and morbidity.[38–42] Approximately 40% of patients with a pelvic fracture may have an associated pelvic vascular injury and hemorrhage is the leading cause of mortality in 60% of cases.[26,39–41,43] Rapid detection and assessment of pelvic vascular injury afforded by the shorter acquisition times and increased spatial resolution of MDCT are useful for properly triaging critically injured trauma patients.[30,31,38,40,42]

Experience at the authors' institution has demonstrated that pelvic CTA can be integrated into requisite torso trauma imaging in the multi-trauma setting, thus providing critical information, such as detection of various types of arterial injuries and differentiation between arterial and venous sources of hemorrhage.[42] Pelvic CTA images are acquired from the iliac crests to the greater trochanters and the authors have found that a standard 23-second delay after the start of contrast injection is optimal for imaging the central pelvic arteries. Bolus triggering software and the test injection method can be used in special circumstances, such as in the elderly population or those with a compromised cardiovascular system, where transit time is expected to be longer than in average patients. In polytrauma patients, pelvic CTA is immediately followed by chest CTA and then by CT of the abdomen and pelvis in the portal venous phase (70 seconds). In addition, CT protocols at most large trauma centers include a delayed phase acquired at 5 to 7 minutes after injection of intravenous contrast. This triphasic CT protocol of the pelvis is reserved for the most severely traumatized patients (ie, those whose portable radiograph of the pelvis demonstrates a fracture with disruption of the pelvic ring) (see Fig. 5). In order to reduce the total radiation dose delivered, the early (angiographic) and delayed phases are acquired with a low radiation dose technique.

Imaging Findings and Clinical Implications

Vascular injuries that may be seen on pelvic CTA include active arterial hemorrhage, pseudoaneurysm, arteriovenous fistula, dissection, occlusion, and venous injury.[26,40,42,44–46] The most common injury and significant source of morbidity and mortality is active arterial extravasation. Active arterial hemorrhage is seen as an area of extraluminal contrast on the arterial phase, which enlarges with time, into the portal venous and delayed phases (see Fig. 5).[30,40,44,46] Pelvic CTA allows for accurate differentiation between arterial and venous injury.[42,45,46] This has significant therapeutic implications.

On a portal venous phase image, an arterial hemorrhage should have a higher attenuation than from a venous source, but significant overlap makes this distinction difficult.[42,45,46] Contrast extravasation seen on a portal venous phase image is defined as an arterial hemorrhage if it is present on the earlier, arterial phase image (Fig. 7). An arterial source of hemorrhage often dictates further intervention, usually in the form of DSA with embolization if the hemorrhage is ongoing. The authors have found a positive correlation between the size of the arterial hemorrhage and the need for subsequent intervention. The larger the hemorrhage, the greater the likelihood an intervention required.[42]

Contrast extravasation seen on a portal venous phase image but not on the earlier arterial phase image is more likely venous in nature.[42,45,46] Venous hemorrhage can often be managed successfully with pelvic stabilization without the need for coil embolization or surgical intervention, unlike arterial hemorrhage, which usually requires direct therapy with embolization. Differentiating and characterizing the type of pelvic vascular injury rapidly and accurately is essential in these severely injured patients.

CTA OF THE EXTREMITIES

Historically, DSA was the primary imaging modality for assessing the vascular integrity of the extremity in trauma patients.[47–49] CTA, however, has increasingly become an invaluable tool in the detection and characterization of extremity vascular injuries.[47,48,50–56] More recently, faster CT acquisition times and the development of longer CT tables that allow the acquisition of whole-body CT digital radiographs have led to the development of more complex and robust protocols in the multitrauma setting, including the integration of extremity CTA into torso trauma imaging with a single injection of contrast material.

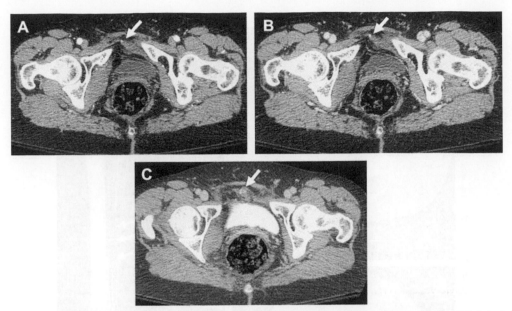

Fig. 7. Active pelvic hemorrhage in a 57-year-old woman involved in a motor vehicle collision. (A) Arterial, (B) venous, and (C) delayed-phase CT images demonstrate a small focal region of active arterial hemorrhage (arrows), which enlarges over time, in a patient with multiple pelvic fractures. Based on the size of the hemorrhage and clinical status of the patient, the arterial hemorrhage was successfully treated conservatively.

Imaging Findings and Clinical Implications

CT imaging findings in extremity arterial injury may be classified into direct and indirect signs. Direct signs are highly specific CT findings of arterial injury and often necessitate immediate endovascular or surgical intervention.[47,52,57] Direct signs of injury include active contrast extravasation, visualization of a pseudoaneurysm, occlusion, abrupt vessel narrowing, intimal defect, dissection, and early venous opacification (likely signifying arteriovenous fistula) (Figs. 8 and 9). Indirect signs of vascular injury represent findings in soft tissues and should increase the suspicion for occult vessel injury. These findings include shrapnel less than 5 mm from a neurovascular bundle, intramuscular hematoma, and a projectile tract in close proximity to a blood vessel. Isolated focal arterial narrowing on CTA poses a diagnostic dilemma because several entities, including dissection, vascular spasm, and external compression from injured soft tissues and hematoma, may present in this fashion. Severe vascular spasm is the most mischaracterized lesion and can mimic a vascular occlusion.[47]

With blunt or penetrating trauma, the clinical findings suggestive of vascular extremity injury can be classified into hard and soft signs. The specific signs of arterial injury are the hard signs, which include pulsatile hemorrhage, distal ischemia, pulse deficit, bruit or thrill, and expanding hematoma. The presence of these hard signs often mandates urgent intervention because they are highly associated with a vascular injury.[47,48,52,58] Less specific signs of vascular injury are termed soft signs and include unexplained hypotension, small stable hematoma, proximity of an injury to a major blood vessel, abnormal ankle-brachial index, and associated nerve injury. These soft signs typically warrant observation and evaluation with CTA may provide valuable information to surgeons, avoiding unnecessary surgical exploration or minimizing delay before treatment is initiated.[47,52,57]

In many large trauma centers, conventional angiography is now used as a second-line diagnostic test when diagnosis of vascular injury on CTA is inconclusive. In patients with focal arterial narrowing at CTA, selected patients may undergo DSA to differentiate true vascular injuries, such as dissection or occlusion, from vascular spasm. Alternatively, if arterial narrowing is presumed secondary to vasospasm, further clinical observation and repeat CTA are often warranted.[47,48] DSA also provides the means for therapeutic endovascular intervention for injuries, such as pseudoaneurysm or arteriovenous fistulae.[47,48] In patients who are likely to have substantial image degradation on CT secondary to metallic shrapnel from gunshot wounds, DSA may be the initial imaging

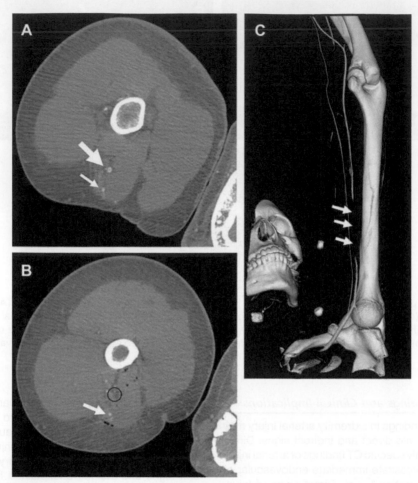

Fig. 8. Brachial artery occlusion in a 34-year-old man who was stabbed in the left upper extremity. Axial CT image proximal to the injury (*A*) demonstrates a patent brachial artery (*large arrow*) and an incidental finding of a high origin of the radial artery (*small arrow*). Distal (*B*) to the injury, the brachial artery is not visualized in the expected location (*open circle*). The radial artery (*arrow*) is again visualized (*B*). The volume-rendered (*C*) image demonstrates a segmental occlusion of the brachial artery. The CT scan was acquired with the patient in the prone position with the affected extremity above the patient's head.

study of choice when there is a high pretest probability of injury.

CTA OF THE HEAD AND NECK

Blunt and penetrating traumatic arterial injuries of the neck have traditionally been assessed by catheter angiography. The high number of negative examinations and the risks associated with catheter angiogram, however, have prompted the use of noninvasive techniques. MDCT angiography is sensitive and specific for the evaluation of carotid and vertebral artery injuries.[58–61] Cerebrovascular injuries occur in 1.2% to 2.7% of blunt trauma patients but up to 25% of patients who have suffered penetrating injuries.[60,62–64] High morbidity

and mortality rates are most commonly attributed to cerebral and cerebellar infarction. Early detection and characterization of traumatic vascular injuries of the neck leads to earlier initiation of medical or interventional treatment.[60,64–68]

CTA may be limited to a study of the carotid and vertebral circulation or be used in tandem with whole-body thoracoabdominal imaging. In the latter circumstance, a single bolus of contrast material is used for the image acquisition, which begins at the level of the aortic arch and extends to the vertex, including the circle of Willis, with subsequent study of the thorax abdomen and pelvis. Axial, coronal, and sagittal maximum intensity projection (MIP) reconstructions are routinely generated for interpretation.

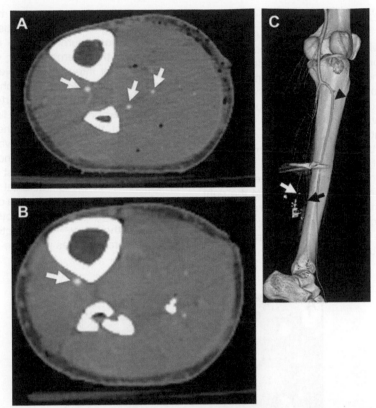

Fig. 9. Lower-extremity vascular injury in a 25-year-old man who sustained multiple gunshot wounds. Axial CTA image proximal to the fibular fracture (A) shows patent vasculature of the leg (arrows). At the level of the fibular fracture, an axial CT image (B) demonstrates only a patent anterior tibial artery (arrow) with occlusion of peroneal and posterior tibial arteries. There is a metallic bullet fragment in the posterior compartment. A volume-rendered Image (C) shows occlusion of the distal posterior tibial (white arrow) and peroneal (black arrow) arteries and patency of the anterior tibial artery (arrowhead). Note the metallic bullets remaining in the soft tissues.

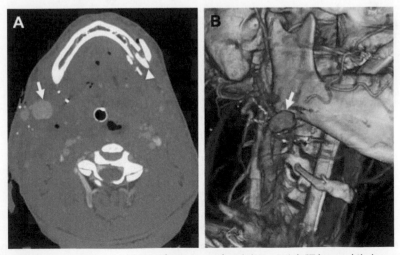

Fig. 10. Pseudoaneurysm in an 18-year-old man from a gunshot injury. Axial CT image (A) shows a pseudoaneurysm (arrow) of the facial artery with irregular contour. Note the left mandibular fracture (arrowhead). Volume-rendered (3-D) reformatted image (B) demonstrates the well-defined collection of contrast material (arrow) consistent with a pseudoaneurysm.

Imaging Findings and Clinical Implications

Interpretation of cerebrovascular CTA requires a thorough knowledge of vascular anatomy and anatomic variations as well as an understanding of the arterial and venous flow dynamics. Flow direction may not be readily apparent on CTA images. Retrograde flow or arteriovenous shunting is inferred by evaluating the relative degree of vessel opacification and caliber size.

Symmetric caliber size and enhancement of the vessels is important in the head and neck, but normal asymmetry in the caliber of the vertebral arteries is a common occurrence; often the right side is smaller than the left. The internal jugular vein caliber is commonly asymmetric; often the right side larger is than the left.[69] Asymmetric filling of the internal jugular veins is often seen with rapid scanning and should not be misdiagnosed as occlusion or thrombus. This is usually caused by slower venous return from the extracranial soft tissues into the internal jugular vein and slower flow in the left internal jugular vein secondary to compression of the brachiocephalic vein by the aortic arch or brachiocephalic artery.

With acute aortic dissection, a linear intraluminal filling defect that represents the intimal flap is usually identified. In cerebral vascular imaging, however, an intimal flap may not be evident in smaller caliber vessels. The most common finding of dissection in the extracranial and intracranial carotid and vertebral arteries is a crescent-shaped intramural hematoma with smooth narrowing and tapering of the artery.[64] A transection of the carotid and vertebral arteries may be seen on CTA;

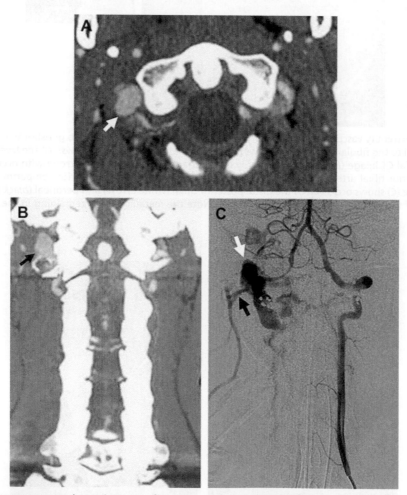

Fig. 11. Pseudoaneursym and arteriovenous fistula in a 42-year-old man from a gunshot injury. Axial (*A*) and coronal (*B*) CT images demonstrate a pseudoaneurysm of the right vertebral artery at the level of C1 (*arrow*). Catheter angiogram image of the left vertebral artery injection (*C*) shows a multilobulated pooling of contrast material (*white arrow*) secondary to the right vertebral artery injury, and early filling of the venous system (*black arrow*).

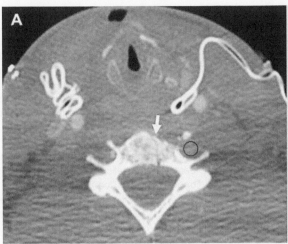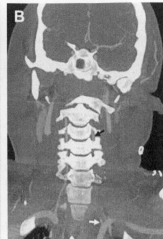

Fig. 12. Vertebral artery occlusion from a gunshot injury in a 28-year-old man. Axial (*A*) CT image shows fractures of the C6 vertebral body (*arrow*) with opacification of the right vertebral artery and lack of opacification of the left vertebral artery (*open circle*). Coronal (*B*) CT image demonstrates occlusion of the proximal left vertebral artery (*white arrow*) with distal reconstitution at C3-C4 level (*black arrow*).

however, patients with dissections are usually unstable and require immediate intervention before imaging is considered. As in other body parts, pseudoaneurysms are characterized by extraluminal collections of contrast material (**Figs. 10** and **11**). Arteriovenous fistulas are characterized by early venous filling (see **Fig. 11**), and partial or complete thrombus results in intramural filling defects. Definitive characterization of the underlying injury in cases of segmental arterial narrowing or occlusion may be challenging in neck CTA, as well as in other areas, given the overlap in imaging findings for traumatic dissection, occlusion, and vascular spasm (**Fig. 12**).

Patients involved in multitrauma are assessed for life-threatening thoracoabdominal injuries requiring immediate attention while a rigid neck collar is placed on them to prevent exacerbation of potential cervical spine and vascular injuries. MDCT allows accurate assessment of the cervical/cerebral vasculature without interfering with the evaluation of thoracoabdominal trauma.

Prior to the advent of MDCT, there was a median delay of 11 days before neurologic sequelae from traumatic carotid/cerebral vascular injury became manifest.[60] In appropriately selected patients, anticoagulation may be initiated to prevent thromboembolic stroke and other neurologic sequelae.[60,65,67,68,70] Anticoagulation may be contraindicated in patients who require emergent surgical intervention for other injuries. In patients with isolated penetrating or blunt carotid/cerebral vascular trauma, specific CTA findings are usually sufficient to determine the need for and type of subsequent therapy: conservative with or without anticoagulation, endovascular intervention, or surgery.[60,65,70] If CTA is inconclusive or if clinical findings are not congruent with the CTA findings, however, a catheter angiogram should be recommended, because this remains the standard of reference.[70]

SUMMARY

Currently, with widely available MDCT technology, the first-line assessment of vascular injury in trauma patients is CTA. CTA affords a rapid, accurate, noninvasive method of detecting vascular injury and appropriately triaging patients to receive the requisite intervention, when necessary. With careful attention to technique and an understanding of commonly encountered vascular injuries in trauma, high-quality, diagnostic CTAs offer an invaluable tool in the imaging evaluation of injured patients.

REFERENCES

1. Kaewlai R, Avery LL, Asrani AV. Multidetector CT of blunt thoracic trauma. Radiographics 2008;28: 1555–70.
2. Steenburg SD, Ravenel JG, Ikonomidis JS, et al. Acute traumatic aortic injury: imaging evaluation and management. Radiology 2008;248:748–62.
3. Dyer DS, Moore EE, Ilke DN, et al. Thoracic aortic injury: how predictive is mechanism and is chest computed tomography a reliable screening tool? A prospective study of 1,561 patients. J Trauma 2000;48:673–82.

4. Melton SM, Kerby JD, McGiffin D, et al. The evolution of chest computed tomography for the definitive diagnosis of blunt aortic injury: a single-center experience. J Trauma 2004;56:243–50.

5. Wong H, Gotway MB, Sasson AD, et al. Periaortic hematoma at diaphragmatic crura at helical CT: sign of blunt aortic injury in patients with mediastinal hematoma. Radiology 2004;231:185–9.

6. Mirvis SE, Shanmuganathan K. Diagnosis of blunt traumatic aortic injury 2007: still a nemesis. Eur J Radiol 2007;64(1):27–40.

7. Dosios TJ, Salemis N, Angouras D, et al. Blunt and penetrating trauma of the thoracic aorta and aortic arch branches: an Autopsy Study. J Trauma 2000; 49(4):696–703.

8. Fabian TC, Richardson JD, Croce MA, et al. Prospective study of blunt aortic injury: multicenter trial of the american association for the surgery of trauma. J Trauma 1997;42(3):374–83.

9. Azizzadeh A, Keyhani K, Miller CC III, et al. Blunt traumatic aortic injury: initial experience with endovascular repair. J Vasc Surg 2009;49(6):1403–8.

10. Hunt JP, Baker CC, Lentz CW, et al. Thoracic aorta injuries: management and outcome of 144 patients. J Trauma 1996;40(4):547–56.

11. Alkadhi H, Wildermuth S, Desbiolles L, et al. Vascular emergencies of the thorax after blunt and iatrogenic trauma: multi–detector row CT and three-dimensional imaging. Radiographics 2004; 24:1239–55.

12. Bashar AH, Kazui T, Washiyama N, et al. Stanford type a aortic dissection after blunt chest trauma: case report with a reflection on the mechanism of injury. J Trauma 2002;52:380–1.

13. Garzon G, Fernandez-Velilla M, Marti M, et al. Endovascular stent-graft treatment of thoracic aortic disease. Radiographics 2005;25:S229–44.

14. Therasse E, Soulez G, Giroux MF, et al. Stent-graft placement for the treatment of thoracic aortic diseases. Radiographics 2005;25:157–73.

15. Saad NE, Saad WE, Davies MG, et al. Pseudoaneurysms and the role of minimally invasive techniques in their management. Radiographics 2005;25:S173–89.

16. Brown KE, Eskandari MK, Matsumura JS, et al. Short and midterm results with minimally invasive endovascular repair of acute and chronic thoracic aortic pathology. J Vasc Surg 2008;47(4):714–22.

17. Bartone AS, Schena S, D'Agostino D, et al. Immediate versus delayed endovascular treatment of post-traumatic aortic pseudoaneurysms and type B dissections: retrospective analysis and premises to the upcoming european trial. Circulation 2002; 106:I-234–40.

18. Kuhlman JE, Pozniak MA, Collins J, et al. Radiographic and CT findings of blunt chest trauma: aortic injuries and looking beyond them. Radiographics 1998;18:1085–106.

19. Ben-Menachem Y. Avulsion of the innominate artery associated with fracture of the sternum. AJR Am J Roentgenol 1988;150(3):621–2.

20. Stuhlfaut JW, Soto JA, Lucey BC, et al. Blunt abdominal trauma: performance of CT without oral contrast material. Radiology 2004;233:689–94.

21. Roberts JL, Dalen RK, Bosanko CM, et al. CT in abdominal and pelvic trauma. Radiographics 1993; 13:735–52.

22. Katz DS, Hon M. CT angiography of the lower extremities and aortoiliac system with a multi–detector row helical CT scanner: promise of new opportunities fulfilled. Radiology 2001;221:7–10.

23. Foley WD. Special focus session: multidetector CT: abdominal visceral imaging. Radiographics 2002; 22:701–19.

24. Steenburg SD, Ravenel JG. Multidetector computed tomography findings of atypical blunt traumatic aortic injuries: a pictorial review. Emerg Radiol 2007;14(3):143–50.

25. Daly KP, Ho CP, Persson DL, et al. Continuing medical education: traumatic retroperitoneal injuries: review of multidetector CT findings. Radiographics 2008;28:1571–90.

26. Hamilton JD, Kumaravel M, Censullo ML, et al. Multidetector CT evaluation of active extravasation in blunt abdominal and pelvic trauma patients. Radiographics 2008;28(6):1603–16.

27. Frauenfelder T, Wildermuth S, Marincek B, et al. Nontraumatic emergent abdominal vascular conditions: advantages of multi–detector row CT and three-dimensional imaging. Radiographics 2004; 24:481–96.

28. Michaels AJ, Gerndt SJ, Taheri PA. Blunt force injury of the abdominal aorta. J Trauma 1996; 41(1):105–9.

29. Yoon W, Jeong YY, Kim JK. CT in blunt liver trauma. Radiographics 2005;25:87–104.

30. Yao DC, Jeffrey RB Jr, Mirvis SE, et al. Using contrast-enhanced helical CT to visualize arterial extravasation after blunt abdominal trauma. AJR Am J Roentgenol 2002;178(1):17–20.

31. Murakami AM, Anderson SW, Soto JA, et al. Active extravasation of the abdomen and pelvis in trauma using 64MDCT. Emerg Radiol 2009;16(5):375–82.

32. Anderson SW, Varghese JC, Lucey BC, et al. Blunt splenic trauma: delayed-phase CT for differentiation of active hemorrhage from contained vascular injury in patients. Radiology 2007;243:88–95.

33. Nosher JL, Chung J, Brevetti LS, et al. Continuing medical education: visceral and renal artery aneurysms: a pictorial essay on endovascular therapy. Radiographics 2006;26:1687–704.

34. Fang JF, Chen RJ, Wong YC, et al. Classification and treatment of pooling of contrast material on computed tomographic scan of blunt hepatic trauma. J Trauma 2000;49:1083–8.

35. Harris AC, Zwirewich CV, Lyburn ID, et al. CT findings in blunt renal trauma. Radiographics 2001;21:S201–14.

36. Kawashima A, Sandler CM, Corl FM, et al. Imaging of renal trauma: a comprehensive review. Radiographics 2001;21:557–74.

37. Fanney DR, Casillas J, Murphy BJ. CT in the diagnosis of renal trauma. Radiographics 1990;10:29–40.

38. Falchi M, Rollandi GA. CT of pelvic fractures. Eur J Radiol 2004;50(1):96–105.

39. Brasel KJ, Pham K, Yang H, et al. Significance of contrast extravasation in patients with pelvic fracture. J Trauma 2007;62(5):1149–52.

40. Yoon W, Kim JK, Jeong YY, et al. Pelvic arterial hemorrhage in patients with pelvic fractures: detection with contrast-enhanced CT. Radiographics 2004;24(6):1591–605 [discussion: 605–6].

41. Eastridge BJ, Starr A, Minei JP, et al. The importance of fracture pattern in guiding therapeutic decision-making in patients with hemorrhagic shock and pelvic ring disruptions. J Trauma 2002;53:446–51.

42. Anderson SW, Soto JA, Lucey BC, et al. Blunt trauma: feasibility and clinical utility of pelvic CT angiography performed with 64–detector row CT. Radiology 2008;246:410–9.

43. Ryan MF, Hamilton PA, Chu P, et al. Active extravasation of arterial contrast agent on post-traumatic abdominal computed tomography. Can Assoc Radiol J 2004;55(3):160–9.

44. Shanmuganathan K, Mirvis SE, Sover ER. Value of contrast-enhanced CT in detecting active hemorrhage in patients with blunt abdominal or pelvic trauma. AJR Am J Roentgenol 1993;161(1):65–9.

45. Kertesz JL, Anderson SW, Murakami AM, et al. Detection of vascular injuries in patients with blunt pelvic trauma by using 64-channel multidetector CT. Radiographics 2009;29:151–64.

46. Uyeda J, Anderson SW, Kertesz J, et al. Pelvic CT angiography: application to blunt trauma Using 64MDCT. Abdom Imaging 2009 May 21. [Epub ahead of print].

47. Rieger M, Mallouhi A, Tauscher T, et al. Traumatic arterial injuries of the extremities: initial evaluation with MDCT angiography. AJR Am J Roentgenol 2006;186:656–64.

48. Soto JA, Munera F, Morales C, et al. Focal arterial injuries of the proximal extremities: helical CT arteriography as the initial method of diagnosis. Radiology 2001;218:188–94.

49. Gakhal MS, Sartip KA. CT angiography signs of lower extremity vascular trauma. AJR Am J Roentgenol 2009;193:W49–57.

50. Seamon MJ, Smoger D, Torres DM, et al. A prospective validation of a current practice: the detection of extremity vascular injury with CT angiography. J Trauma 2009;67(2):238–43 [discussion: 243–4].

51. Anderson SW, Foster BR, Soto JA. Upper extremity CT angiography in penetrating trauma: use of 64-section multidetector CT. Radiology 2008;249:1064–73.

52. Pieroni S, Foster BR, Anderson SW, et al. Use of 64-row multidetector CT angiography in blunt and penetrating trauma of the upper and lower extremities. Radiographics 2009;29:863–76.

53. Inaba K, Potzman J, Munera F, et al. Multi-slice CT angiography for arterial evaluation in the injured lower extremity. J Trauma 2006;60:502–7.

54. Foster BR, Anderson SW, Soto JA. CT angiography of extremity trauma. Tech Vasc Interv Radiol 2006;9:156–66.

55. Busquets AR, Acosta JA, Colon E, et al. Helical computed tomographic angiography for the diagnosis of traumatic arterial injuries of the extremities. J Trauma 2004;56:625–8.

56. Fleiter TR, Mervis SE. The role of 3D-CTA in the assessment of peripheral vascular lesions in trauma patients. Eur J Radiol 2007;64:92–102.

57. McCorkell SJ, Harley JD, Morishima MS, et al. Indications for angiography in extremity trauma. AJR Am J Roentgenol 1985;145:1245–7.

58. Fishman EK, Horton KM, Johnson PT. Multidetector CT and three-dimensional CT angiography for suspected vascular trauma of the extremities. Radiographics 2008;28:653–65.

59. Stuhlfaut JW, Barest G, Sakai O, et al. Impact of MDCT angiography on the use of catheter angiography for the assessment of cervical arterial injury after blunt or penetrating trauma. AJR Am J Roentgenol 2005;185:1063–8.

60. Mutze S, Rademacher G, Matthes G, et al. Blunt cerebrovascular injury in patients with blunt multiple trauma: diagnostic accuracy of duplex doppler US and early CT angiography. Radiology 2005;237(3):884–92.

61. Munera F, Soto JA, Palacio DM, et al. Penetrating neck injuries: helical CT angiography for initial evaluation. Radiology 2002;224:366–72.

62. Berne JD, Reuland KS, Villarreal DH, et al. Sixteen-slice multi-detector computed tomographic angiography improves the accuracy of screening for blunt cerebrovascular injury. J Trauma 2006;60(6):1204–9.

63. Schneidereit NP, Simons R, Nicolaou S, et al. Utility of screening for blunt vascular neck injuries with computed tomographic angiography. J Trauma 2006;60(1):209–15.

64. Sliker CW. Blunt cerebrovascular injuries: imaging with multidetector CT angiography. Radiographics 2008;28:1689–708.

65. Miller PR, Fabian TC, Bee TK, et al. Blunt cerebrovascular injuries: diagnosis and treatment. J Trauma 2001;51(2):279–86.

66. Eastman AL, Muraliraj V, Sperry JL, et al. CTA-based screening reduces time to diagnosis and stroke rate

in blunt cervical vascular injury. J Trauma 2009;
67(3):551–6.

67. Cothren CC, Biffl WL, Moore EE, et al. Treatment for
blunt cerebrovascular injuries. equivalence of anticoagulation and antiplatelet agents. Arch Surg
2009;144(7):685–90.

68. Cothren CC, Moore EE, Biffl WL, et al. Anticoagulation
is the gold standard therapy for blunt carotid injuries
to reduce stroke rate. Arch Surg 2004;139(5):540–6.

69. Sakai O, Nakashima N, Shibayama C, et al. Asym-
metrical or heterogeneous enhancement of the
internal jugular veins in contrast-enhanced CT of
the head and neck. Neuroradiology 1997;39(4):
292–5.

70. Schroeder JW, Baskaran V, Aygun N. Imaging of
traumatic arterial injuries in the neck with an
emphasis on CTA. Emerg Radiol 2009;17(2):
109–22.

Pediatric Computed Tomographic Angiography: Imaging the Cardiovascular System Gently

Jeffrey C. Hellinger, MD[a],*, Andres Pena, MD[b],
Michael Poon, MD[c], Frandics P. Chan, MD PhD[d],
Monica Epelman, MD[e]

KEYWORDS

- Pediatrics • Cardiovascular disease
- Computed tomographic angiography
- Multidetector-row computed tomography
- Ultra-low dose radiation exposure

Cardiac and vascular disease in pediatric patients encompasses a broad spectrum of pathology. The majority of this pathology is congenital, resulting in alterations in gross and histologic structural morphology. Acquired pathology, however, is not uncommon; etiologies are often related to underlying systemic disease; surgical, endovascular, or procedural interventions; and blunt and penetrating trauma. Whether congenital or acquired, timely recognition and management of disease is imperative, as hemodynamic alterations in blood flow, tissue perfusion, and cellular oxygenation can have profound effects on organ function, growth and development, and quality of life for the pediatric patient.

Cardiovascular imaging plays a central role in diagnosis, treatment planning, and surveillance in this patient population. Non-invasive options include radiography, echocardiography, vascular ultrasound, magnetic resonance imaging (MRI) and angiography (MRA), computed tomographic angiography (CTA), single photon emission computed tomography (SPECT), and positron emission tomography (PET) CTA. Invasive catheter angiography (CA) remains the standard reference for all diagnostic modalities.

In considering which modality to use, it is important for the well being of the pediatric patient, to base decisions upon the benefits and risks of the examination. In general, non-invasive imaging is employed prior to invasive techniques, with selective use of the radiation modalities. Committing to a policy of safety first, leads to several salient questions regarding the application of state of the art computed tomography (CT) in assessment of pediatric cardiovascular disease, particularly in

---

A revised version of this article can be found online at: www.radiologic.theclinics.com.

[a] Cardiovascular Imaging and The 3D Imaging Laboratory, Department of Radiology, The Children's Hospital of Philadelphia, University of Pennsylvania School of Medicine, Philadelphia, PA, USA
[b] Department of Radiology, The Children's Hospital of Philadelphia, University of Pennsylvania School of Medicine, Philadelphia, PA, USA
[c] Advanced Cardiovascular Imaging, Department of Radiology, Stony Brook University School of Medicine, Stony Brook, NY, USA
[d] Cardiovascular Imaging, Department of Radiology, Lucile Packard Children's Hospital, Stanford University School of Medicine, Palo Alto, CA, USA
[e] Neonatal Imaging, Department of Radiology, The Children's Hospital of Philadelphia, University of Pennsylvania School of Medicine, Philadelphia, PA, USA
* Corresponding author.
E-mail address: jeffrey.hellinger@yahoo.com

light of the advancements in cardiovascular MRI and MRA: What is the role of CTA in evaluating pediatric cardiovascular disease? Which patients are suitable candidates and what are appropriate indications for these patients? What radiation dose reduction strategies are available to achieve low radiation exposure while maintaining high diagnostic image quality?

The answers to these questions center on technology and imaging technique. Ensuring safe CTA practice and "gentle" as low as reasonably achievable (ALARA) pediatric imaging requires the cardiovascular imager to have strong working knowledge of CTA technical principles and clinical utilization balanced with sound understanding of pediatric cardiovascular anatomy, pathology, and pathophysiology. From this vantage point, CTA can be a useful adjunct along with the other modalities.

To assist the reader attain success in these endeavors, this review article presents a summary of dose reduction methodologies available to achieve 1–3 mSv low dose and submillisievert ultra-low dose radiation exposures in pediatric CTA (Fig. 1). Discussion points and recommendations are based upon 1550 consecutive exams performed over 39 months directly by or under the supervision of the lead author at the Children's Hospital of Philadelphia using a single source 64-channel Sensation multidetector-row computed tomography (MDCT) scanner (Siemens Medical Solutions, Malvern, PA, USA).[1] In the first portion of this review, CTA technical principles are discussed with an emphasis on dose reduction methodologies and safe contrast medium delivery strategies. Recommended parameters for currently available MDCT scanners are summarized in vendor-defined tables, while recommended radiation and contrast medium parameters are summarized in respective weight-based tables. In the second part of this work, an overview of pediatric CTA clinical applications is presented, illustrating low-dose and ultra-low dose techniques.

IMAGING OPTIONS: COMPLEMENTARY MODALITIES

Chest radiography is a valuable modality in the initial investigation of suspected congenital heart disease. Assessment of visceral—atrial situs, systemic veins, cardiac apex and chamber size, aortic arch sidedness and contour, pulmonary vascularity, and the axial skeleton readily can direct the working diagnosis, initial management, and further work-up. Recognition of the position and course of support devices can also aid in this process. Radiography provides similar useful information when investigating the peripheral vascular system, guiding early treatment and subsequent advanced imaging. When more detailed imaging is required, first-line considerations are echocardiography (heart, coronary arteries, pulmonary vasculature, thoracic aorta, intra-thoracic systemic veins) and vascular ultrasound (peripheral vascular system). Both afford non-invasive assessments of morphology, function, and flow without radiation or potentially nephrotoxic or allergenic contrast medium. From a workflow perspective, they are widely available, can be performed rapidly at the bedside or in the outpatient setting, and have low cost. With current technology and algorithms, real-time two dimensional (2D) gray scale and color Doppler images, spectral tracings, and CINE-loops are acquired

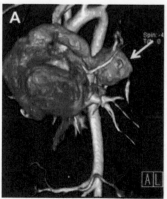
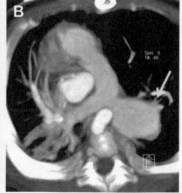
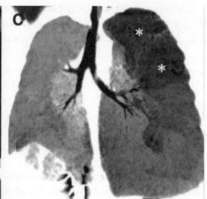

Fig. 1. A 3-month-old patient with increasing respiratory distress and a history of tetralogy of Fallot, absent pulmonary valve, and left pulmonary artery aneurysm (post plication). (A) Left anterior oblique volume-rendered (VR) image and (B) maximum intensity projection (MIP) axial image demonstrate a residual, large left pulmonary artery aneurysm (yellow arrows). (C) Minimum intensity projection (MinIP) image reveals hyperexpansion and air trapping in the left upper lobe (asterisk) secondary to aneurysm compression on the left upper lobe bronchus (red arrow).

from multiple projections and regions to depict segments of cardiac anatomy and vascular territories. Three dimensional (3D) techniques are available, providing true volumetric data and enhancing morphologic evaluations. These modalities are limited by operator skill, the acoustic window, and spatial display. Regarding the acoustic window, coils, surgical clips, stents, catheters, and pacing wires, along with large body habitus, soft tissue edema, soft tissue scar, chest or abdominal wall deformities, pleural effusions, ascites, lung disease, and enteric and colonic gas all may negatively impact the ability to identify and interpret structures with reasonable confidence. As the intrinsic nature of this technology limits the ability to depict complete anatomical structures and vascular territories in a single display and in relation to adjacent structures, interpretation and application is based upon a virtual summation of the individual images and CINE loops.

At the other end of the imaging spectrum, from echocardiography and vascular ultrasound, is catheter angiography. While it only generates 2D projectional images in standard operation, catheter angiography affords real-time angiographic flow, imaging cardiovascular structures with the highest temporal resolution. In addition, this modality provides real-time in-vivo hemodynamic data analysis. Current state of the art angiographic equipment offers 3D cardiovascular and soft tissue reconstructions, improving clinical utility, decreasing exam time, and potentially decreasing radiation exposure. Nonetheless, as it is invasive with inherent risks of injury, exposes patients to radiation and iodinated contrast, and in most instances, requires moderate conscious sedation or general anesthesia, advanced diagnostic cardiovascular evaluation in pediatrics depends upon the selective, complementary use of non-invasive cardiovascular MRI (CVMR), CT (CVCT), SPECT and PET-CTA. Pediatric cardiac and peripheral vascular catheter angiography is reserved for either (1) diagnostic problem-solving for issues not answered by the other modalities, and (2) endovascular interventions. CVMR and CVCT are the main alternative considerations to catheter angiography, given their ability to comprehensively evaluate morphology, function, and flow (indirect with CVCT). SPECT and PET-CTA are relegated to a selective third tier role, given their potential high radiation exposures relative to CVMR and state-of-the-art CVCT. In addition, while PET-CTA provides evaluation of cardiac and vascular morphology and function, SPECT (cardiac and pulmonary) is restricted to functional information. When faced with the decision to image with either CVMR or CVCT, CVMR should always be given priority as it utilizes no radiation or iodinated contrast medium. In addition, CVMR directly assesses function and hemodynamics with superior temporal resolution, but without the burden of additional radiation. Non-cardiovascular structures can be evaluated, however, additional sequences may be required and depending on the region imaged and hydrogen content, resolution may be less ideal than with CT (ie. airway and lungs). Volumetric CVCT is utilized selectively based upon the intrinsic limitations of MRI and advantages of CT (Table 1). For each requested exam, the imaging team should affirm one or more of these criteria, offsetting the risks of radiation and iodinated contrast medium exposures. From a MRI perspective, CVCT is indicated when MRI is not available; MRI is contraindicated (ie, incompatible medical devices); patient physical restrictions preclude obtaining an MRI; MRI is non-diagnostic (ie, ferromagnetic materials - coils, clips, stents, prosthetic valves); or MRI has a high pre-test probability for yielding a non-diagnostic exam (Fig. 2). CT advantages include flexible availability, short exam times, ease of patient access (for critical management), high patient tolerance, and high spatial resolution. In addition, non-cardiovascular structures are evaluated simultaneously during the same acquisition with robust detail (Figs. 3 and 4). As listed in Table 1, CT advantages are applied to support the appropriate use of CTA in the following circumstances: the high sedation or

Table 1 Pediatric CTA: appropriate criteria	
MR Imaging Limitations	**CT Advantages**
MR imaging is not available	High conscious sedation or general anesthesia risk patient
MR imaging is contraindicated	Assess noncardiovascular structures
Patient physical restrictions	Higer spatial resolution is necessary for diagnosis
MR imaging is nondiagnostic	Mandatory emergent imaging
High pretest probability for a nondiagnostic MR imaging	

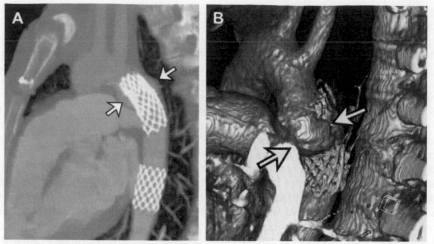

Fig. 2. A 15-year-old patient post bare stent placement for juxtaductal coarctation and complex congenital heart disease. (*A*) MIP image depicts a stent in the midthoracic aorta . Stent migration occurred during stent deployment. A second stent was successfully deployed (*white arrows*). (*B*) VR image shows an eccentric pseudoaneurysm (*yellow arrows*) located at the superior margin of the proximal stent.

general anesthesia risk patient; co-assessment of non-cardiovascular structures; requirement for higher spatial resolution; and emergent imaging.

CTA TECHNIQUE: SEEKING ALARA

Pediatric CTA is readily performed on first (4–16 channels), second (20–64 channels), and the latest third (128–320 channels)-generation MDCT scanners. Protocols are organized by anatomical regions and designed based upon the cardiovascular territories and pathologies to be imaged (Table 2). For each protocol, achieving a high

quality CT angiogram with reduced radiation exposure requires technical consideration of the minimally necessary coverage (field of view [FOV]), the table speed, desired spatial and contrast resolution, targeted radiation exposure, and acceptable noise. Acceptable noise, and thus how low radiation can be targeted, will vary among readers and patient care providers. It is important to reach a balance, as excessive noise may diminish the accuracy of exam interpretation and confidence in using the exam for management decision making. Contrast medium delivery becomes an essential means to accommodate

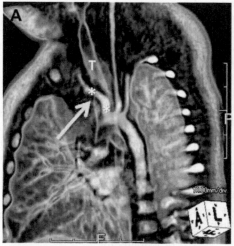
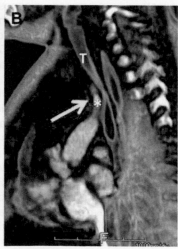

Fig. 3. A 45-day-old patient presenting with acute life-threatening event and stridor on clinical examination. (*A*) Left anterior oblique and (*B*) lateral VR images reveal severe tracheal (T) narrowing (*arrow*) as the innominate artery (*asterisks*) crosses anterior to the airway, needing subsequent aortopexy.

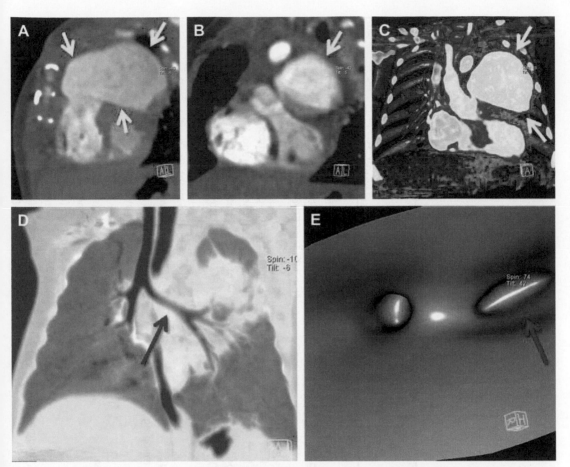

Fig. 4. A 4-week-old girl status post 3 weeks following truncus repair presenting with increasing respiratory distress and increasing opacity in the left upper lobe on chest radiographs (not shown). (A, B) MIP and (C) VR images reveal a large right ventricular outflow pseudoaneurysm (*arrows*) measuring 5 cm in maximal diameter. (D) MinIP and (E) virtual bronchoscopy images show narrowing and effacement of the left main stem bronchus secondary to compression by pseudoaneurysm (*arrows*).

increased noise and maintain a diagnostic contrast to noise ratio (CNR). Ultimately, while there are recommended protocols, selection of the acquisition parameters and the extent of dose reduction strategies are specific to each patient and will depend upon the type of MDCT scanner and its software algorithms (Table 3). For each exam, ancillary dose reduction strategies are an integral factor in preparing patients and selecting the contrast medium protocol (see Table 3).

Patient Preparation

For all requested exams, initial screening needs to first verify that CTA is the best option for the patient and that it is appropriate to proceed forward. The imaging team should also confirm normal renal function and the absence of allergies to iodinated contrast or related products. If

a patient has abnormal renal function and is on hemodialysis or peritoneal dialysis, the exam may be performed prior to scheduled dialysis. If the patient is not on dialysis, MRI with non-gadolinium MRA sequences is recommended. If a CTA is still the preferred modality, adequate hydration and low-osmolarity contrast medium are paramount. If a known or possible contrast allergy is identified, steroid preparation is necessary for the CTA to proceed forward. Patients should be screened for sedation requirements and whether sedation can be achieved by a nursing team or if anesthesiology is required. Alternatively, for neonates, discussion with the primary patient care team should determine if a sucrose-flavored pacifier may lead to a motionless exam.[2] If the study will require ECG-Gating, the heart rate should be obtained to assist in planning the scan and potentially seeking additional preparatory

Table 2
Pediatric CTA Protocols

Protocol	Clinical Applications	Examination Considerations
Cardiac		
Calcium scoring	FH, DM	Isolated examination vs combined with CoCTA
Coronary arteriogram	CA, KD, FH, mapping, post surgery	Retrosp vs prospective ECG-Gating
Coronary venogram	EP mapping	Nongated vs ECG-gating (Retrosp vs Prospective)
Cardiac structure & function		
Right heart	Obstructive CHD lesions (right, left)	Nongated vs ECG-gating (Retrosp vs Prospective)
Left heart	Conotruncal CHD, septation defects	NCA, extended chest coverage, 8–10 min DA
Global	PA/PV Anomalies, Valvular/Myocardial	DA may be nongated vs ECG-gated
	Pericardial Disease, Post-Surgery/EVT	(if ECG-Gated, prospective preferred)
Head and neck		
Cervical arteriogram	Trauma, VM	NCA, extended coverage (ie, chest)
Cerebral arteriogram	AOD, VM, aneurysms, mapping	NCA, PI, delayed venous phase
Cervicocerebral arteriogram	Trauma, AOD, VM, aneurysms, mapping	NCA, PI, extended coverage, delayed venous phase
Cervicocerebral venogram	VOD	NCA, extended coverage (ie, chest)
Chest		
Congenital lung	CPAM, BA, sequestration, PAVM	Coverage to RAs (systemic arterial supply)
Pulmonary AVM	HHT, acquired PAVM	NCA, head/abdomen coverage (HHT), DA
Pulmonary embolism	Venous thromboembolism	Direct or indirect (delayed) CTV
Pulmonary hypertension	Primary and secondary PHTN	NCA, I/E with controlled PEEP ventilation
Thoracic aorta	Congenital/acute AD, vasculitis, trauma, hemoptysis	NCA, ECG-gating (retrosp for wall motion), DA
Thoracic venogram	VOD, SVC syndrome	Direct or indirect CTV

Abdomen-pelvis		
Abdominal aorta	Congenital/acute AD, vasculopathy, trauma	NCA, ECG-Gating (retrosp for wall motion), DA
Mesenteric		
Arteriogram	Acute and chronic mesenteric ischemia	Negative bowel contrast, NCA, Visceral PI
Biphasic	GIB, PLE, portal HTN, masses, mapping, liver Txp	Negative bowel contrast, NCA, PI, DA
Renal		
Native	HTN, vasculitis, masses, mapping, UPJO, trauma	NCA, IVP topogram, delayed CTN/CTU
Transplant	Post-Txp HTN, rejection, trauma	NCA, IVP topogram, delayed CTN/CTU
Iliac IVC venogram	VOD, venous stents	Direct vs indirect CTV, extended coverage
Extremity		
Aortogram with runoff	AOD, vasculitis, trauma, masses, mapping, HDA	NCA, DA^a function (TOS, PAES)
Runoff	Follow-up vasculitis, trauma, masses, mapping	NCA, DA,^{a} kinetic imaging (128–320 channel MDCT)
Indirect venogram	VOD, venous stents, vascular masses, mapping	Targeted vs complete coverage, function (TIS, PAES)
Direct venogram	VOD, venous stents, vascular masses, mapping	Targeted vs complete coverage, function (TIS, PAES)
Whole body	Systemic congenital vasculopathy Acquired vasculopathy	NCA, ECG-gating Retrosp vs Prospective), DA

Abbreviations: AD, aortic disease; AOD, arterial occlusive disease; ARVD, arrhythmogenic right ventricular dysplasia; BA, bronchial atresia; CA, coronary anomalies; CHD, congenital heart disease; CoCTA, coronary CTA; CPAM, congenital pulmonary adenomatoid malformation; CTN, CT nephrogram; CTU, CT urogram; CTV, CT venogram; DA, delayed acquisition; DM, diabetes mellitus; EVT, endovascular; therapy; FH, familial hypercholesterolemia; GIB, GI bleed; HDA, hemodialysis access; HHT, hereditary hemorrhagic telangiectasia; HTN, hypertension; I/E, inspiration/expiration; KD, Kawasaki disease; NCA, noncontrast acquisition; PAES, popliteal entrapment syndrome; PAVM, pulmonary arteriovenous malformation; PEEP, positive end-expiratory pressure; PHTN, pulmonary hypertension; PI, perfusion imaging; PLE, protein-losing enteropathy; PV, pulmonary vein; RAs, renal arteries; Retrosp, retrospective; SVC, superior vena cava; TIS, thoracic inlet syndrome; TOS, thoracic outlet syndrome; Txp, transplant; UPJO, ureteral pelvic junction obstruction; VM, vascular malformation; VOD, venous occlusive disease.
^{a} Elbow to hand or knee to feet for an extremity delayed acquisition.

Table 3
CTA dose reduction strategies

Patient Preparation	Scanner Technology	Acquisition Parameters
Appropriate imaging indications	Dual energy (virtual NCA)	Appropriate coverage
Appropriate gauge PIVC	Iterative reconstruction[a]	Limit number of acquisitions
Shield nonimaged organs	Tube Current Modulation Software • General Automated • Anterior Chest Modulation	Lowest possible voltage (kVp)[c]
	Cardiac ECG-gating • Prospective ECG-gating[b] • ECG-pulsing	Lowest possible amperage (mAs)[c] Shortest possible scan time • high pitch • fast gantry rotation time • thick detector width[d]
		Iodine dose optimization

Abbreviations: NCA, noncontrast acquisition; PIVC, peripheral intravenous catheter.
[a] Raw data reconstruction.
[b] For cardiac function evaluation, retrospective ECG-gating is required.
[c] Consider primary or secondary iterative reconstruction algorithms to improve image quality.
[d] Applicable with adaptive detector configurations.

measures. Finally, if the objective of the exam is to evaluate a transplant kidney, the location of the kidney should be confirmed by reviewing operative notes, recent post-operative imaging (eg, abdominal radiographs, ultrasound), or both.

By nature of the CTA, a peripheral intravenous catheter (PIVC) is required for delivery of contrast medium. The ability to safely administer contrast is directly dependent upon adequate PIVC gauge and placement. Appropriate placement will ensure that relative high flow rates can be achieved to optimize iodine delivery and CNR. Table 4 lists recommended PIVC size and location, according to the CTA protocol and patient weight, with additional guidelines in the table description. In general the largest reasonable PIVC should be placed to accommodate high flow rates. The antecubital location is the preferred access site, given the larger vein size. When this is not feasible, access should be targeted in the forearm or hand. In neonates and infants up to 15 kg, a foot vein is also an alternative. If these sites are not accessible, considerations include an external jugular vein or a centrally placed venous catheter which can accommodate power injection. The exceptions to these rules are patients with renal insufficiency who are candidates for or are on dialysis. The antecubital fossa and cephalic veins are avoided to preserve future hemodialysis surgical access.[3] When imaging through the thorax or neck, access should be in the right upper extremity to limit streak artifact across the aortic arch. If suspected pathology is in the right thorax,

right neck, or right brain, access is gained in the left upper extremity. To assess a known or suspected persistent left superior vena cava, contrast injection is from the left upper extremity. Access for upper extremity CTA and indirect CT venography is in the upper extremity contralateral to the affected side. Access for direct upper extremity CT venography is placed in the ipsilateral hand or forearm. To help comfort pediatric patients during PIVC placement, topical anesthetic, child life support, or both are recommended.

When the patient is placed on the CT gantry table, there are several measures that should be taken to optimize photon delivery and minimize the impact of noise. First, the patent is positioned with the targeted region isocenter in the gantry. This positioning will yield more uniform photon delivery. Next, all external metallic objects should be removed from the expected scan region. The high-density material will limit photon exposure, cause streak artifact, and exacerbate potential increased noise when prescribing low-dose parameters. For chest and abdomen-pelvis CTA, the upper extremities are raised out of the field of view; for head and neck CTA, they are placed at the patient's side. These strategies are aimed at reducing noise from increased soft tissue attenuation. Once the exact position is finalized, nontargeted anatomy susceptible to radiation should be shielded with full lead wraps. Physical barriers should also be placed over the thyroid gland and breast tissue.[4]

Table 4
Pediatric CTA: peripheral IV catheter placement

Protocol	Extremity First	Extremity Second	2–10 kg Location First	2–10 kg Location Second	2–10 kg IV Gauge First	2–10 kg IV Gauge Second	11–30 kg Location First	11–30 kg Location Second	11–30 kg IV Gauge First	11–30 kg IV Gauge Second	31–60 kg Location First	31–60 kg Location Second	31–60 kg IV Gauge First	31–60 kg IV Gauge Second	>60 kg Location First	>60 kg Location Second	>60 kg IV Gauge First	>60 kg IV Gauge Second
Cardiac	RUE	LUE	AC/FA	HD	22	24	AC	FA	20	22	AC	FA	20	22	AC	FA	18	20
Head and Neck																		
Arteriogram	RUE	LUE	AC/FA	HD	22	24	AC	FA	20	22	AC	FA	20	22	AC	FA	18	20
Venogram	R/L vs CLUE		HD	HD	24	24	HD	HD	22	24	AC	FA	20	22	AC	FA	20	22
Chest																		
Arteriogram/ICTV	RUE	LUE	AC/FA	HD	22	24	AC	FA	20	22	AC	FA	20	22	AC	FA	18	20
DCTV	ILUE		HD	HD	24	24	HD	HD	24	24	FA	HD	22	24	FA	HD	20	22
Abdomen-Pelvis																		
Arteriogram/ICTV	R/L UE		AC/FA	HD	22	24	AC	FA	20	22	AC	FA	20	22	AC	FA	18	20
DCTV	R/L LE		FT	FT	24	24	FT	FT	24	24	FT	FT	22	24	FT	FT	22	24
Extremity																		
Upper																		
Arteriogram/ICTV	CLUE		AC/FA	HD	22	24	AC	FA	20	22	AC	FA	20	22	AC	FA	18	20
DCTV	ILUE		HD	HD	24	24	HD	HD	24	24	HD	FA	22	24	HD	FA	20	22
Lower																		
Arteriogram/ICTV	R/L UE		AC/FA	HD	22	24	AC	FA	20	22	AC	FA	20	22	AC	FA	18	20
DCTV	ILLE		FT	FT	24	24	FT	FT	24	24	FT	FT	22	24	FT	FT	22	24
Whole body	RUE	LUE	AC/FA	HD	22	24	AC	FA	20	22	AC	FA	20	22	AC	FA	18	20

First indicates first choice, Second indicates second choice.
If the patient has renal insufficiency, AC and cephalic veins should not be accessed.
With head and neck CTA, if the suspected pathology can be localized, PIVC should be placed contralateral to the affected side.
All UE CTAs require PIVC placement in the UE contralateral to the effected UE, except for UE DCTV.
Patients weighing from 2 to 10 kg: for head and neck, chest, and UE CT arteriograms or ICTV, PIVC can be placed in a foot vein, if access is not achieved in the UE.
Cavopulmonary shunts may require bilateral UE or both UE and LE PIVC access.
Abbreviations: AC, antecubital; CLUE, contralateral UE; DCTV, direct CTV; FA, forearm; FT, foot; HD, hand; ICTV, indirect CTV; ILLE/ILUE, ipsilateral LE/UE; LE, lower extremity; LUE, left upper extremity; PIVC, peripheral IV catheter; R/L, right or left; RUE, right upper extremity; UE, upper extremity.

Acquisition

The objective of CT angiography is to synchronize image acquisition with the delivery of iodine at the peak of arterial or venous enhancement. The quality of the images is characterized by the degree and detail of enhanced cardiac and vascular structures in relationship to background organs and soft tissues. Acquisition parameters are selected to maximize spatial and contrast resolution while minimizing noise and artifacts. The artifacts may include cardiac and arterial pulsation, respiratory motion, patient motion, high density streaks, beam hardening, blooming, and edge pixilation. Achieving these study goals becomes challenging in pediatrics, as the primary objective in pediatric imaging is to image with the lowest possible amount of radiation.

Spatial resolution, as defined by the matrix size, is controlled by the detector width and collimation configuration. Three levels of resolution may be considered: standard resolution, high resolution, and isotropic resolution (Tables 5A–C). The operator should decide prior to scanning, if the maximum spatial resolution is ultimately required for diagnosis as noise and edge pixilation are inversely proportional to the square root of matrix size, such that noise will increase when reducing the detector width.[5] Contrast resolution is directly dependent upon the degree of iodine attenuation and the tube voltage (kVp). MDCT scanners may have up to four voltage options: 80, 100, 120, and 140. Reducing the voltage will increase iodine attenuation as the photons will be closer to the k-edge of iodine (33.2 keV).[6] Reducing the voltage will also yield less radiation dose. Both effects reach a maximum at 80kVp. Whether the voltage is dialed down to improve contrast resolution, reduce radiation exposure, or both, noise will increase.[6]

Based upon the anticipated noise and what the operator feels will be acceptable noise for a given patient weight and size, the operator can manipulate the tube current (mA) and exposure time (seconds) to control the flow of photons and radiation exposure (tube current × exposure time, mAs). Increasing exposure inversely decreases noise by the square root of the exposure, while directly increasing the amount of radiation dose.[7] In accordance with ALARA, however, exposure should be kept as low as possible. Depending on the scanner, this may require sacrificing image quality to a reasonable extent and accepting to interpret studies through noise. To deliver reasonably low radiation exposure, the operator should prescribe the lowest acceptable tube current. Low radiation exposure is also achieved by increasing the gantry rotation speed and the pitch, as the scan time will decrease. The exception to this strategy is with Siemens' MDCT technology whereby tube current is maintained at a constant level independent of the pitch and gantry speed (effective mAs; Siemens Medical Solutions, Malvern, PA, USA). To circumvent this potential increased exposure with increased table speed, the targeted mAs can be set to a lower value or the automated tube current modulation can be de-activated. Of note, if the gantry speed and pitch are reduced to increase exposure, the longer scan times may yield a greater degree of pulsation and motion artifacts. In addition, as pitch decreases to less than 1, overlapping rotations will lead to increased tissue irradiation. The peak effect is seen with retrospective ECG-Gating, in which values can be as low as 0.15 (Siemens Medical Solutions, Malvern, PA, USA).

Protocol Series

A pediatric CTA protocol may have a minimum of three series and up to at least five. To maintain low exposure, protocols should strive for the core minimum. The first series is the required topogram, necessary to prescribe the axial images. To reduce radiation exposure, only a single anterior-posterior topogram should be obtained. The topogram voltage should be set to equal the anticipated voltage for the CTA acquisition in order to utilize automated tube current modulation. The second series is an optional non-contrast acquisition (NCA) with 1–3.0 mm thick images. NCA images can help assess calcifications, endovascular stents, surgical clips, surgical grafts, catheters, bone fragments (ie, trauma), residual intravenous contrast, active bleeding, and hematomas. However, in pediatric patients, this series does not routinely offer benefit. As such, it is acquired on a select basis, depending on the exam indications and patient's history, when the monitoring physician feels high density material may limit image quality and interpretation or may itself be obscured by the contrast medium. If obtained, the FOV should be targeted to the narrowest possible range for recognized (ie, radiographs, topogram) or suspected high density material. If a Calcium Scoring dataset is acquired (ie, familial hypercholesterolemia, diabetes mellitus), 3 mm thick images are acquired using prospective rather than retrospective ECG-gating, given the reduced radiation exposure with prospective ECG-Gating.[8] Pitch is eliminated with prospective ECG-gating, so that tissues are irradiated only once. With dual-energy MDCT scanners, a virtual NCA is possible, also reducing the amount of patient

Table 5A
Pediatric CTA acquisition and reconstruction parameters

MDCT Scanner	Mode	Detector Configuration (channels x mm)	Pitch Routine	Pitch ECG	Gantry Rotation Time (s)	Table Speed Routine (mm/s)	Table Speed ECG (mm/s)	ScanTime Routine (s)	ScanTime ECG (s)	Slice TH (mm)	Slice RI (mm)	Number of Images
4 – Channel												
GE	SR	4 x 2.5	1.5	NA	0.5	30	NA	5.3	NA	2.5	1.5	107
Philips	SR	4 x 2.5	1.5	NA	0.5	30	NA	5.3	NA	2.5	1.5	107
Siemens	SR	4 x 2.5	1.5	0.2	0.5	30	4	5.3	40	2.5	1.5	107
Toshiba	SR	4 x 2.0	1.5	0.23	0.5	24	3.7	7	43.5	2	1.0	160
8 – Channel												
GE	HR	8 x 1.25	1.35	NA	0.5	27	NA	6	NA	1.25	0.8	200
Toshiba	HR	8 x 1.0	1.438	0.23	0.5	23	3.7	7	43.5	1.0	0.8	200
GE	SR	8 x 2.5	1.35	NA	0.5	54	NA	3	NA	2.5	1.5	107
Toshiba	SR	8 x 2.0	1.438	0.23	0.5	46	7.4	3.5	22	2.5	1.0	160
16 – Channel												
GE	IR	16 x 0.625	1.375	0.325	0.5	27.5	6.5	6	25	0.625	0.5	320
Philips	IR	16 x 0.75	1.5	0.24	0.5	36	6	4.4	28	0.75	0.5	320
Siemens	IR	16 x 0.75	1.5	0.33	0.5	36	8	4.4	20	0.75	0.5	320
Toshiba	IR	16 x 0.5	1.438	0.23	0.5	23	3.7	7	43.5	0.5	0.4	400
GE	HR	16 x 1.25	1.375	0.325	0.5	55	13	3	12.3	1.25	0.8	200
Philips	HR	16 x 1.5	1.5	0.24	0.5	72	11.5	2.2	14	1.5	0.8	200
Siemens	HR	16 x 1.5	1.5	0.33	0.5	72	16	2.2	10	1.5	0.8	200
Toshiba	HR	16 x 1.0	1.438	0.23	0.5	46	7.4	3.5	22	1.0	0.8	200

Scan times are for a Z-axis coverage of 160mm. Routine and retrospective ECG-Gated acquisition parameters (detector configuration, pitch, gantry rotation speed) reflect helical scanning. Reconstruction parameters: slice thickness (TH) and reconstruction interval (RI).
Abbreviations: SR, standard resolution; HR, high resolution; IR, isotropic resolution; NA, option not available.

Table 5B
Pediatric CTA acquisition and reconstruction parameters

MDCT Scanner	Mode	Detector Configuration (channels x mm)	Pitch Routine	Pitch ECG	Gantry Rotation Time (s)	Table Speed Routine (mm/s)	Table Speed ECG (mm/s)	ScanTime Routine (s)	ScanTime ECG (s)	Slice TH (mm)	Slice RI (mm)	Number of Images
20 – Channel												
Siemens	IR	20 x 0.6	1.5	0.15[a]	0.33	54.5	5.5	2.9	29	0.75	0.5	320
Siemens	HR	16 x 1.2	1.5	0.49[a]	0.33	87	28.5	1.8	5.6	1.5	0.8	200
32 – Channel												
GE	IR	32 x 0.625	1.375	0.16	0.35	79	9	2	17.5	0.625	0.5	320
Toshiba	IR	32 x 0.5	1.5	0.175	0.4	60	7	2.7	23	0.5	0.4	400
GE	HR	32 x 1.25	1.375	0.26	0.35	157	30	1	5.4	1.25	0.8	200
Toshiba	HR	32 x 1.0	1.5	0.23	0.4	120	18	1.3	9	1.0	0.8	200
40 – Channel												
Philips	IR	40 x 0.625	1.5	0.2	0.4	94	12.5	1.7	13	0.75	0.5	320
Siemens	IR	2 x 20 x 0.6	1.5	0.15[a]	0.33	54.5	5.5	2.9	29	0.75	0.5	320
Philips	HR	32 x 1.25	1.5	0.2	0.4	150	20	1.1	8	1.5	0.8	200
Siemens	HR	16 x 1.2	1.5	0.49[a]	0.33	87	28.5	1.8	5.6	1.5	0.8	200
64 – Channel												
GE	IR	64 x 0.625	1.375	0.16	0.35	157	18	1	9	0.625	0.5	320
Philips	IR	64 x 0.625	1.5	0.2	0.4	150	20	1.1	8	0.75	0.5	320
Siemens	IR	2 x 32 x 0.6	1.5	0.15[a]	0.33	87	8.7	1.8	18	0.75	0.5	320
		(2) 2 x 32 x 0.6[b]	3	0.15	0.33	175	8.7	0.92	18	0.75	0.5	320
Toshiba	IR	64 x 0.5	1.5	0.175	0.4	120	14	1.3	11	0.5	0.4	400
GE	HR	32 x 1.25	1.375	0.26	0.35	157	30	1	5.4	1.25	0.8	200
Philips	HR	32 x 1.25	1.5	0.2	0.4	150	20	1.1	8	1.5	0.8	200
Siemens	HR	24 x 1.2	1.5	0.49[a]	0.33	131	43	1.2	3.7	1.5	0.8	200
		(2) 24 x 1.2[b]	3	0.49	0.33	262	43	0.61	3.7	1.5	0.8	200
Toshiba	HR	32 x 1.0	1.5	0.23	0.4	120	18	1.3	9	1.0	0.8	200

Scan times are for a Z-axis coverage of 160mm. Routine and retrospective ECG-Gated acquisition parameters (detector configuration, pitch, gantry rotation speed) reflect helical scanning. Reconstruction parameters: slice thickness (TH) and reconstruction interval (RI).

Abbreviations: SR, standard resolution; HR, high resolution; IR, isotropic resolution.

[a] Based upon Adaptive Scanning technology

Table 5C
Pediatric CTA acquisition and reconstruction parameters

MDCT Scanner	Mode	Detector Configuration (channels x mm)	Pitch Routine	Pitch ECG	Gantry Rotation Time (s)	Table Speed Routine (mm/s)	Table Speed ECG (mm/s)	ScanTime Routine (s)	ScanTime ECG (s)	Slice TH (mm)	Slice RI (mm)	Number of Images
128 – Channel												
Siemens	IR	2 x 64 x 0.6	1.5	0.15[a]	0.33	175	17.5	0.9	9.2	0.75	0.5	320
Siemens	IR	(2) 2 x 64 x 0.6[b]	3.4	0.17[a]	0.33	396	20	0.4	8.1	0.75	0.5	320
Siemens	HR	32 x 1.2	1.5	0.52[a]	0.33	175	60.5	0.9	2.6	1.5	0.8	200
Siemens	HR	(2) 32 x 1.2[b]	3.4	3.4[a]	0.33	396	396	0.4	0.4	1.5	0.8	200
160 – Channel												
Toshiba	IR	160 x 0.5[c]	1.5	0.151	0.4	300	30	0.5	5.3	0.5	0.4	400
Toshiba	HR	80 x 1.0[c]	1.5	0.184	0.4	300	37	0.5	4.3	1.0	0.8	200
256 – Channel												
Philips	IR	(2) 128 x 0.625[b]	1.5	0.14	0.27	444	41.5	0.4	3.9	0.625	0.5	320
Philips	HR	(2) 64 x 1.25[b]	1.5	0.18	0.27	444	53	0.4	3	1.25	0.8	200
320 – Channel												
Toshiba	IR	320 x 0.5[v]	NA	NA	0.35	NA	NA	0.175	1.25	0.5	0.25	640
Toshiba	IR	160 x 0.5[c]	1.5	NA	0.4	300	NA	0.5	NA	0.5	0.4	400
Toshiba	HR	80 x 1.0[c]	1.5	NA	0.4	300	NA	0.5	NA	1.0	0.8	200

Scan times are for a Z-axis coverage of 160mm. Routine and retrospective ECG-Gated acquisition parameters (detector configuration, pitch, gantry rotation speed) reflect helical scanning with exception to the 320 x 0.5mm detector configuration. The 320 x 0.5mm configuration reflects volumetric scanning (v) in which pitch is eliminated. Reconstruction parameters: slice thickness (TH) and reconstruction interval (RI).

Abbreviations: SR, standard resolution; HR, high resolution; IR, isotropic resolution; NA, option not available.
[a] Based upon Adaptive Scanning technology
[b] Dual Source MDCT scanner
[c] Pending US Food and Drug Administration clearance.

radiation exposure.[9] The third series is a low dose timing acquisition (bolus tracking or automated triggering) which is essential for precise synchronization of cardiovascular enhancement and image acquisition. By nature of the CTA, all protocols require the fourth series, in which the contrast enhanced angiographic images are obtained. Precise attention to technical detail is essential to avoid repeating this series. The FOV should not extend beyond the anatomical region(s) of interest. When imaging in the thorax, unless extended coverage is required, every effort must be made to exclude the thyroid glands and the liver, spleen, and/or kidneys as these are the most radiosensitive organs in the neck and abdomen, respectively. For evaluation of cardiac morphology on second and third generation MDCT scanners, routine non-ECG-gated spiral acquisitions can reliably generate high resolution diagnostic images, free of motion. First generation scanners tend to have a greater extent of cardiac and vascular pulsation artifact, such that ECG-gating may be required to optimize image quality. In general, ECG-gating is reserved for evaluation of the coronary arteries, cardiac function, and valvular morphology. For patients undergoing coronary artery evaluation, who do not require functional evaluation and have heart rates between 50–60 beats per minute, prospective ECG-gating is recommended for the reduced radiation dose.[9] Retrospective ECG-gating, with superior temporal resolution, is utilized in all other cases. Retrospective ECG-gating will provide multiphase reconstructions for dynamic 4-dimensional (4D) display of atrial, ventricular, septal, and valvular structure and function. The fifth series is an optional delayed post-contrast acquisition. This phase is also only acquired under select circumstances. Examples include a delayed venous phase following the arterial phase (ie, biphasic abdominal CTA; indirect UECTV) and in evaluation of suspected vasculitis, vascular masses, and hemorrhage. When monitoring an upper or lower extremity CTA or a whole body CTA, if the acquisition gets ahead of the contrast bolus, an immediate delayed phase can be obtained.

CTA Parameters

Tables 5A, 5B, and 5C list recommended pediatric CTA acquisition (detector configuration, pitch, gantry speed) and reconstruction (slice thickness, reconstruction interval) parameters using the three generations of MDCT systems for phantom 160 mm non-ECG-Gated and retrospective ECG-Gated scans. Recommended weight-based voltage and tube currents for the anatomical-based protocols are shown in Table 6.

Across all three generation of scanners, a unifying theme for pediatric CTA is maximizing table speed. This reduces the scan duration and exposure time and overall radiation exposure.

Table 6
Pediatric CTA radiation exposure parameters

Weight (kg)	kVp	Cardiac ECG-Gated	Cardiac Non-ECG-gated	Head and Neck	Chest	Abdomen-Pelvis	Extremity	Whole Body
<20	80	50	15	20	15	15	15	15
21–30	80	75	20	25	20	20	20	20
31–40	80	100	25	35	25	30	30	25
41–50	80	125	30	45	30	40	40	30
51–60	80	150	35	55	35	50	50	40
61–70	80	175	40	65	40	60	60	50
71–80	80	200	50	75	50	70	70	60
81–90	100	250	60	85	60	80	80	70
91–100	100	300	70	95	70	90	90	80
101–110	100	350	80	105	80	100	100	90
111–120	100	375	90	125	90	120	120	100
120–140	100	400	100	150	100	150	150	120

Reference mAs (column group header spanning Cardiac ECG-Gated, Cardiac Non-ECG-gated, Head and Neck, Chest, Abdomen-Pelvis, Extremity, Whole Body)

Recommended parameters are based upon applications with a 64-channel sensation MDCT scanner (Siemens Medical Solutions, Malvern, PA, USA). Contrast optimization is essential for high SNR and image quality. Weight based contrast injection protocols are shown in Table 7.

For non-gated acquisitions, it also reduces potential pulsation and motion artifacts. Maximizing table speed is achieved by three mechanisms. The first is to apply the fastest available gantry rotation speed. The second is to use the highest appropriate pitch with helical scanning. Routine, non-ECG-gated pitch values range up to 1.4–1.5 for the majority of vendors. Dual source technology can achieve a pitch of 3 and 3.4 for 64- and 128-channel scanners, respectively (Siemens Medical Solutions, Malvern, PA, USA). In some of the early model scanners, too high of a pitch will lead to slice broadening and an increase in effective slice thickness, with current technology, however, vendors have made pitch independent of spatial resolution. For helical retrospective ECG-gating, to maximize temporal resolution, pitch values of less than 1 are the rule for most scanners. Coronary imaging requires the lowest "cardiac mode" pitch values, while function-only evaluations utilize the highest "cardiac mode" pitch value to reduce radiation exposure. For most scanners, the pitch is dialed in by the operator. However, software algorithms are available for adaptive pitch selection based upon the heart rate. The third mechanism to maximize table speed reflects one of the central elements of advanced MDCT technology: wider collimation coverage as a result of increased detector rows. This culminates with state of the art non-helical volumetric scanning (Toshiba American Medical Systems, Tustin, CA, USA). With adaptive collimation (first and second generation scanners), increased detector width can also be used to increase the collimation.

For most protocols, the number of detector rows is exploited for the benefit of spatial resolution, reduced radiation, or both, based upon the MDCT scanner, coverage and exam requirements. For example, with non-ECG-gated acquisitions on a 4-channel system, a 4 × 2.0 mm or 4 × 2.5 mm detector configuration is recommended (see Table 5A). 2.0–2.5 mm images are reconstructed with a soft kernel at 1.0–1.5 mm increments, yielding an effective slice thickness of 3.0 mm (Standard Resolution [SR]). With an 8-channel system, a High Resolution (HR) technique (8 × 1.0 mm, 8 × 1.25 mm) is used to scan similar coverage in duration comparable to SR acquisitions (see Table 5A). Datasets are reconstructed every 0.8 mm into 1.0–1.25 mm thick images. Table speed can be increased (for radiation reduction) by using a SR mode, with the penalty for reduced spatial resolution. In a 16–channel system, similar coverage is now possible with Isotropic Resolution (IR), improving spatial detail. Datasets are generated using submillimeter collimations

(16 × 0.5 mm, 16 × 0.625 mm, 16 × 0.75 mm) in durations similar to the 4–channel SR and 8–channel HR modes, but with approximately 2 to 3 times the number of reconstructed images (see Table 5A). If isotropic resolution is not crucial for diagnosis, 16-channel CT angiograms are acquired with a HR mode (16 × 1.0 mm, 16 × 1.25 mm or 16 × 1.5 mm), reducing the scan duration, noise, radiation exposure, and the number or reconstructed images.

With 20 to 320-channel systems (see Tables 5B, 5C), non-ECG-gated exams are also acquired in either high or isotropic resolution modes. The table speeds are progressively faster as compared to 16-channel systems, yielding reduced scan durations and radiation exposure times per similar coverage. This is directly proportional to the number of detector-rows and the collimation coverage per gantry rotation. For second generation (20-64 channels; see Table 5B) systems, both adaptive and matrix configurations are available such that for most scanners through 40 mm of collimation, HR will further increase the table speed. Despite the time savings, reducing the tube current remains the principle strategy to achieve low exposure, potentially sacrificing image quality if dialed down too low. Beginning with 64-channel systems, iterative reconstruction software algorithms are an alternative to filtered-back projection to reduce noise in the raw data and optimize image quality when prescribing a low tube current and other dose reduction strategies.[10] Third generation scanners (128–320 channels; see Table 5C) have matrix configurations only. For helical scanning, IR and HR modes will yield equal table speeds, which are significantly faster as compared to those for first and second generation scanners. This translates into the ability to attain sub-second scan durations with isotropic resolution; exposure times are substantially reduced without loss in image detail. Volumetric scanning will also yield sub-second scanning and reduced exposure time. The exposure time savings for both helical and volumetric scanning can be used to dial up the tube current to an acceptable low exposure level with the goal of reducing noise. Alternatively, noise reduction algorithms can be applied to keep the tube current low and maximize the complete ALARA benefits of the third generation MDCT scanners.

Recommended weight-based voltage and tube current parameters in Table 6 are presented as a guideline with the understanding that parameters may alter depending upon the MDCT scanner; contrast delivery protocol; patient positioning; presence of metallic devices, stents, surgical clips, wires, and other high density material; and ultimately, the preference of the imager, primary care provider, or both. When adjusting either voltage or the tube current, the operator should keep in mind that radiosensitivities are greatest for the neonate, followed subsequently by the infant, toddler, young child, and lastly, the adolescent. Automated tube current modulation software should be used in all pediatric CT angiograms to account for variable attenuation in the Z-axis.[8] ECG-dependent tube current modulation is utilized when appropriate in the majority of retrospective ECG-gated CT angiograms.[11] The exception may be the large body-habitus patient with suboptimal heart rate control. For neck and/or chest coverage, anterior tube current modulation can be selected on Siemens' MDCT scanners to decrease breast and thyroid exposure (Siemens Medical Solutions, Malvern, PA, USA).

Contrast Medium Delivery

As noise increases, to achieve a constant CNR for a given cardiovascular territory (contrast resolution), the intracardiovascular iodine attenuation (density) must increase. In addition to decreasing the voltage, the other means to increase iodine attenuation is to directly increase the iodine content in the targeted territory. However, the amount of iodine that can be safely delivered is limited by a patient's body weight and renal function. Thus, the strategy is to deliver an appropriate weight-based amount of iodine (iodine dose) at an appropriate, relatively fast rate (iodine flux) and acquire images when the iodine reaches peak accumulation in the targeted territory. This task is best achieved with a power injector.

Synchronization

Automated bolus tracking software or a test bolus injection is required to determine the transit time for iodine to travel from the injection site to the targeted cardiovascular structure(s) (contrast medium transit time). For both techniques, 10 mm thick images are acquired at 80 kVp and the lowest reasonable tube current to view the images. With the test bolus technique, the time to peak enhancement is determined at a reference level in serial axial images and then pre-selected as the minimum diagnostic delay. With automated tracking, reference vessel attenuation is monitored in near real-time. Once the pre-determined threshold opacification (100–150 HU) is achieved at the reference level, the scan is initiated after a short diagnostic delay. Of the two options, we recommend automated triggering to achieve synchronization as an extended monitoring delay

can be prescribed based upon the injection rate and flow, such that only 1 to 2 monitoring slices may be necessary until the targeted threshold is reached, thereby keeping the additional radiation low. In comparison to a test-bolus injection, the actual time to trigger the scan is longer with automated triggering secondary to inherent interscan and image reconstruction delays, in addition to the diagnostic delay. Depending on the scanner, the minimum scan delay may range between 2 and 8 seconds.

Injection Parameters

Table 7 details recommended weight-based contrast medium injection protocols for low and ultra-low dose pediatric CT angiography, with the goal of optimizing iodine delivery. Depending upon the weight of the patient, iodine dose may range between 400–600 mg iodine per kilogram (1.3–2.0 ml/kg for 300 mg iodine/ml concentration), while average iodine flux may range between 0.23–1.9 g Iodine per second (0.8–6.2 ml/sec for 300 mg iodine/ml concentration). For all acquisitions, injection protocols are tailored to the specific patient and exam conditions, by adjusting the contrast medium concentration (300–370 mg iodine per millimeter), injection rate, injection volume, and/or injection duration based upon the patient's body weight, cardiac function, the scan distance, table speed, the targeted acceptable noise, and the PIVC. If the desired injection rate exceeds the tolerable limit for the accessed vein, the iodine concentration, the injection duration, or both should be increased to maintain the required iodine dose. Prior to injecting contrast, a saline "test" infusion is recommended at the designated CTA flow rate to assess the PIVC access and confirm that the exam can proceed safely.

Early generation CTA injection protocols were based upon the concept that the injection duration should equal the scan duration. This concept still applies for *slow* MDCT acquisitions (≤30 mm/second table speed) as with 4-channel SR, 8-channel HR, and 16-channel IR acquisition modes (Table 5A).[12] Vascular flow is well synchronized with the transit of contrast throughout the acquisition, achieving uniform enhancement. With *fast* MDCT acquisitions (>30mm/sec table speed, Tables 5A–C), if the injection duration is set to equal the scan duration, an insufficient amount of iodine will be delivered and an increased amount of injected contrast will not contribute to imaging, unless there is a delayed phase. The scan will extend through the targeted territories ahead of the majority of the contrast bolus, resulting in suboptimal enhancement.

Table 7
Pediatric CTA weight-based contrast medium injection protocols

Weight (kg)	Scan Delay (s)	Iodine Dose[a] (g)	Iodine Flux[a] (g/s)	300 mg I/mL CM		350 mg I/mL CM		370 mg I/mL CM	
				Volume[a] (mL)	Rate[a] (mL/s)	Volume[a] (mL)	Rate[a] (mL/s)	Volume[a] (mL)	Rate[a] (mL/s)
2–5	t_{CMT}+InD+DxD	600 mg I/kg 2.1	65 mg I/s/kg 0.23	2 mL/kg 7	0.22 mL/s/kg 0.8	1.7 mL/kg 6	0.19 mL/s/kg 0.7	1.6 mL/kg 5.7	0.18 mL/s/kg 0.6
6–10	t_{CMT}+InD+DxD	600 mg I/kg 4.8	60 mg I/s/kg 0.48	2 mL/kg 16	0.20 mL/s/kg 1.6	1.7 mL/kg 14	0.17 mL/s/kg 1.4	1.6 mL/kg 13	0.16 mL/s/kg 1.3
11–15	t_{CMT}+InD+DxD	600 mg I/kg 7.8	55 mg I/s/kg 0.72	2 mL/kg 26	0.18 mL/s/kg 2.4	1.7 mL/kg 22	0.16 mL/s/kg 2.0	1.6 mL/kg 21	0.15 mL/s/kg 1.9
16–20	t_{CMT}+InD+DxD	600 mg I/kg 10.8	50 mg I/s/kg 0.90	2 mL/kg 36	0.17 mL/s/kg 3.0	1.7 mL/kg 31	0.14 mL/s/kg 2.6	1.6 mL/kg 29	0.14 mL/s/kg 2.4
21–30	t_{CMT}+InD+DxD	500 mg I/kg 12.5	45 mg I/s/kg 1.13	1.7 mL/kg 42	0.15 mL/s/kg 3.8	1.4 mL/kg 36	0.13 mL/s/kg 3.2	1.35 mL/kg 34	0.12 mL/s/kg 3.0
31–40	t_{CMT}+InD+DxD	500 mg I/kg 17.5	40 mg I/s/kg 1.4	1.7 mL/kg 58	0.13 mL/s/kg 4.7	1.4 mL/kg 50	0.11 mL/s/kg 4.0	1.35 mL/kg 47	0.11 mL/s/kg 3.8
41–50	t_{CMT}+InD+DxD	500 mg I/kg 22.5	35 mg I/s/kg 1.58	1.7 mL/kg 75	0.12 mL/s/kg 5.3	1.4 mL/kg 64	0.10 mL/s/kg 4.5	1.35 mL/kg 61	0.095 mL/s/kg 4.3
51–60	t_{CMT}+InD+DxD	500 mg I/kg 27.5	30 mg I/s/kg 1.65	1.7 mL/kg 92	0.10 mL/s/kg 5.5	1.4 mL/kg 79	0.09 mL/s/kg 4.7	1.35 mL/kg 74	0.08 mL/s/kg 4.5
61–70	t_{CMT}+InD+DxD	500 mg I/kg 32.5	26 mg I/s/kg 1.69	1.7 mL/kg 108	0.09 mL/s/kg 5.6	1.4 mL/kg 93	0.07 mL/s/kg 4.8	1.35 mL/kg 88	0.07 mL/s/kg 4.6
71–80	t_{CMT}+InD+DxD	500 mg I/kg 37.5	23 mg I/s/kg 1.73	1.7 mL/kg 125	0.08 mL/s/kg 5.8	1.4 mL/kg 107	0.066 mL/s/kg 4.9	1.35 mL/kg 101	0.06 mL/s/kg 4.7
81–90	t_{CMT}+InD+DxD	450 mg I/kg 38.3	21 mg I/s/kg 1.79	1.5 mL/kg 128	0.07 mL/s/kg 5.95	1.3 mL/kg 109	0.06 mL/s/kg 5.1	1.2 mL/kg 103	0.057 mL/s/kg 4.8
91–100	t_{CMT}+InD+DxD	450 mg I/kg 42.8	19 mg I/s/kg 1.81	1.5 mL/kg 143	0.06 mL/s/kg 6.0	1.3 mL/kg 122	0.054 mL/s/kg 5.2	1.2 mL/kg 116	0.05 mL/s/kg 4.9
101–120	t_{CMT}+InD+DxD	400 mg I/kg 44	17 mg I/s/kg 1.87	1.3 mL/kg 147	0.057 mL/s/kg 6.2	1.14 mL/kg 126	0.05 mL/s/kg 5.3	1.1 mL/kg 119	0.046 mL/s/kg 5.0
121–140	t_{CMT}+InD+DxD	400 mg I/kg 52	15 mg I/s/kg 1.95	1.3 mL/kg 173	0.05 mL/s/kg 6.5	1.14 mL/kg 149	0.04 mL/s/kg 5.3	1.1 mL/kg 141	0.04 mL/s/kg 5.3

Parameters are weight-based (2 to 140 kg) to optimize intravascular iodine delivery. Contrast medium transit time (CMT) is established with automated triggering or bolus timing. When automated triggering is used, the overall scan delay and injection duration are increased by a value equivalent to the inherent delay (InD) of automated triggering (ie, 2–8 s). A variable diagnostic delay (DxD) is added with the goal that the combined scan delay and the scan duration equal the injection duration. The result is that the delivery of contrast medium and the scan duration will end together. For extremity CTA, the diagnostic delay is extended, such that the scan is completed approximately 3–5 seconds after the injection is completed. The iodine dose (400–600 mg I/kg) and flux are optimized with flexible injection rates and contrast medium volumes and concentrations. High concentration contrast medium (CM) allows for reduced volumes and injection rates. For all injections, saline flush follows the second phase of contrast medium.

[a] Average.

For pediatric CTA, where fast imaging is a prerequisite to achieve low and ultra-low dose radiation exposures, it is imperative to increase the diagnostic delay such that the scan duration and injection durations end simultaneously (Table 7). For patients with high heart rates, the operator may choose a slightly shorter diagnostic delay so that the acquisition is completed 2–3 seconds ahead of the contrast infusion, ensuring contrast delivery throughout the acquisition. For extremity and whole body CTA, the extended scan delay will be the difference between the actual scan time and an anticipated scan duration when coverage is made at a table speed of 30 mm/s. In this instance, for a given iodine dose, the injection duration is adjusted by a combination of decreasing the rate of injection and increasing the volume of contrast medium, such that the injection duration will match the sum of the extended scan delay and the actual scan time. At the operator's discretion, the scan delay can be extended by an additional 5 seconds. In this case, the scan will end after the infusion of contrast, increasing the prospect that contrast medium will reach the digital arteries. The pitfall with these strategies is venous contamination. The benefit however, is dose reduction for the pediatric patient.

Injection parameters for indirect CTV, whether obtained as a primary or delayed acquisition, follows those of the arterial phase, as the goal is to get contrast rapidly into the targeted region. It is essential to apply an appropriate delay so that the acquisition is optimized, with the majority of contrast in the veins. With direct CTV, low injection rates (0.8–2 mL/s) are applied over an extended delay to optimize uniform enhancement using venous first pass and recirculation phases.

Saline Flush

Infusion of saline following the contrast medium injection improves contrast utilization and reduces perivenous streak artifacts. It should be applied as a means to utilize the full volume of contrast, prolong the peak of injection, and improve image quality.[13] While there are various methods to deliver the saline, a dual-chamber power injector is most reliable. The saline volume (6–40 ml) varies depending upon the injection tubing length and body weight. The rate of injection should equal the contrast injection rate.

Image Analysis

Display and interpretation of CT angiograms are most efficient with primary use of advanced workstation visualization techniques and secondary review of the source images (Table 8). In all instances, it is essential to use flexible angiographic window and level settings, including a wide window setting to account for noise, vascular calcification, and high contrast attenuation. Regarding the workflow, source data is acquired as two-dimensional (2D) transverse images and transferred to a picture archiving and communication system (PACS) for viewing and storage. Workstations are integrated into PACS or exist as separate systems (thin client servers or stand-alone units). Only thin section datasets (angiographic and non-contrast acquisitions) need transfer to the workstation. The size of datasets impacts transmission, display, and interpretation and depends upon the coverage, reconstruction interval, and the use and percentage of multiphase reconstructions. Optional non-contrast and delayed images, and any additional angiographic phases and series reconstructions further add to potential "data overload".

Effective use of the workstation visualization techniques requires that they are applied in a complementary manner according to their strengths. This may occur through real-time workstation interrogation with user defined interaction or with protocol driven static post-processed images which are generated on the workstation and sent to PACS for review along with the source images. As listed in Table 8, 3D volume rendering (VR) and 2D maximum intensity projection (MIP) techniques provide angiographic overviews. They require sliding thin-slabs or pre-rendering editing to remove bone and other anatomical structures which may obscure vascular visualization. 2D multiplanar (MPR) and curved planar (CPR) reformations are most beneficial for analysis of structural detail, namely cardiac morphology and vessel lumens and walls. MPR may be applied real time on the workstation using multiple planes. Alternatively, batch thin-section coronal and sagittal reformations are generated for review. Similarly, CPR may be applied as rotating longitudinal sections on the workstation or as static coronal and sagittal longitudinal sections. Minimum intensity projection (MinIP) and Ray-sum (thick MPR) have limited applications in CT angiography. MinIP is useful to show cardiac valves, airways, air-trapping, and abnormal non-pulmonary air collections. Ray-sum is applied to generate radiographic-like images for structural overview. Depending on the nature of ECG-gating, cardiac 4D datasets can be viewed with VR, MPR, MIP, and/or MinIP.

Findings identified using the advanced visualization techniques are confirmed on the source images. Source images are also essential to

Table 8
Advanced visualization techniques

	Display	Principal Use	Advantages	Disadvantages
MPR	2D	• Structural Detail • Quantitative analysis	• "Slice" through dataset in coronal, sagittal, and oblique projections • Real-time multiplanar interrogation • Simplify image interpretation	• Limited spatial perception
CPR	2D	• Structural Detail • Centerline Display • Simplify MPR	• Single anatomic display • Longitudinal cross-sectional anatomic display	• Operator dependent
Ray-Sum	2D	• Structural Overview	• "Slice" through dataset in axial, coronal, sagittal, and oblique projections • Real-time multiplanar interrogation • Radiograph-like display	• Loss of structural detail with increased slab thickness

MIP	2D	• Structural Overview
		• Angiographic Display
			• "Slice" through dataset in axial, coronal, sagittal, and oblique projections
			• Real-time multiplanar interrogation
			• Improved depiction
			  - small-caliber vessels
			  - poorly enhanced vessels
			• Communicate findings
				• Anatomic overlap (vessels, bone viscera) with increased slab thickness
				• Visualization degraded by high-density structures (ie, bone, calcium, stents, coils)
				• Loss of structural detail with increased slab thickness
				• Limited grading of stent lumens

MinIP	2D	• Structural Overview • Tracheobronchial Airway	• "Slice" through dataset in axial, coronal, sagittal, and oblique projections • Real-time multiplanar interrogation • Depict low-density structures • Communicate findings	• Anatomic overlap • Loss of structural detail with increased slab thickness
VR	3D	• Structural Overview • Angiographic Display	• "Slice" through dataset in axial, coronal, sagittal, and oblique projections • Real-time multiplanar interrogation • Depict structural relationships • Accurate spatial perception • Communicate findings	• Opacity-transfer function dependent • Anatomic overlap • Loss of structural detail with increased slab thickness

Abbreviations: 2D, 2-dimensional; 3D, 3-dimensional; CPR, curved planar reformation; MIP, maximum intensity projection; MinIP, minimum intensity projection; MPR, multiplanar reformation; VR, volume rendered.

assess image quality and exclude artifacts. Review may proceed with the original transverse sections, the coronal and sagittal reformations, or both. PACS review of non-cardiovascular structures is facilitated by generating 3–5 mm thick axial reconstructions. Alternatively, the coronal and sagittal reformations may be used. Quantitative analysis is readily performed on current workstations and PACS. Workstations offer automated, semi-automated, and manual algorithms and tool sets to generate standard 2D and volumetric data, calculate cardiac chamber volumes and ejection fraction, and analyze tissue perfusion. PACS analysis is restricted to 2D measurements.

Practice Quality Improvement

Quality assurance policies and procedures are necessary for a pediatric CVCT program. The objectives are to ensure safe radiation practice, safe contrast delivery, acceptable and reliable image quality, appropriate technologist skills, and accurate physician interpretation. Technologists performing and physicians performing and interpreting pediatric CVCT should meet established guideline requirements for CTA practice, including knowledge of dose reduction strategies. Physicians should have additional expertise in pediatric cardiovascular anatomy, pathology, and pathophysiology. Physicians responsible for supervising practice quality improvement (maintaining and updating protocols; administering quality assurance initiatives; providing training to team members) should have additional skills in protocol design, monitoring radiation exposure, and measuring image quality. Team leaders should be well versed in and incorporate where appropriate, the most up to date CT and workstation technologies and contrast administration procedures.

Periodic review of examinations and individual protocols, addresses the prescribed parameters, exam coverage, radiation output, absorbed patient radiation dose, image noise, and contrast administration. Review of the images objectively addresses noise related artifacts, quality of enhancement, and overall CNR. Subjective feedback should be obtained from both readers and patient care providers. Follow-up should be obtained with technologists, nursing teams, and patient care providers. to investigate any known or unknown adverse outcome related to contrast administration. When appropriate, protocols should be revised and additional training obtained.

Regarding assessment of radiation, the output is available for each scan, reported by vendors as the CT Dose Index volume (CTDIvol) and Dose Length Product (DLP). CTDIvol, measured in mGy, represents the average radiation dose per scan volume for a standardized phantom. The DLP, measured in mGy · cm, is the product of the CTDIvol and scan length. DLP is directly proportional to the radiation output and the scan coverage. While CTDIvol and DLP provide a measure of CT radiation output, neither are a measure of absorbed effective (organ) patient radiation dose. Two practical means to calculate pediatric absorbed effective dose (mSv) include CT dosimetry simulation software (ie, ImPACT CT Patient Dosimetry Calculator; ImPACT, London, United Kingdom) and DLP conversion (using factors based upon the body size and region(s) scanned).[14] With both methods, additional age conversion factors are applied to account for the inversely proportional organ radiosensitivity.

CLINICAL APPLICATIONS: ILLUSTRATIONS IN ALARA

Pediatric CVCT interpretation and structured reporting has three components: image quality, cardiovascular structure and function, and non-cardiovascular structure and function.

The main objective of assessing image quality is to recognize one or more artifacts which may hinder image display, interpretation, or both. Readers should acknowledge the presence of motion, excessive noise, suboptimal enhancement, metallic densities (eg, streak artifact), and large calcifications (eg, blooming and streak artifacts). In addition, it is recommended that readers acknowledge whether the exam retains diagnostic quality or is partially or completely non-diagnostic as a result of the artifact(s).

All cardiovascular anatomy included in the scan volume requires systematic review. This includes anatomy primary and secondary to the clinical indications. Evaluation begins with the establishment of thoracic and abdominal Situs. While this has greater importance in the setting of known or suspected congenital heart disease, segmental anatomical review will ensure recognition of unsuspected abnormal and anomalous structures and connections.

Depending upon the CTA technique, cardiac review may include the pericardium (thickness, effusions); atria and ventricles (connections, orientation, size, and configuration); myocardium (thickness, enhancement, function), inter-atrial and inter-ventricular septae (defects, shape, function/oscillation); valves (leaflet morphology, function); and veno-atrial (inflow) and ventricular – arterial (outflow) connections (anomalies, obstruction/patency). 4D datasets afford qualitative and quantitative evaluation of cardiac function. Chamber function (ventricular, atrial) is characterized with regards to both global and regional wall motion (ie, normal, hypokinetic, akinetic, dyskinetic). Valve function is described based upon the degree of global aperature and coaptation and individual leaflet motion. On dedicated cardiac exams, 2D chamber major and minor dimensions should routinely be measured. When retrospective ECG-Gating is performed, ventricular volumes and ejection fractions should be quantified. On non-cardiac protocol CT angiograms, when cardiac chamber size and morphology are recognized to be abnormal, 2D chamber dimensions should be measured and reported.

Coronary and peripheral vascular review addresses ostial location, caliber, and patency as well as the course, caliber, contour, luminal patency, and branching pattern of the post-ostial proximal, mid, and distal segments for each particular vascular tree. Pathology may include anomalous origins, course and connections (arterial–arterial, arterial–venous); wall thickening; vasospasm; stenosis; occlusion; tortuosity; ectasia; aneurysms; pseudoanrurysms; dissection; and traumatic injury. It is recommended to analyze and report stenoses with quantitative and qualitative descriptions as follows: less than 25% (minimal), 25–49% (mild), 50–69% (moderate); 70–99% (severe); occluded. Recording and reporting vascular measurements is recommended for arterial and venous anatomy essential to the exam indications and for any additional recognized abnormal territory.

Non-cardiovascular review may detect both expected and unexpected findings. These findings are useful to provide additional understanding of a patient's cardiovascular disease. In addition, findings may provide alternative diagnoses, enhancing or altering patient management. For each cardiovascular territory imaged, end organs should be evaluated for perfusion, viability, and function. In a retrospective review of 300 pediatric patients with congenital heart disease, Malik and colleagues reported an 82% prevalence of non-cardiovascular findings; 74% of the study population had significant non-cardiovascular findings, with an incremental clinical value of 39%.[15]

Cardiac

Routine and ECG-gated cardiac CTA is most frequently applied to evaluate congenital heart disease (Figs. 5–8). Right sided obstructive lesions, left sided obstructive lesions, conotruncal abnormalities, pulmonary vein anomalies, and coronary anomalies are all common applications (see Table 2). In the author's practice, it is most prevalent in patients who also require airway and lung evaluation, are high sedation risks patients, or have post-operative metallic devices precluding MRI. For select disease states, calcium scoring and coronary venography can be performed.

Head and Neck

Head and neck CVCT can rapidly evaluate the cervicocerebral arteries and veins (see Figs. 7–8). Applications include trauma, vascular malformations, aneurysms, arterial occlusive disease, venous occlusive disease, and vascular mapping (see Table 2). In the author's experience, it is most commonly applied in the trauma setting and the post-operative patient (eg, vascular malformations, aneurysms). The increased coverage and more rapid table speeds with the third generation MDCT scanners, may afford the ability to safely perform pediatric CT brain perfusion at low radiation exposure, expanding potential CTA applications for pediatric neurovascular disease.

Chest

Chest CT angiography is utilized to assess the pulmonary arteries, pulmonary veins, thoracic aorta, and central systemic veins (Figs. 9–11). Clinical applications include congenital lung lesions (sequestration, bronchial atresia, congenital pulmonary adenomatoid malformation), primary and secondary pulmonary hypertension, pulmonary arteriovenous malformations (congenital and acquired), venous occlusive disease, venous thromboembolism (pulmonary embolism), congenital aortic arch disease (coarctation; vascular rings, slings, and anomalies), aortopathies (congenital and acquired), acute aortic disease (dissection, traumatic injury), and hemoptysis (see Table 2). Chest CTA is most beneficial as a one-stop shop for comprehensive airway, lung, and cardiopulmonary evaluation (ie, patients with pulmonary hypertension, Fig. 3). Dynamic inspiration—expiration acquisitions with targeted inflation pressures can be incorporated to assess airway disease (eg, tracheobronchomalacia), lung volumes, and global and regional pulmonary function. In this instance, the NCA is acquired during inspiration and the CTA phase at expiration. In all other applications, chest CTA typically consists of only the angiographic phase. Additional exam considerations are listed in Table 2.

Abdomen-Pelvis

Abdominal–pelvis CTA can be applied to evaluate the abdominal aorta, inferior vena cavae (IVC), and

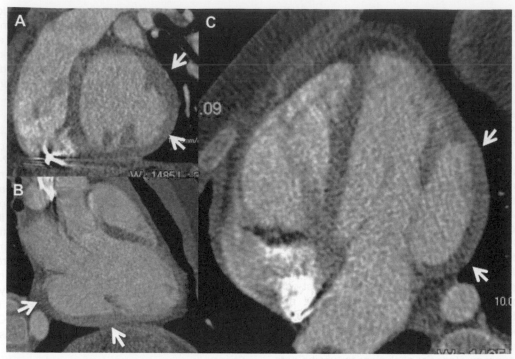

Fig. 5. A 12-year-old boy with possible left ventricular aneurysm on echocardiography. (*A*) Four-chamber, (*B*) short-axis, and (*C*) 3-chamber view reveal a broad-based left ventricular diverticulum (*arrows*) along the midlateral and posterior basilar wall, with a saccular component extending posterior and inferior to the basilar left ventricle and the left atrium. Examination was performed with retrospective ECG-gating and low-dose technique. mSv = 1.5.

iliac, mesenteric, and visceral arteries and veins (see Table 2; Figs. 12–14). Aortic applications include abdominal coarctation, vasculopathies (congenital and acquired), trauma, dissection, and post-endovascular or surgical surveillance. Coverage typically extends partially or completely through the iliac arteries in a single arterial phase acquisition. Rarely a targeted noncontrast (eg,

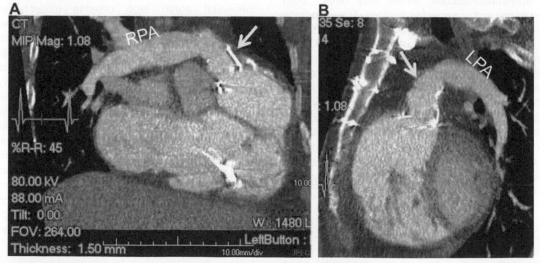

Fig. 6. An 18-year-old man status post tetralogy of Fallot repair with a valve-graft from right ventricle to pulmonary conduit. Oblique images for the right pulmonary artery (*A, RPA*) and left pulmonary artery (*B, LPA*) show patent conduit (*arrows*), RPA and LPA. Examination was performed with retrospective ECG-gating and low-dose technique. mSv = 1.0.

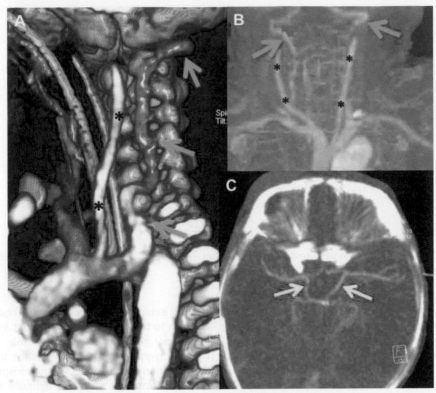

Fig. 7. PHACE syndrome with congenital absence of the bilateral internal carotid arteries (ICA). (*A*) Lateral VR, (*B*) frontal MIP through the neck, and (*C*) axial MIP through the circle of Willis reveal that intracranial circulation is dependent on dominant posterior vertebral artery circulation (*green arrows*) with flow across bilateral posterior communicating arteries (*yellow arrows*). Green arrows demonstrate prominent vertebral arteries. Asterisks show bilateral common carotid arteries without ICA segments.

coarctation-assess for calcium; post-intervention) or delayed (eg, vasculopathies – wall enhancement) acquisition may be required. Mesenteric CTA can be utilized to assess acute and chronic mesenteric ischemia, gastrointestinal bleeding, portal hypertension, protein losing enteropathy, mesenteric and visceral masses, vascular mapping, and pre- and post-operative liver transplant vascular anatomy. Coverage typically includes the entire abdomen and pelvis.

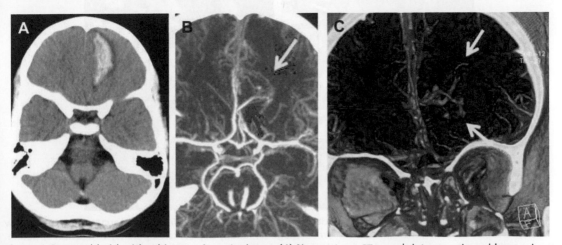

Fig. 8. A 5-year-old girl with a history of meningismus. (*A*) Noncontrast CT reveals intraprenchymal hemorrhage in the left frontal lobe. (*B*) MIP and (*C*) VR images show a left frontal parasagittal arteriovenous malformation (AVM) (*yellow arrows*) fed by a frontopolar branch from the left A2 segment (*red arrow*). mSv = 0.22.

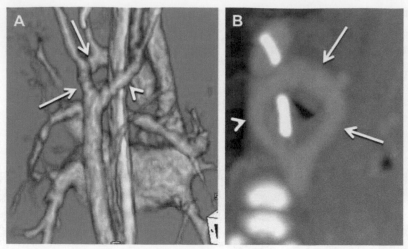

Fig. 9. An 11-month-old female with respiratory difficulties. (A) VR and (B) MIP images reveal an intact double aortic arch (arrows). mSv = 0.77.

Depending upon the exam indications, coverage may be restricted to only target the abdomen or pelvis. When evaluating acute and chronic mesenteric ischemia, a single arterial phase is usually sufficient. For all other applications, a biphasic acquisition with arterial and portal venous phases, is standard. Coverage on the portal venous phase may be extended to the IVC – atrial junction. Renal CTA is most commonly applied to evaluate renovascular hypertension. Additional applications include vasculitis, uretero-pelvis junction obstruction, renal masses, vascular mapping, and traumatic injury. Coverage for native renal arteries should extend from the thoracolumbar junction through to the mid pelvis to account for potential accessory renal arteries which may be found from as high as the phrenic arteries to a low as the common iliac arteries. Renal transplant recipients may undergo a CTA to evaluate the arterial and venous anastomoses as well as the respective transplant arterial and venous segments in the settings of post-operative hypertension, possible or known rejection, and trauma. Coverage is targeted to the transplant kidney (eg, pelvis CTA). Direct and indirect CT venography is performed for diagnosis and surveillance of iliac and/or IVC

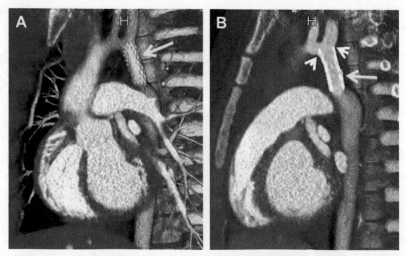

Fig. 10. A 16-year-old boy with a history endovascular stent placement for aortic coarctation (A, B; yellow arrows). Despite the noise, the thin-slab VR lumen image (B) readily depicts stent patency with intact structure. The posterior margin of the stent extends to the left subclavian artery origin, while the anterior margin extends vertically into the distal native transverse arch (B, arrow heads) resulting in approximate 40% area reduction of the distal arch. mSv = 0.28.

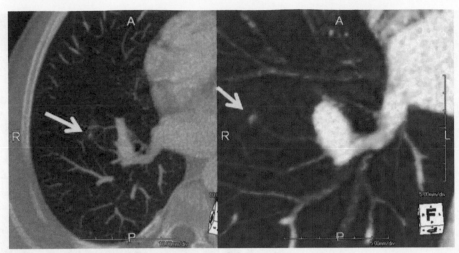

Fig. 11. An 8-year-old boy with a family history of hereditary hemorrhagic telangiectasia and a positive echocardiogram for a pulmonary AVM. Low-dose CTA detected a single 3-mm pulmonary AVM with arterial inflow and venous outflow (*arrows*). mSv = 0.21.

venous occlusive disease. It is most beneficial for assessment of iliac or IVC venous stent patency and for evaluation of IVC filter positioning and clot burden prior to removal of an IVC filter.

Upper and Lower Extremities

CT angiography can evaluate arterial occlusive disease, vasculitis, venous occlusive disease, trauma, vascular masses, and hemodialysis access in the upper and lower extremities. In addition, it is a useful for vascular mapping (see **Table 2; Fig. 15**). Coverage may include the complete extremity vascular tree or a targeted region. Dynamic functional evaluation is possible for both upper (eg, thoracic inlet and outlet syndromes) and lower (eg, popliteal entrapment syndrome) extremity disease. With first and second generation MDCT scanners, these protocols require two contrast injections for two separate acquisitions. With the rapid scan durations afforded by third generation scanners, low dose dynamic kinetic imaging is possible. In the future, delivering a single contrast bolus during kinetic imaging may enhance functional extremity CT angiography.

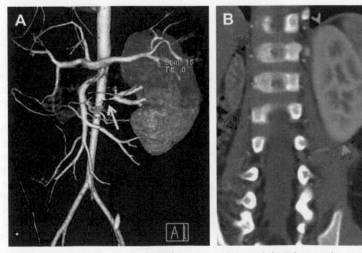

Fig. 12. A 4-year-old boy with hypertension and mid-aortic syndrome. (*A*) VR image shows show high-grade ostial and postostial renal artery stenosis over 6.0 mm (*yellow arrow*), and there is mild diffuse narrowing of the inframesenteric abdominal aorta. (*B*) Multiplanar reformatted image reveals a significant discrepancy in size and enhancement of the kidneys. The right kidney (*red arrowheads*) is atrophic and poorly enhancing. The right renal artery is not opacified and likely occluded (image not shown). The left kidney demonstrates compensatory hypertrophy (*blue arrowheads*).

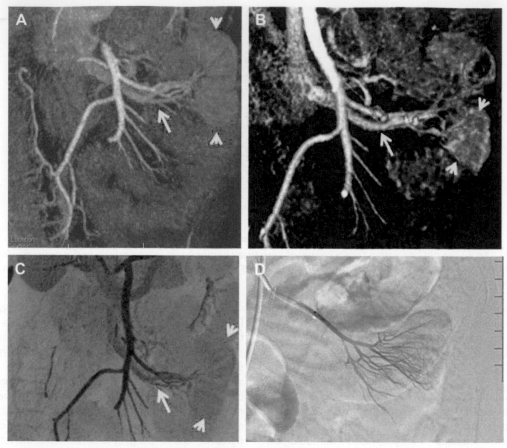

Fig. 13. An 18-year-old man with recurrent gastrointestinal bleeding and worsening anemia. (A) MIP, (B) VR, and (C) inverted MIP images reveal proximal jejunal angiodysplasia evidenced by an early draining vein (*arrow*) and a faint blush (*arrowheads*) of the involved bowel loop. (D) Corresponding conventional angiography image performed for preoperative coil localization confirms the findings.

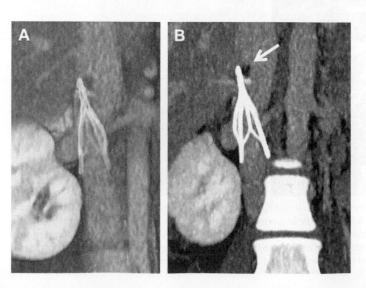

Fig. 14. A 14-year-old girl with a history of psoas abscess and deep venous thrombosis (DVT) status post inferior vena cava (IVC) filter placement. Indirect CTV was performed to evaluate for residual DVT and assess IVC filter position before retrieval. (A) VR and (B) MIP images demonstrate the retrievable filter within the IVC with rightward angulation and extension into the wall at L1 level. A small amount of residual eccentric clot on the left side of the cone is identified (*arrow*).

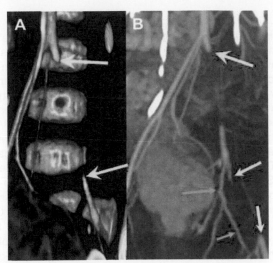

Fig. 15. A 2-year-old female presenting with decreased left pedal pulses post left femoral catheterization. (*A*) VR and (*B*) MIP images show long segment occlusion of the left common iliac and external iliac arteries (*yellow arrows*) reconstituted at the common femoral artery via internal iliac system collaterals (*green arrows*).

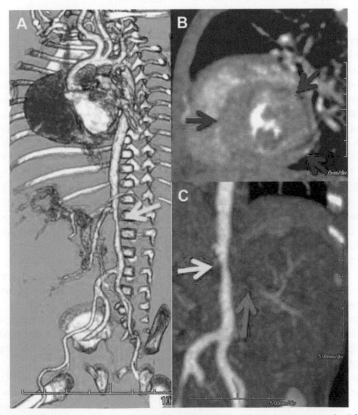

Fig. 16. A 10-day-old patient with hyperkalemia and hypertension. (*A*) VR image reveals diffuse, irregular luminar narrowing of the abdominal aorta (*yellow arrow*) consistent with mid-aortic syndrome. (*B*) Short-axis MIP image demonstrates moderate to severe left ventricular hypertrophy (*red arrows*). (*C*) Left anterior oblique MIP view of the abdominal aorta demonstrates no opacification of the ostial and postostial segments of the left renal artery (*blue arrow*), reflective of severe high-grade stenosis versus complete occlusion.

Whole Body

Global imaging of the entire or nearly the entire peripheral vascular system is often necessary in pediatric patients to evaluate known or suspected systemic congenital vasculopathies (Fig. 16). These vasculopathies may affect large, medium, or small arteries, veins, or both in one or more vascular territories. They include syndromic disorders impacting angiogenesis (eg, Hereditary Hemorrhagic Telangectasia) and structural integrity (eg, Marfan, Ehlers-Danlos, Loeys-Dietz, Willims-Beuren, PHACE Syndromes) as well as disorders leading to autoimmune inflammation (eg, Takayasu Arteritis, Giant Cell Arteritis, Polyarteritis Nodosa). Acquired pathology in multiple territories, as in the setting of mycotic aneurysms, dissection, and poly trauma, may also warrant a multi-vascular territory imaging approach.

In considering which diagnostic angiographic modality to use to address the global imaging needs, both whole body MRA (WB-MRA) and whole body CTA (WB-CTA) should clearly be considered prior to invasive catheter angiography since patient risk is directly proportional to the number of catheter manipulations, vascular territory interrogations, and the procedural time. With current technology, WB-CTA is a reasonable consideration over WB-MRA, as CTA can achieve and maintain robust 3D image quality, uniformly across a large Z-axis coverage acquisition (ie, complete peripheral vascular system), in the shortest possible exam duration and with minimal to no sedation or general anesthesia requirements. For complete WB-CTA coverage, scanning proceeds in a cranio-caudad direction, from the vertex of the head through to the feet, with the patient's arms positioned at their side. Targeted coverage includes imaging through, but not limited to portions of the head and neck; chest, abdomen and pelvis; and upper extremities and lower extremities (Fig. 16).

As WB-CTA exposes multiple radiosensitive organs, judicious considerations of the exam appropriateness, extent of coverage, and radiation acquisition parameters remain paramount. For a given pediatric patient size, the coverage and the selection of voltage and tube current parameters will depend highly upon the MDCT scanner. Reasonably acceptable low radiation exposure and ultra-low dose exposure are both achieved with 64-channel technology. The lower exposure times afforded by the third generation MDCT scanners provide the opportunity to routinely achieve ultra-low dose exposures when prescribing similar voltage and tube current parameters (see Table 6).

SUMMARY

Complimentary, "gentle" use of CVCT can enhance the diagnosis and management of the pediatric patient with cardiovascular disease. Given the intrinsic dependence upon radiation, utilizing this modality in pediatric patients mandates a commitment to dose reduction strategies, striving for ALARA in each CVCT examination. Recommended protocols for current state of the art MDCT scanners incorporate these dose reduction strategies. For each patient, preparatory steps are essential, including individual review of the risks, benefits, and alternatives to CVCT. The pediatric CTA protocols are uniquely designed to maximize the table speed, image at the lowest possible voltage, and use the lowest possible weight-based tube current. Weight-based contrast medium protocols are important to maximizing iodine delivery, achieving high CNR, and maintaining high image quality in presence of increased noise. As the MDCT technology continues to rapidly evolve, these strategies will provide a framework for adapting future technology.

REFERENCES

1. Hellinger JC, Poon M, Epelman M. Pediatric 64-Channel CT Angiography: Technical and Clinical Applications in 1550 Consecutive Examinations. JACC 2010;55(16):A201.
2. Blass EM, Hoffmeyer LB. Sucrose as an analgesic for newborn infants. Pediatrics 1991;87:215–8.
3. National Kidney Foundation. K/DOQI clinical practice guidelines for vascular access, 2000. Am J Kidney Dis 2001;37(Suppl 1):S137–81.
4. Fricke BL, Donnelly LF, Frush DP, et al. In-plane bismuth breast shields for pediatric CT: effects on radiation dose and image quality using experimental and clinical data. AJR Am J Roentgenol 2003; 180(2):407–11.
5. Goodsitt MM, Johnson RH. Precision in quantitative CT: impact of x-ray dose and matrix size. Med Phys 1992;19(4):1025–36.
6. Huda W, Ogden KM, Khorasani MR. Effect of dose metrics and radiation risk models when optimizing CT x-ray tube voltage. Phys Med Biol 2008;53(17): 4719–32.
7. Kalender WA, Wolf H, Suess C, Gies M, et al. Dose reduction in CT by on-line tube current control: principles and validation on phantoms and cadavers. Eur Radiol 1999;9(2):323–8.
8. Shuman WP, Branch KR, May JM, et al. Prospective versus retrospective ECG gating for 64-detector CT of the coronary arteries: comparison of image

quality and patient radiation dose. Radiology 2008; 248(2):431–7.

9. Sommer WH, Graser A, Becker CR, et al. Image quality of virtual noncontrast images derived from dual-energy CT angiography after endovascular aneurysm repair. J Vasc Interv Radiol 2010;21(3): 315–21.

10. Prakash P, Kalra MK, Pigumarthy SR, et al. Radiation dose reduction with chest computed tomography using adaptive statistical iterative reconstruction technique: initial experience. J Comput Assist Tomogr 2010;34(1):40–5.

11. Poll LW, Cohnen M, Brachten S, et al. Dose reduction in multi-slice CT of the heart by use of ECG-controlled tube current modulation ("ECG pulsing"): phantom measurements. Rofo 2002; 174(12):1500–5.

12. Fleischmann D, Rubin GD. Quantification of intravenously administered contrast medium transit through the peripheral arteries: implications for CT angiography. Radiology 2005;236(3):1076–82.

13. Lee CH, Goo JM, Bae KT, et al. CTA contrast enhancement of the aorta and pulmonary artery: the effect of saline chase injected at two different rates in a canine experimental model. Invest Radiol 2007;42(7):487–90.

14. Huda W, Ogden KM, Khorasani MR. Converting dose-length product to effective dose at CT. Radiology 2008;248(3):995–1003.

15. Malik A, Hellinger JC, Gruber P, Epelman M. Prevalence of non-cardiovascular findings in pediatric MDCT angiography performed for evaluation of congenital heart disease [abstract]. Presented at RSNA; 2009.

Index

Note: Page numbers of article titles are in **boldface** type.

A

Radiol Clin N Am 48 (2010) 469–475
doi:10.1016/S0033-8389(10)00049-7

radiologic.theclinics.com

Moving?

Make sure your subscription moves with you!

To notify us of your new address, find your **Clinics Account Number** (located on your mailing label above your name), and contact customer service at:

Email: journalscustomerservice-usa@elsevier.com

800-654-2452 (subscribers in the U.S. & Canada)
314-447-8871 (subscribers outside of the U.S. & Canada)

Fax number: 314-447-8029

Elsevier Health Sciences Division
Subscription Customer Service
3251 Riverport Lane
Maryland Heights, MO 63043

*To ensure uninterrupted delivery of your subscription, please notify us at least 4 weeks in advance of move.

Printed and bound by CPI Group (UK) Ltd, Croydon, CR0 4YY

03/10/2024

01040358-0012